Principles of
BONE X-RAY DIAGNOSIS

Third Edition

GEORGE SIMON, M.D., F.R.C.P., F.F.R.

Lately Radiologist, St. Bartholomew's Hospital, London; Demonstrator in Radiological Anatomy, St. Bartholomew's Hospital, London; Curator of the Radiological Museum and Teacher of Radiology, The Institute of Diseases of the Chest, University of London; Tutor in Radiology, University College Hospital, London; formerly Director, X-ray Department, Brompton Hospital, London

BUTTERWORTHS

ENGLAND: BUTTERWORTH & CO. (PUBLISHERS) LTD.
                LONDON: 88 Kingsway, WC2B 6AB

AUSTRALIA: BUTTERWORTHS PTY. LTD.
                SYDNEY: 586 Pacific Highway, 2067
                MELBOURNE: 343 Little Collins Street, 3000
                BRISBANE: 240 Queen Street, 4000

CANADA: BUTTERWORTH & CO. (CANADA) LTD.
                TORONTO: 14 Curity Avenue, 374

NEW ZEALAND: BUTTERWORTHS OF NEW ZEALAND LTD.
                WELLINGTON: 26–28 Waring Taylor Street, 1

SOUTH AFRICA: BUTTERWORTH & CO. (SOUTH AFRICA) (PTY) LTD.
                DURBAN: 152–154 Gale Street

First Edition 1960
Second Edition 1965
Third Edition 1973

Suggested U.D.C. Number 616·71–073·75

ISBN 0 407 36319 X

Text set in 11/12pt. Monotype Times New Roman, printed by letterpress,
and bound in Great Britain at The Pitman Press, Bath

Principles of

BONE X-RAY DIAGNOSIS

Contents

Preface to the Third Edition

In this third edition much of the original text has been used, but some changes of order have been made to give a more logical approach to the description of the bone changes seen in various diseases. New knowledge has entailed additions to the text, and Chapter 6 on widespread and regional reduction in bone density has been completely rewritten, the clinical and pathophysiological aspects being under the care of N.J.Y. Woodhouse, Lecturer in Medicine at King's College Hospital, London, who takes full responsibility for the views now put forward.

Fifty-five new illustrations have been chosen for the same reasons as the additional ones in the second edition (*see below*).

LONDON, 1973   GEORGE SIMON

Preface to the Second Edition

In this second edition much of the original text has been used, a few errors corrected, and some new knowledge incorporated. Some alterations of order or wording have been made with the object of making the principles of bone x-ray diagnosis clearer or easier to memorize.

Altogether 52 new illustrations have been chosen either to show the x-ray appearances of some particular lesion or to clarify the principles described in the text, while new blocks have been made from some of the original radiographs to improve the clarity and general quality of illustrations considered inadequate in this respect. In a few instances the original illustration has been replaced by one showing a similar lesion, but with greater clarity for the purpose of the reproduction. Two radiographs of the skull have been included since in each the lesion was sufficiently gross to be easily seen in the reproduction.

LONDON, 1965   GEORGE SIMON

Acknowledgements

I wish to acknowledge the help and encouragement I have received from all the clinicians whose cases have enabled me to learn something about the various abnormalities which may be seen in a radiograph.

I am also particularly indebted to Dr. A. D. Thomson, Director of Pathology, Royal Masonic Hospital, formerly of the Middlesex Hospital and Lecturer in Pathology to the D.M.R. course, for his advice on the pathological matter in this book, and for his contribution to the pathological descriptions incorporated into the text.

I wish to thank Dr. A. G. Stansfeld and Dr. R. J. R. Cureton of the Department of Pathology, St. Bartholomew's Hospital, for reviewing the histological material of the cases illustrated, and when necessary reporting again on the sections of many of the cases, particularly the bone tumours and developmental defects. Some of the cases were first seen in the 1935–1945 period, and it was felt essential to check the histological diagnoses made at the time in the light of recent advances in bone pathology, particularly to confirm and grade the cases of osteoclastoma, and separate them from the variants, and to review those cases labelled "Ewing's" tumour.

I wish to thank Dr. G. DuBoulay of St. Bartholomew's Hospital for contributing the material, much of it original, for the section on "A transradiant area in the vault of the skull", and Dr. J. H. Middlemiss of Bristol for his contribution on "Madura foot".

The illustrations are reproduced from radiographs of patients passing through the x-ray departments of St. Bartholomew's Hospital and the Brompton Hospital with the exception of Fig. 76 (Thiemann's disease) kindly sent to me from Perth, Australia, by Dr. R. D. McKellar-Hall and Dr. A. L. Frazer, and Fig. 227 (hydatid cyst) sent to me from South Africa by Dr. A. S. Kimmel.

The illustrations are from photographs prepared from the original radiographs by D. F. Kemp in the photographic department of the Institute of Diseases of the Chest, the Brompton Hospital.

The references given are only a faint indication of my debt to the work of others. Most of the references are key ones which themselves refer to the work of others on that particular subject.

I wish to thank Mr. J. N. Aston and Mr. Charles Manning for their advice on some of the orthopaedic clinical problems related to radiology.

I also wish to thank the Department of Medical Illustration of St. Bartholomew's Hospital for the care with which they prepared photographs of the radiographs for the new illustrations.

The new blocks for the third edition were prepared from prints made by the Department of Medical Illustration, St. Bartholomew's Hospital, London, the Department of Medical Photography, the Royal Marsden Hospital, and the National Heart Hospitals, London.

The original radiographs for Fig. 53 were kindly supplied by Dr. Philip Jacobs, Birmingham; those for Figs. 28 and 29 by Dr. W. J. Alexander, Montreal; and those for Figs. 13 and 15 by Dr. F. H. Doyle, London.

The chart in Fig. 154*a* is reproduced by kind permission of the authors and Editor from *Clinical Radiology* (1967), Vol. 18, p. 103, and the chart in Fig. 154*b* by kind permission of the author and Editor from *Clinics in Endocrinology and Metabolism*, Vol. 1, p. 143 (published by W. B. Saunders Co.).

Fig. 204 is reproduced from Woodhouse, Doyle and Joplin (1971) by courtesy of the Editor of *Lancet*.

Introduction

The value of grouping x-ray material according to the type of x-ray shadow rather than the clinical disease label was established in *Principles of Chest X-ray Diagnosis* (Simon, 1956), and a similar method has been followed in this book. In a radiograph of the chest, changes in the pulmonary vessel pattern and the position of the interlobar fissues, mediastinal contents or diaphragm singly or together form important aids to the diagnosis, and in a radiograph of a bone a parallel consideration is the balance between absorption, sclerosis and periosteal new bone. A study of this balance, together with the size, shape and position of the lesion, in any given case may help to reduce the list of possibilities to a less formidable number, or to indicate the need for biochemical, endocrine, histological, haematological or bacterial investigations which might not otherwise be done, and which might lead to the correct diagnosis, or even to give the correct diagnosis out of hand before it could be established clinically.

The amount of material available for the book was found to be very large and, in spite of a very generous allocation of illustrations by the publishers, it has not been possible to include a radiograph to illustrate every condition described. The objective has been to select examples which illustrate the principles of bone x-ray diagnosis rather than to make a complete catalogue of all the conditions referred to. This also accounts for the mixture of common conditions and rarities.

When possible the radiographs have been reproduced full size or even slightly enlarged, and to this end large lesions in large bones have been avoided if alternative radiographs showing similar conditions in bones of smaller surface area have been available. For this reason and because of difficulties in satisfactorily reproducing the radiographs, few skull lesions are shown.

Limitations of space and numbers of illustrations forbade the inclusion of certain specialized investigations such as arteriography in the differential diagnosis of malignant bone tumours from relatively innocent conditions, and arthrography either by air or by opaque contrast media. Nor has there been space to illustrate the appearances seen after the many orthopaedic operative procedures commonly practised.

The various biochemical and haemotological values quoted throughout the book, especially in the captions to figures, are all from the Department of Pathology, St. Bartholomew's Hospital. The lists of normal values drawn up by that department appear on pages 220–222 for reference.

Definition of Terms

The meanings of certain words used in this book are defined below.

Decalcification
Synonyms.—Decreased bone density, under-mineralization, bone resorption.

All these terms are somewhat unsatisfactory since they imply specific mechanisms. They are used in this book in the radiological sense only, implying that a part of the bone shadow is rendered less radio-opaque or is invisible.

The term decalcification does not mean halisteresis and does not preclude the simultaneous removal of other elements than calcium. It describes neither the mechanism nor the inciting cause of the calcium loss, and is meant only as a descriptive term for the x-ray appearances. It is a term in general use, and no objection to it was raised by Cooke (1955) so long as it was understood that it did not mean simple halisteresis. It seems preferable to the term deossification. It is often the result of resorption, a process defined by McLean (1956) as "putting into solution of a complicated structure in such a fashion that it disappears, its end products entering the blood stream". This process is possibly brought about by something the osteoclasts do. The rôle of the osteoclasts in the removal of the matrix, collagen fibrils and calcium phosphorus complex crystals in day-to-day remodelling and in pathological bone removal is discussed by Pritchard (1956) and Hancox (1956).

Decreased bone density
A purely descriptive term applying solely to the radiographic appearance and not implying any specific mechanism or particular element of bone affected.

Erosion
Circumscribed area with loss of trabecular pattern and/or a part or full width of the cortex; local area with loss of bone density.

E.S.R.
Erythrocyte sedimentation rate. All figures are for 1 hour (Westergren).

Generalized
Lesions not necessarily in all bones but not confined to a local region, for instance one bone or one extremity.

Hodgkin's disease
Synonyms.—Lymphadenoma; lymphoid follicular reticulosis; lymphogranuloma.

Periostitis
Radiographic descriptive term to indicate a line or band-like shadow parallel to the cortex suggesting periosteal new bone. Shadow the same whether the result of inflammation from infection, a haematoma or neoplastic cellular deposits. It may be induced by a regional circulatory defect or by some lesion in the thorax, small intestine or liver.

Rose–Waaler test
Synonym.—S.C.A.T.

A positive Rose–Waaler test regardless of whether it was done as a sheep cell agglutination test or a modification with polystyrene latex.

Sclerosis

Descriptive term for increase of bone density whatever the cause.

Transradiancy

Synonym.—Radiolucency.

The term is used in preference to translucency since x-rays are somewhat different from light rays. The meaning is similar and refers to a relative transradiancy compared, for instance, with that of adjacent areas of bone.

Transradiant area

Synonym.—Translucent area.

Relatively transradiant area.

1—Alterations in Bone Shape

The shape of a bone, as seen in a radiograph, may be altered in four ways. First in the length–breadth relationship, the bone being relatively wide and of normal or perhaps decreased length (Fig. 1) or relatively narrow and of normal or increased length (Fig. 5). Such changes are symmetrical and generalized throughout most or all of the skeleton in achondroplasia or osteogenesis imperfecta, regional in arachnodactyly (*see* page 10), and isolated in various other conditions such as a collapsed vertebra (Fig. 40) or craniocleidodysostosis (Fig. 17).

A second alteration in the contour of the bone is produced by over-emphasis or under-emphasis of certain normal curves, narrow regions or protuberances, seen for instance in acromegaly (Fig. 14*a*); a third by an abnormal local bony protuberance such as an exostosis (Fig. 33); and a fourth by the bowing or flattening of a bone because of its abnormal softness. Bowing may be seen in a congenital condition such as osteogenesis imperfecta, or in any of the numerous acquired lesions causing osteoporosis or osteomalacia described in Chapter 6 under "widespread decrease in bone density" or in Chapter 9 under "Paget's disease". Flattening of vertebral bodies is common whenever softening occurs as a result of either a general loss of calcium or a local destructive bone lesion.

Alterations in bone shape may be seen associated with a normal bone architecture in, for instance, acromegaly and the lesser manifestations of achondroplasia; or with an altered bone architecture, as in osteogenesis imperfecta and bone atrophy following severe muscular paralysis, in which conditions the long abnormally narrow bones have a thin cortex and the trabeculae in the spongy bone are very tenuous or invisible. Bowing of a bone, for instance in Paget's disease, is associated with an abnormally wide cortex and an abnormal crissc-ross trabecular pattern.

ALTERATIONS IN LENGTH–BREADTH RELATIONSHIP

SHORT AND WIDE—ACHONDROPLASIA

A decrease in the length of the long bones of the limbs with a relative increase in the width of the shaft is characteristic of achondroplasia. The changes are usually most obvious in the humeri, femora and tibiae and are symmetrical on both sides. The relative increase in width tends to be greatest towards the two ends of the bones, resulting in a "dumb-bell" appearance (Fig. 1).

The bones of the hands, especially the metacarpals, are abnormally short, the fingers tend to diverge and the hand appears trident-shaped. The base of the skull is short and the normal-sized vault appears relatively large with the bridge of the nose flattened.

The vertebral column in many cases appears normal apart from excessive lordosis, but in others the lesions are more severe and characteristic changes are present (Caffey, 1958). In the lower lumbar region the vertebral bodies are reduced in width and the pedicles of L. 4 and 5 are closer together than those of L. 1 and 2 (Fig. 2). At all levels the anterior–posterior width of the spinal canal is reduced in the lateral view owing to the short pedicles. The dorsal surface of the vertebral body is concave, and in some cases the antero-posterior width is reduced, the shape being otherwise fairly normal, while in others the anterior aspect shows a rounded bullet-shaped end rather similar to the tongue-shaped deformity of chondro-osteodystrophy (*see* page 40).

The pelvis may be square in shape with the triradiate cartilage almost on a level with the lower margin of the sacro-iliac joint (Fig. 3).

The bone structure may be normal, especially in the less severe manifestations. During childhood the appearance of the epiphyseal regions may be normal, the centres of ossification becoming visible and the epiphyseal discs uniting at the normal average age. The ossific centre at the lower end of the femur may be normal in structure but tends to be deeply set in the metaphysis, which may show an angled distal concavity opposite the epiphysis (Figs. 1 and 4). In more severe manifestations with a defect of epiphyseal structure the appearances are virtually those of chondro-osteodystrophy (*see* page 40).

The diagnosis is usually obvious from inspection of the patient with his short limbs and relatively normal trunk.

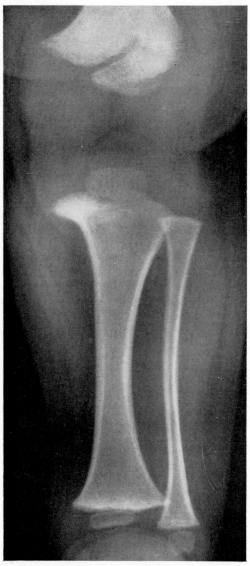

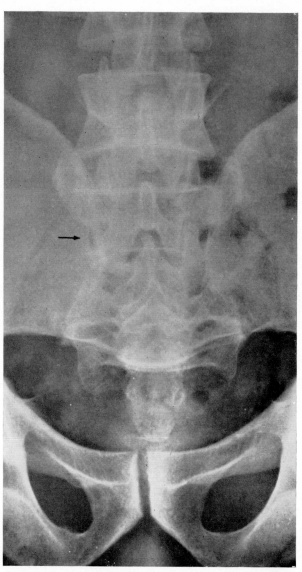

FIG. 1.—Achondroplasia. Male aged 2 years. Tibia short and ends splayed out giving a dumb-bell appearance. Cortical and trabecular structure normal. Similar changes in all the long bones, symmetrical on both sides. Skull normal.

FIG. 2.—Achondroplasia. Male aged 41 years. Fifth lumbar vertebra (opposite arrow) is very narrow and low in position in relation to pelvis. Wide disc space. In lateral view A–P diameter was small. Other bones wide and short as in Fig. 1.

Pathology

The condition is a developmental defect and affects all the bones formed in cartilage. On pathological examination a failure of the zone of proliferating cartilage can be seen, thus there is little growth in length of the shaft of the long bones. However, the epiphyseal bone at each end of the shaft develops normally to produce the characteristic "dumb-bell" appearance as is shown in Fig. 1.

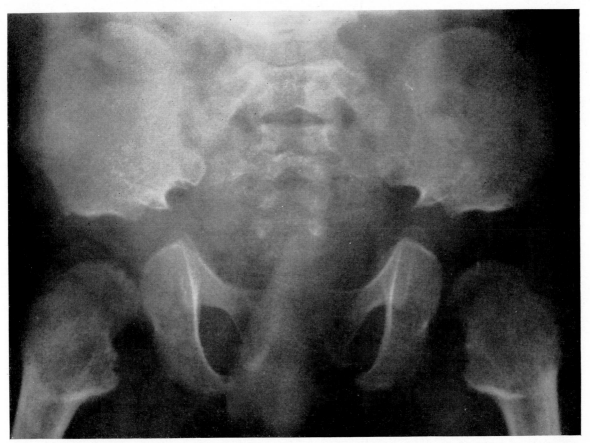

FIG. 3.—Achondroplasia. Female aged 1 year. Narrow L. 4–5. Square shape of ilia; acetabular cartilage high. Horizontal upper rim of acetabulum. Poorly developed upper femoral epiphysis. The lower one was similar to that in Fig. 4. Humeri and femora short and wide.

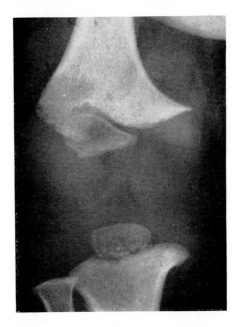

FIG. 4.—Achondroplasia. Child aged 2 years. Lower femoral epiphysis deeply set in distal concave notch of metaphysis.

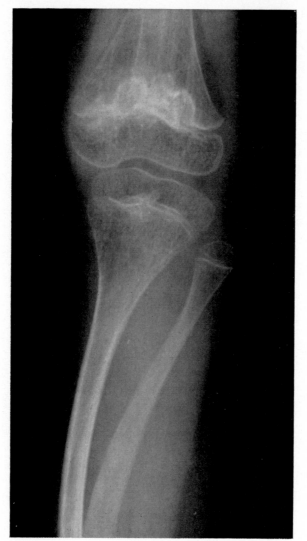

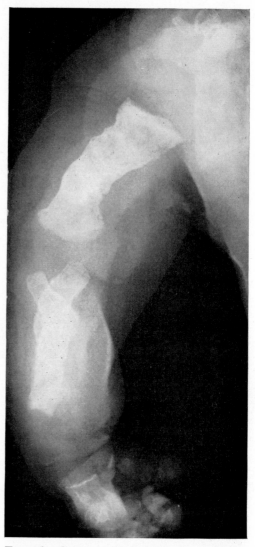

FIG. 5.—Osteogenesis imperfecta. Female aged 9 years. Long bones in knee region very narrow and bowed with thin cortex and few trabeculae. A few thickened trabecular strands above lower femoral epiphysis. Similar changes in all the long bones. Vault thin. Triradiate pelvis. Spontaneous fractures, many united in bad positions.

FIG. 6.—Osteogenesis imperfecta. Stillborn male aged about 38 weeks. Histologically very little bone, and fracture of the few trabeculae.

CHONDRO-OSTEODYSTROPHY

The appearances in chrondro-osteodystrophy are described in detail under "developmental defects" (page 40). In some cases with this diagnosis the epiphyses appear normal or nearly normal but there remains the characteristic widening of the femoral necks, the rather square-shaped pelvic bones and tongue-shaped vertebral bodies with irregular upper and lower margins.

LONG AND THIN—OSTEOGENESIS IMPERFECTA (FRAGILITAS OSSIUM)

Abnormally thin bones which therefore appear relatively long in relation to their width are seen in osteogenesis imperfecta (Fig. 5). The trabecular pattern may be absent or very small, thin and incomplete, and the cortex is also very thin. In some cases a few rather thick trabeculae are formed in long strands running irregularly across the remaining uncalcified cancellous bone, and these give the bones a multiloculated cystic appearance. Epiphyseal development is fairly normal as regards the age of appearance and fusion of the epiphyses and the general form of each epiphyseal centre, but the deficiency of the trabecular pattern within the epiphysis becomes obvious with growth.

Spontaneous fractures are common and usually unite (Fig. 7). They often occur without being diagnosed at the time and, because no treatment is given, union is apt to occur in a faulty position with resultant angular deformity. In the course of time the angulation tends to get smoothed out, leaving a residual bowing which is very similar to the deformity resulting from softening of the bone. In addition there may be some softening which itself contributes to the deformity.

Sometimes, especially in a patient in whom the changes are well marked pre-natally, the bones are abnormally wide and short instead of narrow and long (Fig. 7), thus simulating the appearances in achondroplasia. This seems to be due to compression fractures producing a concertina-like deformity (Fig. 6). The cortical thinning and absence of trabeculae are well marked and will indicate the diagnosis.

Vertebral flattening is common, the bodies being too narrow vertically relative to their antero-posterior width (Fig. 8). The end plates may be wider than normal and stand out unduly clearly against the adjacent under-mineralized cancellous bone of the vertebral body. In the skull the vault may be rather enlarged, thin and poorly ossified, and wormian bones are often conspicuous. The epiphyseal line in osteogenesis imperfecta is normal but the resulting bone formation, although orderly, is deficient in quantity. Thus the cortical bone is thin and the trabeculae are narrow and widely spaced to produce a bone which is deficient in strength.

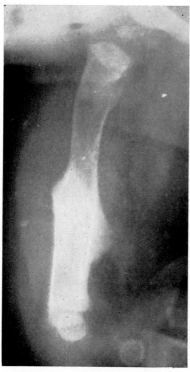

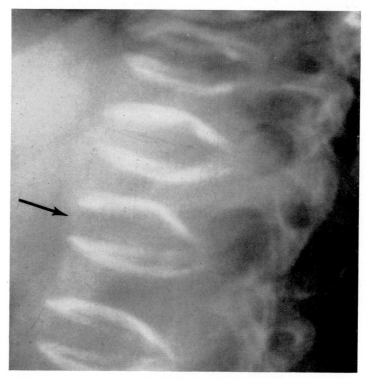

FIG. 7.—Osteogenesis imperfecta. Female aged 3 months. Femur wide and short, apparently due to concertina-like compression. Abundant calcified callus from united fracture in middle third. Vault thin and poorly ossified. Blue sclerotics; no F.H.

FIG. 8.—Osteogenesis imperfecta. Female aged 12 years. Poor ossification of the vertebral bodies, only the end plates showing as white line shadows (arrow points to a disc space). Bodies flattened. Long bone similar to Fig. 5.

In osteogenesis imperfecta the fundamental defect appears to be a failure of maturation of collagen beyond the reticulin stage, and the bone matrix is immature and disorganized. The epiphyseal cartilages appear normal. The skin is thin and the blue sclerotics suggest that the condition is a connective tissue disorder. McKusick (1966) lists it under heritable disorders of connective tissue and finds that there is disorganization of a defective collagen matrix in the bone. In this respect he suggests fibrodysplasia ossificans progressiva as likely, and the following as also coming within this group with the disorder limited to one variety of connective tissue:

Achondroplasia (pages 439–441)
Alkaptonuria (page 271)
Chondro-osteodystrophy (pages 235–399)
Fibrodysplasia ossificans progressiva (pages 400–415)
Homocystinuria (page 15)
Hurler–Hunter syndrome (pages 325–399)
Marfan (pages 38–149)
Multiple exostoses (page 457)
Osteogenesis imperfecta (pages 230–270)
Osteopetrosis (page 444)
Osteopoikilosis (page 415)

In all of these there are some bones with an abnormal shape except for osteopetrosis, in which the shape is normal but the density is altered.

MUSCULAR PARALYSIS

In extensive muscular paralysis with greatly diminished movements of the body and diminished stresses on the bones, most of the bones undergo a disuse atrophy or, if the patient is young, fail to develop, with the result that they are abnormally narrow and therefore appear abnormally long. The trabecular pattern is deficient or absent and the cortex is thin (Fig. 9). There is some resemblance to the appearances

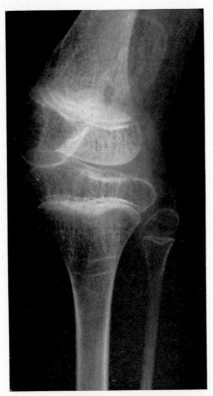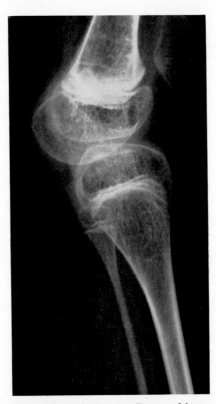

FIG. 9.—Old poliomyelitis with bone atrophy. Female aged 11 years. Bones of knee region very narrow. Thin cortex, loss of many trabeculae with compensatory widening of remaining ones giving a coarse pattern near bone ends and absence of trabeculae towards the middle third. Rotational deformity with femur facing forwards naturally, while ankle faces laterally. Paralysis lower limb since baby. Hand bones normal.

seen in lesser manifestations of osteogenesis imperfecta, but the diagnosis will be apparent from the clinical history and the clinical evidence of flaccid or spastic paralysis, the former often being due to poliomyelitis.

As a result of the abnormal stresses or absence of stresses other alterations in bone shape are common. There may be an increase in the angle between the femoral neck and shaft (coxa plana). Torsion deformity of a long bone may appear after a number of years if the limb is habitually placed in an abnormal position. For instance, if the foot is always kept well everted, in the course of time the femur will alter its shape so that eventually a posterior-view radiograph will show the femoral neck in its normal position and the lower femoral condyles and the patella in a lateral position.

If the muscular disorder is more limited in extent, the bone changes will be confined to one or two regions but never to a single bone.

EXAGGERATION OF SIZE—ACROMEGALY

The diagnosis of acromegaly may be obvious from inspection of the patient, but a doubtful case may be confirmed by a radiograph showing enlargement of the sella, thinning of the posterior clinoid processes, possibly elevation of the anterior clinoid processes and depression of the floor of the fossa (Figs. 10 and 11). If the depression is only on one side, it may pass undetected in the plain radiograph

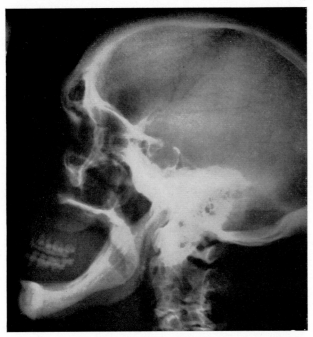

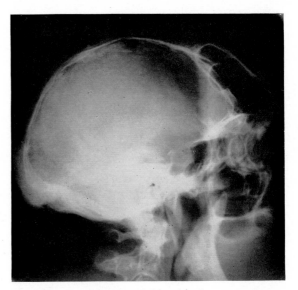

FIG. 10.—Acromegaly. Female aged 40 years. Large sella with thinning of the dorsum sellae and depression of the floor. Large frontal sinuses. Vault thick in frontal area. Anterior angle of mandible increased.

FIG. 11.—Acromegaly. Enlarged sella. Huge frontal sinuses; vault thick in occipital area.

(Fig. 12), but can be clearly seen in the lateral view tomogram (Fig. 13). There are often characteristic changes in the shape of the phalanges, mandible, skull and vertebrae.

The terminal phalanges may be rather spade-like in shape because of an exaggerated tufting of the tips (Fig. 14a). The other phalanges may be increased in size and there may be an undue prominence of the lateral ridges and protuberances normally seen projecting from the shafts. There may also be marginal protuberances or lipping of the phalangeal joint margins, but no diminution of the joint spaces. Excessive growth of part of the head of a metacarpal may lead to a local prominence giving a beak-like deformity (Fig. 14b). This may be the only obvious change. It is reminiscent of the deformity due to erosion sometimes seen in rheumatoid arthritis (see Fig. 309b).

The heel pad thickness can be measured in a lateral view radiograph (Fig. 15). Usually it is less than 23 mm. in normal males and 21·5 mm. in normal females (Steinbach and Russell, 1964; Kho, Wright and

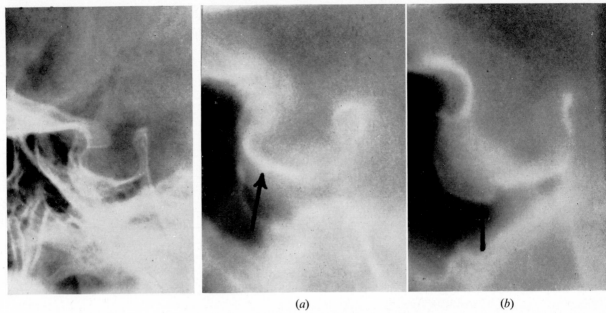

(a)   (b)

FIG. 12.—Acromegaly. Male aged 65 years. Plain lateral view of sella. Diagnosis uncertain.

FIG. 13.—(a) Sella: lateral view tomogram of left side; 11 cm. Same case as in Fig. 12. Floor intact (opposite arrow). (b) Same case, left side, 11·9 cm. Line of floor bulging downwards and forwards (opposite arrow).

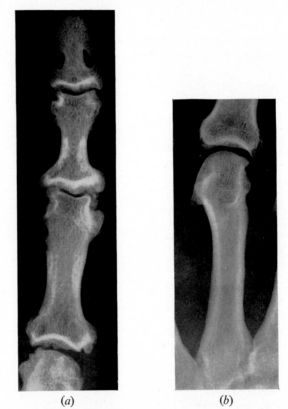

(a)   (b)

FIG. 14.—(a) Acromegaly. Female aged 40 years. Tufting of the terminal phalanges, exaggeration of the joint marginal angles and other bony ridges. Six years' amenorrhoea; enlargement of the hands and the lower jaw. Same case as in Fig. 10. (b) Acromegaly showing beak-like deformity of head of third metacarpal due to overgrowth of bone. Similar changes in all metacarpals except those of thumb.

Doyle, 1970), but in a patient with clinically obvious acromegaly it is more than this. Unfortunately there is no simple way of obtaining a true lateral view, and some normal people have a thick heel pad, so that in clinically doubtful cases the evidence from this measurement is often uncertain and changes in the sella are likely to be more helpful.

The mandible in a lateral view may appear lengthened, with relative elongation of the horizontal ramus and an increase in the angle from the usual near right angle to something more obtuse (Fig. 10). The frontal sinuses are usually very large with forward bulging of the anterior wall (Fig. 11). In many cases there are exaggerations of vault structure which, while not abnormal, are not seen as frequently in normal people: there may be hyperostosis frontalis; the vault may be thickened through widening

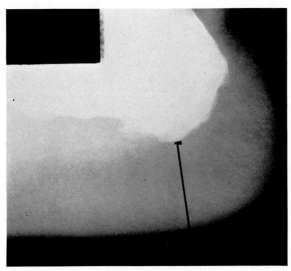

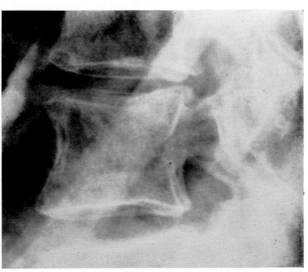

FIG. 15.—Acromegaly. Male aged 50 years. Obvious clinical features. Heel pad thickness 31 mm. (normal < 23 mm. in males, 21·5 mm. in females).

FIG. 16.—Acromegaly. Dorsal vertebra; lateral view showing new bone laid down on anterior and posterior surfaces of the body of the vertebra. Vertebral body large; all dorso-lumbar spine affected.

of the diploic bone; or there may be loss of bone definition in the vault, the two tables and the diploic bone producing a single homogeneous shadow either grossly widened (sometimes exceeding 3 centimetres) or of the normal width. All these changes may be seen in different parts of the vault in a single patient.

A late change sometimes seen is a relative increase in the antero-posterior diameter of the vertebral bodies partly due to the deposition of new bone in front of the original cortex. This original cortex may remain identifiable as a distinct linear shadow lying deep to the new bone (Fig. 16) or may eventually become indistinguishable from the new bone. Marginal lipping out of proportion to any diminution of the disc spaces may also be seen.

In response to the hypersecretion of growth hormone there is a hypertrophy of many organs, especially affecting the connective tissues. The periosteum is also stimulated to lay down new bone, producing the irregular thickening of the bones well seen in the radiograph. If facilities are available, the diagnosis can be established with some certainty by measuring the level of growth hormone.

REGIONAL ALTERATIONS IN SHAPE

Regional alterations in the shape of the bones may be divided into those caused by a congenital growth defect and those caused by a disease process. They may be seen in different sites in one patient, as in craniocleidodysostosis, or confined to one region such as the hands, feet or vertebrae. The diagnosis of a congenital defect is usually easy, especially if the deformity has been noticed since infancy and there is no skin scarring to suggest an old inflammatory lesion. The main distinguishing feature in a radiograph is the relatively normal trabecular pattern of the deformed bone.

CONGENITAL GROWTH DEFECTS

Ill-formed clavicles—craniocleidodysostosis

In craniocleidodysostosis there is incomplete development of both clavicles, the bone on each side being represented by a short ill-formed fragment (Fig. 17). Other regional bone deformities are often present: the mandibles are often deformed and since dentition is delayed, many unerupted teeth may be seen; the fontanelles in the skull may be wide open; in some patients the terminal phalanges are small and stunted. The bones formed from membrane are chiefly affected, whereas in achondroplasia (*see* page 1) it is the bones formed from cartilage.

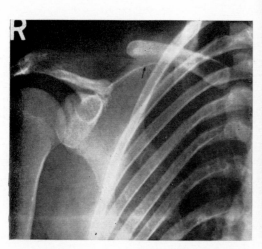

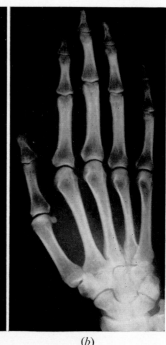

(a)   (b)

FIG. 17.—Craniocleidodysostosis. Male aged 28 years. Clavicle represented by central bony fragment (above arrow). Distal parts of terminal phalanges of fingers and toes absent.

FIG. 18.—Marfan (arachnodactyly). (a) Normal control; metacarpal index 6·0. (b) Marfan; metacarpal index 8·2. Female aged 38 years with dilated ascending aorta.

Long fingers—arachnodactyly (Marfan syndrome)

In archnodactyly the bones of the fingers are unduly long in relation to their width (Fig. 18). This elongation, which is often more obvious clinically than radiologically, can be proved by measurements. The length of each metacarpal (excluding the thumb) is measured, and the width of each one at its mid point (Fig. 18). The figures are added up and the total of the length is divided by the total of the widths to to give the metacarpal index. In a normal person this is usually less than 8; in arachnodactyly it is usually more than this and is often between 7·9 and 8·4. In some cases the height of each lumbar vertebral body is increased relative to its anterior–posterior diameter in a lateral view (Fig. 19), and the body may show a deep concavity of the posterior surface. In a posterior view the transverse processes may be very long.

These increases in bone length may be the only changes seen in arachnodactyly, or may be associated with other congenital defects such as dislocation of the lenses of the eyes and a high arched palate. Commonly there is an abnormality of the aortic wall leading to aneurysmal dilatation of the ascending aorta and aortic incompetence, or aortic incompetence may arise if the lesion affects the aortic valve cusps. Sometimes there is prolapse of the leaflet of the mitral valve.

The histology of the aortic wall shows a characteristic abnormality with fragmentation of the elastic pattern of the media and sometimes disappearances of the fibres. If there is cystic degeneration, the elastic fibres tend to be reflected round the cystic space rather than interrupted by it. Because of these histological features, McKusick (1966) considers that the Marfan syndrome falls into the category of heritable disorders of connective tissue.

Short wide hands

Short wide hands with short metacarpals are seen in the so-called trident hand (*see* Fig. 68), in chondro-osteodystrophy in association with defective ossification of the epiphyses, and with less epiphyseal deformity in achondroplasia.

Microdactyly, especially of the thumbs, is seen in fibrodysplasia ossificans progressiva (*see* Fig. 69).

A short scaphoid will tilt the thumb laterally. When associated with an atrial septal defect, this is known as the Holt–Oram syndrome (Fig. 20). The fourth metacarpal is abnormally short and its head lies below a line joining the ends of the third and fifth metacarpals. There may be fusion of the ends of the radius and ulna, or the radius may only partially develop. It is as if the organizer on the radial side only were defective. The fourth metacarpal is also short in some cases of ovarian agenesia (Turner's syndrome).

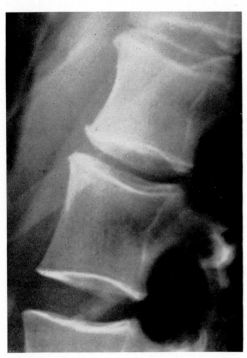

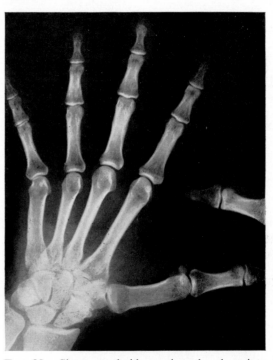

FIG. 19.—Marfan. Lateral view of lumbar spine. Vertebral height excessive in relation to antero-posterior diameter. Same case as in Fig. 18*b*.

FIG. 20.—Short scaphoid, so that thumb points laterally. Fourth metacarpal is short and lies below a line joining heads of third and fifth metacarpals. Male aged 35 years who also had an atrial septal defect (Holt–Oram syndrome).

Spondylo-epiphyseal dysplasia

Thickening of the end plates by a heaping up of bone on the superior and inferior surfaces of the vertebral bodies (Fig. 21) is seen in a rare heritable anomaly known as spondylo-epiphyseal dysplasia. It is often associated with severe osteoarthritis of the hips, and this may be secondary to some protrusio acetabulae. If seen in childhood, there are fragmented epiphyses. The fourth and fifth fingers may be short.

Deformed tarsals—club foot

A regional abnormality of the shape of the bones is seen in the more severe manifestations of club foot (talipes equino-varus) (Fig. 22). In this condition it must be realized that owing to the peculiar position in which the foot is held, an ordinary lateral view is not possible; often the tarsal bones are viewed rather foreshortened, and the degree of deformity may thus be hard to assess. It may also be hard to determine whether the foot deformity is due to the abnormal shape of the bones, or whether the bone deformity is the result of the persistently abnormal position of the foot.

Gross failure in the development of the hands or feet

Gross failure in the development of the hand or foot as a whole, as in claw hand or webbed fingers and toes, will involve gross alterations in the shape of the bones as well as the obvious soft tissue deformities. When plastic reconstruction operations are under consideration, radiographs may be of value to show which bones are missing and which fused and what are the particular alterations in shape of the individual bones.

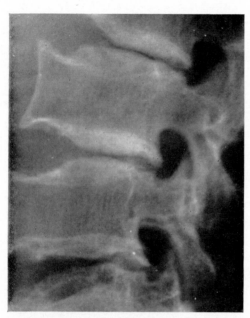

FIG. 21.—Spondylo-epiphyseal dysplasia tarda. Lumbar vertebra; lateral view showing heaping up of bone on posterior half of superior and inferior surfaces. Male aged 34 years with recent hip pain. Deformed femoral head and severe osteoarthritis.

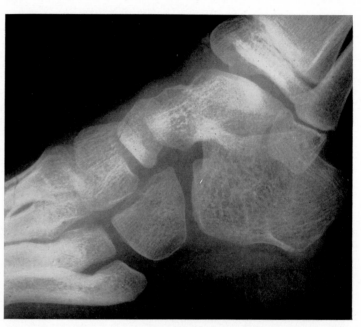

FIG. 22.—Talipes equino-varus (club foot). Female aged 8 years. Deformed shape of tarsal and metatarsal bones. Foot turned inwards and patient walks with heel off ground. Steindler operation and correction.

Congenital wedge-shaped and supernumerary vertebra

A vertebral body may appear wedge-shaped in a posterior-view radiograph and there may be an additional (supernumerary) vertebra which is usually incomplete and often only a hemi-vertebra (Fig. 23). These congenital growth defects may be discovered incidentally from, for instance, a routine chest radiograph, or they may be found to be the underlying cause of a scoliosis for which treatment has been sought.

The trabecular pattern is quite regular and almost normal in contrast to the coarsened or otherwise grossly affected trabecular pattern seen in vertebrae deformed by disease even after the original lesion has healed. In the upper cervical or dorsal region, tomograms may be more useful than plain radiographs for demonstrating the exact anatomy of the deformed vertebrae.

Spina bifida

Another common vertebral developmental deformity is non-fusion of the neural arch or spina bifida. This may consist only of a narrow transradiant band running vertically through the spinous process (Fig. 24), or there may be a much wider gap over the sacrum (Fig. 24), with the lateral bone masses demarcated by a well-defined medial margin. In some cases the two unfused masses with their surrounding cortex are seen end-on as ring shadows medial to the ring shadows of the pedicles. Spina bifida may be the only radiological change, or it may be associated with abnormalities of shape in the bodies such as

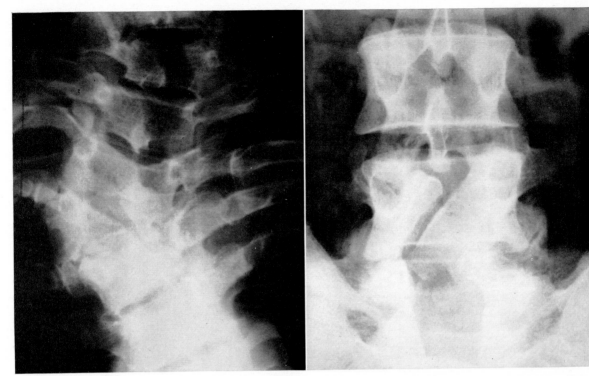

FIG. 23.—Congenital wedge-shaped vertebra. Female aged 40 years. The third thoracic vertebra is wedge-shaped with its left side undeveloped. Normal trabecular structure. Scoliosis convex to right. Asymptomatic.

FIG. 24.—Spina bifida. Male aged 25 years. Transradiant band across shadow of the fourth and fifth lumbar vertebrae and upper part of the sacrum marking the extent of the defect in the neural arch.

a wedge-shaped vertebra. There may be an associated diastematomyelia, a condition in which a central bony spur projects forwards into the region of the spinal canal, the spur often resulting in a mid-line oval shadow different in shape from the spinous processes seen above and below (Fig. 25). Spina bifida is most common in the lower lumbar region, but is also seen in the cervico-dorsal and dorso-lumbar junctional areas. It may be of no clinical significance or it may be associated with gross neurological lesions or with a meningocoele.

Fusion of vertebral bodies

Congenital fusion of two or more vertebral bodies is sometimes seen in the cervical region (Klippel–Feil) and sometimes in the mid-dorsal or lumbar region.

Not only is there no disc space between the two bodies, but there is often bony fusion of the posterior parts near the bases of the spinous processes, with considerable alteration in the shape of the vertebrae (Fig. 26). In such gross manifestations the nature of the lesion is obvious, but when the fusion is confined to the vertebral bodies without gross alteration in form, distinction must be made from fusion resulting from an inflammatory process. In congenital fusion the trabecular pattern is quite normal. It may extend in an even manner across the zone of fusion, or a horizontal line may mark the position of a rudimentary end plate.

In the Klippel–Feil type of defect the neck is abnormally short as in Fig. 26, but in other types fusion may occur with some elongation of the neck. In either case the fusion may be in the upper or lower cervical region (Figs. 26 and 27).

REGIONAL DEFORMITIES DUE TO DISEASE

Deformity of vertebral bodies

A regional deformity in the lumbo-dorsal spine may be the only bone abnormality, as in some cases of kyphosis, or it may be associated with a generalized abnormal development of the epiphyses in such conditions as hypothyroidism in a child (cretin) or chondro-osteodystrophy (*see* page 40).

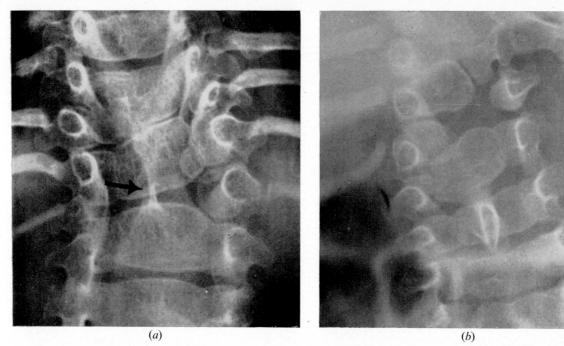

(a)   (b)

FIG. 25.—(a) Diastematomyelia. Female aged 18 months. Central bony spur (opposite arrow) L. 1. Fragmentary wedge vertebra D. 12 left side, and spina bifida lower dorsal vertebrae. Poorly developed disc space. On myelography central defect in contrast medium by bony spur. (b) Wedge-shaped hemivertebra D. 10, spina bifida and probable diastematomyelia.

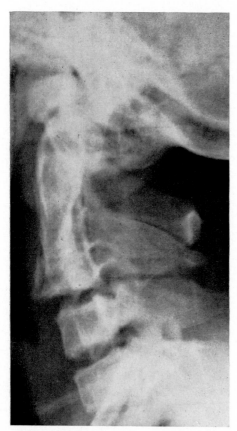

FIG. 26.—Congenital fusion of upper cervical vertebrae. There is a long segment of bone representing the upper cervical vertebrae with no disc spaces, and the lower vertebrae are normal.

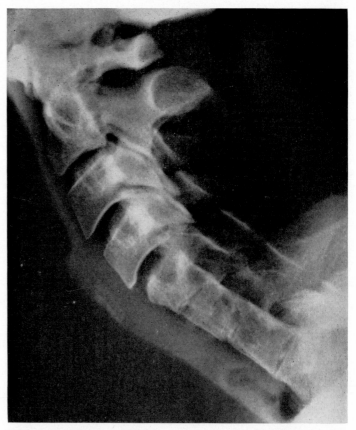

FIG. 27.—Congenital fusion lower cervical vertebrae. Female aged 38 years. Upper 4 vertebrae normal. Neck long. Asymptomatic. Disc spaces can still be identified by lines of end plates.

14

Kyphosis

Slight or moderate wedge-shaped deformity of several adjacent vertebrae in the thoracic region is seen in persons with long-standing kyphosis, and is generally the result of the faulty posture and not its cause. It is seen particularly in elderly persons with or without a poor calcium content of the bones, and may be in the region D. 4–6 or at a lower level. Vertebral wedging is also common in young adults in the D. 9–12 region with a normal structure of the bones. In some cases there is some irregularity of the end plates, but whether this is related to the cause or is secondary to the postural defect is often uncertain. The condition is usually asymptomatic and is a common finding in routine lateral-view chest radiographs even in athletic students and nurses. For scoliosis *see* page 34.

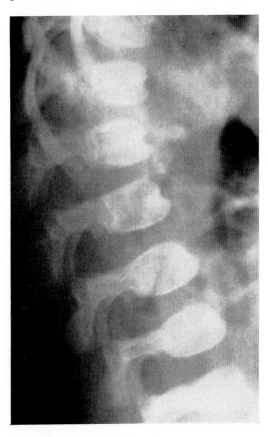

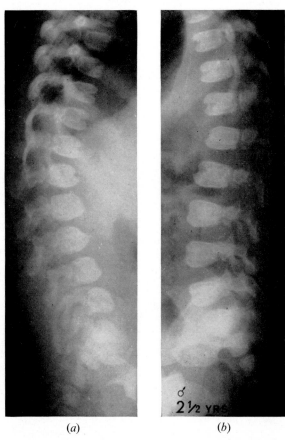

(a)   (b)

FIG. 28.—Cretin aged 2 years. Poor maturation of vertebrae. Rounded anterior end of L. 3. No ossification centres in femoral heads, similarly to case in Fig. 62.

FIG. 29.—(a) Cretin: female aged 6 months. Poorly developed vertebral bodies. Delayed growth. Good response to thyroid extract. (b) Cretin aged 2½ years. L. 2 poorly formed.

Cretinism

An alteration in the shape of some of the vertebral bodies in the dorso-lumbar region, with an apparent deficiency of the anterior part of the body of the vertebra, is seen in some cretinoid children (Figs. 28 and 29). The ill-formed anterior part tends to have a rather ragged margin, and the degree of wedge-shaped collapse is much less than would be expected from the apparent bone deficiency; the disc spaces are normal. The other bone changes seen in hypothyroidism are described under "endocrine epiphyseal defects" (*see* pages 39 and 44).

Faulty modelling of the long bones

Faulty modelling of the long bones, particularly the lower ends of the femora, may result in the bones being abnormally wide just proximal to the articular condylar expansion, producing a rather flask-shaped appearance.

This change is seen particularly in Gaucher's disease and is associated with a thin trabecular pattern and a thin cortex described under "widespread reduction in bone density" (*see* page 100). The patient often presents with swelling of the abdomen due to splenomegaly. Histological examination of the bone reveals bone resorption due to multiple accumulations of Gaucher cells. These are large cells with darkly staining nuclei and an abundant hyaline or reticulated cytoplasm containing the lipoid substance, cerebroside.

Faulty modelling may also be present in polyostotic fibrous dysplasia, when it is associated with the cyst-like or granular hazy appearance of the cancellous bone described under "well-demarcated trans-radiant area within a bone" (*see* Figs. 207 and 210*b*).

A similar widening of the lower ends of the femora may be seen in the haemoglobinopathies, and is associated with a coarsened trabecular pattern (*see* page 108).

Faulty modelling is also seen in some cases of osteopetrosis (*see* Fig. 101 and page 59), but is rather overshadowed by the extraordinary appearance of the dense structureless bone.

Deformity following epiphyseal damage

Following epiphyseal damage the rate of growth may be slowed down with consequent shortening (Fig. 30), and the direction of growth in length of a long bone may be altered with consequent deformity. Damage to the lower epiphysis of the radius, for instance, may cause the lower end of the bone to become bowed anteriorly (Madelung deformity).

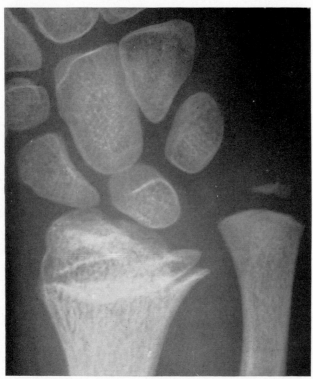

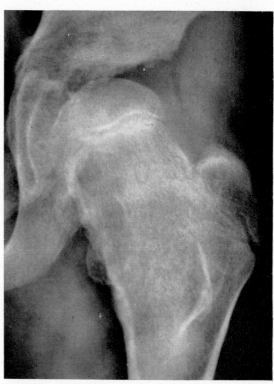

Fig. 30.—Post-traumatic growth defect of the radius. Female aged 6 years. Deformed shape of radial epiphysis, and failure of radius to grow as fast as the ulna. Injury some years before. Other wrist normal.

Fig. 31.—Exostoses causing deformity of femora neck. Male aged 16 years. Similar appearances in the other femur, and pointed exostoses from most of the major long bones similar to Fig. 33 only longer.

In the case of two adjacent long bones such as the tibia and fibula or the radius and ulna, interference with the growth of one will lead to relative overgrowth of the other. This frequently leads to marked bowing of the longer bone (Fig. 34).

Local enlargement of the bones of a limb

Local giantism or enlargement of the bones of a limb may occur with a local circulatory disorder such as an arterio-venous fistula, or a haemangiomatous or lymphangiomatous condition. It may also occur in neurofibromatosis (Charters, 1957).

LOCAL BONY PROTUBERANCE

EXOSTOSIS

Another alteration of bone shape is produced by an abnormal local bony protuberance projecting out from the cortex as exemplified by an exostosis. The protuberance may be sessile with a flat or rounded outer edge, or it may be pointed with an end which curves round away from the epiphysis. In either case its trabecular structure will be similar to that of normal cancellous bone and will merge into the normal cancellous bone beneath. It will also have a dense linear covering of cortical bone which is

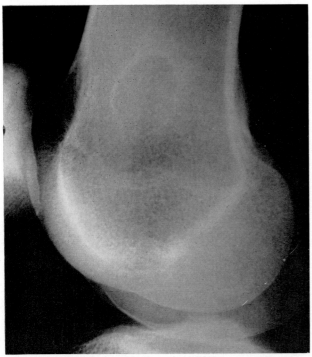

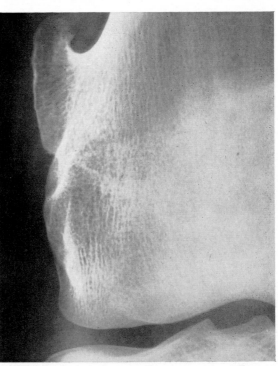

FIG. 32.—Exostosis of the femur (lateral view) showing a 2 cm. hair-line oval shadow in the middle of the femur just above the condyles. Male aged 21 years. Lump noticed on outer side since age of 15 years with little change in size.

FIG. 33.—Same case as in Fig. 32 (posterior view). Bony protuberance with outer linear cortical shadow and inner linear (trabecular) shadows continuous with those of the bone beneath.

continuous with the normal cortex beyond the limits of the protuberance. If there is a cap of cartilage, this is usually uncalcified and invisible in the radiograph, as is the covering of thick periosteum which is frequently present. Exostoses of both kinds vary in size from a few millimetres to several centimetres as regards both their base on the parent bone and their height from it.

Any bone may be the site of an exostosis, including the vertebrae or skull, ribs or scapulae. A single flat bony projection is most common on the lateral aspect of the middle third of the humerus, and a single rather more rounded projection on the posterior wall of a frontal sinus. A local, rather pointed bony projection may follow local trauma such as a stab wound. It may be the result of a local tear of the periosteum and the consequent loss of any restraining action by this structure on local cell proliferation.

Multiple, rather flatter projections from many bones, some pointed and some flat or rounded, are seen in multiple exostosis.

A local change of shape may occur as the result of an adjacent exostosis, or the change of shape may be due to a local cartilage growth defect or to the exostosis itself. In this case the cause of the abnormal shape may not be obvious. A flat exostosis on either side of the femoral neck, for instance, may merely give the bone the appearance of an irregular increase in width (Fig. 31), and one just below on the upper third of the shaft may give the appearance of a raised lesser trochanter. Flat projections on the neck of the humerus may also result in a rather broad and deformed humeral head which to the superficial glance will not suggest an exostosis. These appearances may be mistaken for chondro-osteodystrophy unless the more obvious forms of exostosis are present in other bones.

If a sessile or a short pointed exostosis is seen end-on it may appear as a ring shadow in the radiograph (Fig. 32), the ring representing the cortex seen *en face*, and will simulate a cystic condition. However, a view at right angles will probably show the bony projection quite clearly (Fig. 33).

An exostosis may grow towards a neighbouring bone and produce a pressure erosion in it. The eroded bone retains its structure and an intact cortical layer over the indentation facing the exostosis.

Another consequence of an exostosis may be faulty growth in length of the affected bone. An exostosis of the lower end of the ulna may cause a defect in its growth so that the distal end is deformed

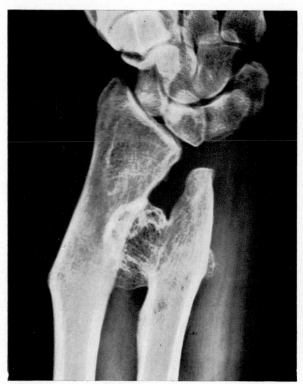 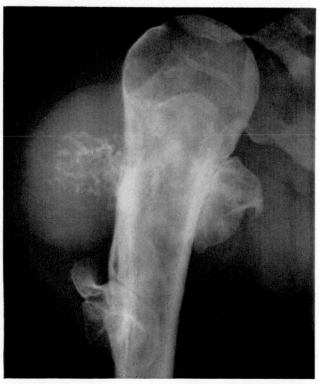

FIG. 34.—Exostosis of the ulna with growth defect. Female aged 48 years. Ulna relatively short and radius therefore bowed. Sessile exostosis ulna 2 cm. proximal to its deformed pointed distal end. Pointed exostoses similar to Fig. 33 from all the major long bones. Also growth defect upper end of the fibula because of a large exostosis.

FIG. 35.—Chondroma, lipoma and exostosis. Female aged 29 years. Medially the shadow with an outer line of cortex and an inner trabeculated appearance suggests an exostosis. Upper laterally there is a low-density shadow with dense spots representing calcifications in the chondroma; another exostosis below it. Ten years lump on arm slowly enlarging. Removal of chondroma with lipoma over it.

partly by the bony projection of the exostosis and partly by the lesion interfering with epiphyseal growth, so that the distal end of the bone is ill-formed and abnormally short. Since the radius may grow at a normal rate, it will be relatively lengthened and as a result may be bowed over the shorter ulna (Fig. 34).

In multiple exostoses all these x-ray changes may be seen together. A single patient, for instance, may have sessile and pointed exostoses in the knee region, deformities due to localized overgrowths in the region of the femoral necks and stunting of growth in an ulna with overgrowth of a radius.

Nothing is known for certain of the cause of an exostosis other than that it may follow periosteal damage or trauma. McKusick (1966) considers that multiple exostoses should be grouped with heritable disorders of connective tissue, and found disorganization of a defective collagen matrix in the bone. In most cases it is probable that the cartilage of the epiphysis develops in an irregular manner for some unknown reason and displaced nests of cartilage give rise to the exostosis. They are often apparent in infancy, but grow larger to their more characteristic shape in later childhood or adolescence and then cease to increase in size at the time of general epiphyseal fusion.

External Chondroma

An ecchondroma, if it is purely cartilaginous, may be invisible in a radiograph except for a puckering out of the cortex at its base. More often extensive calcification takes place in the cartilage, which then casts a massive amorphous shadow without a recognizable trabecular pattern (Fig. 35). Sometimes the part of the projection closest to the bone shows a trabecular pattern while the opacity further out is mottled, so that an osteochondroma can be diagnosed. The distinction is really one of degree, since the most bony-looking protuberance often has a cartilaginous cap which may be invisible in the radiograph, while an amorphous shadow of a calcifying chondroma may be found to have bony elements in it on histological examination.

In a case of multiple exostoses (diaphyseal aclasis) chondromata, osteochondromata and "classical" pointed and sessile exostoses may all be present at varying sites in the same patient. Most of the prominences will be of the more bony type, while many of the larger examples of calcifying chondromata are single.

There is a tendency for the larger calcifying chondromata to undergo a focal malignant change to chondrosarcoma. The transition to this stage may not be manifest radiologically, though any change in the size or density of the shadow after adolescence should always suggest this possibility (Fig. 36).

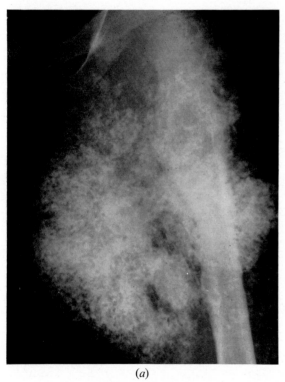

(a)

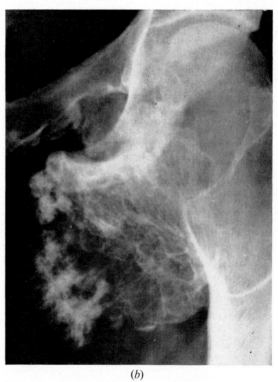

(b)

Fig. 36.—(a) Chondrosarcoma on chondroma. Male aged 23 years. Dense spots in a huge calcifying chondroma of the femur. Lump in thigh recently enlarging. Biopsy: chondrosarcoma. Typical pointed exostoses similar to Fig. 33 from all the major long bones, and growth defect of the ulna as Fig. 34. Condition familial, but no other sarcomata in other members of the family as yet. (b) Ossifying chondroma. Female aged 27 years, sister of patient illustrated in (a). No sarcoma as yet. Pointed exostoses similar to Fig. 33.

LOCAL BONE DEFICIENCY

Developmental deficiency

A developmental deficiency of the middle third of a long bone may result in a tapering type of deformity with gross narrowing of the centre of the shaft. There may even be a complete gap in the bone with a pseudo-arthrosis separating the two tapering halves. This appearance is seen in the tibia in some cases of neurofibromatosis, when it presumably represents an associated developmental defect and is not the result of a local neurofibroma. The tibia may develop normally at first, and the developmental abnormality may grow later and cause the area of bone absorption. A similar condition is seen occasionally in a case of fibrous dysplasia. The developmental nature of this deformity will be apparent if characteristic lesions are seen in other bones.

Acquired conditions

The same deformity from an acquired condition, such as trauma or an infection, is more likely to be isolated. In the absence of any history the presence of overlying skin damage may suggest the cause.

Deficiencies at the end of a bone of the hands or feet are seen in some cases of arthritis (*see* arthritis mutilans, page 195) and in some trophic or vascular lesions. Among the vascular lesions may be included the absorption of the tip of a terminal phalanx in diffuse systemic sclerosis (scleroderma) (Fig. 248) when this is the result of the thickened sclerodermatous tissue constricting the vessels.

In hyperparathyroidism the tips of the terminal phalanges may become so undermineralized that they cease to be visible in the radiograph, but they may reappear after treatment of the underlying cause (Figs. 203 and 204)—*see* page 120.

COLLAPSE OF A SINGLE VERTEBRA

A vertebra which appears in the radiograph to be evenly flattened or flattened anteriorly and therefore wedge-shaped will either be collapsed or have failed to develop into its normal shape. If the cause is not obvious clinically, it may be suggested by certain radiographic features, particularly the appearance of the adjacent disc spaces, the presence or absence of a paravertebral low-density shadow, any structural changes in the collapsed vertebra, and the presence of osteoporosis of the spinal column as a whole (*see* page 113).

Normal disc space with a collapsed vertebra of normal density will suggest a traumatic collapse or a developmental defect, while normal disc spaces with decreased density of the vertebral body from bone erosion will suggest a xanthomatous deposit, a benign tumour, a secondary deposit, or a hydatid cyst (in areas where the disease is endemic). A collapsed vertebra with increased density and either a normal or a reduced disc space would suggest a vascular lesion—in an older child, of unknown aetiology, or in an adult a complication of trauma.

If the collapsed vertebra is associated with narrowing or complete loss of the disc space, the condition will usually be tuberculous, although a similar combination may be seen in a pyogenic or brucella infection (Fig. 41). An associated paravertebral low-density shadow is most likely to be seen with a tuberculous infection, and the collapse is commonly wedge-shaped. In even collapse from an extensive secondary deposit, the disc space may be narrowed if the disc herniates into the destroyed vertebra. A similar change may occur in osteochondritis.

A dense rather structureless vertebral body, which is also wider than normal although somewhat flattened, will suggest Paget's disease (Figs. 120 and 121).

The presence of widespread osteoporosis of all the vertebrae is difficult to detect (*see* page 113), and the presence of a single collapsed vertebra as the sole change is unusual but may occur. A slightly reduced height of one or two other vertebrae, nearby but not necessarily adjacent, may pass undetected, but if found would suggest osteoporosis.

VERTEBRAL OSTEOCHONDRITIS

Vertebral osteochondritis with collapse (Calvé)

In a young child with trivial symptoms, a collapsed vertebral body with a normal disc space may be the result of an osteochondritis as suggested by Calvé (1925). The number of cases in which pathological material has been available is very small, so there is some doubt whether the collapse results from a vascular lesion with aseptic necrosis of the bone, or whether in fact it is the result of an indolent form of tuberculosis as suggested by Fenyes and Zoltan (1959), or more probably a xanthomatous granuloma (histiocytosis x) which neither progresses locally nor exhibits other manifestations later.

The collapse may be even but is usually more marked anteriorly, producing a wedge-shaped deformity. Such a vertebra plana in a child (Fig. 37), when the cause is unproved, may be observed radiologically to improve after some years, indicating that the lesion is quiescent and not interfering with growth, so that eventually the vertebral body may appear almost normal (Fig. 38) (Fripp, 1959).

Vertebral osteochondritis with disc intrusion

Whereas in young children an osteochondritis of the vertebral body may result in gross collapse but with a normal disc space as described above (Fig. 37), in an older child the lesion may affect only a part of the vertebral body, so that there is only slight wedge-shaped collapse. In many cases there is some protrusion of the intervertebral disc into the affected part of the vertebral body, so that there is also slight narrowing of the disc space (Fig. 39). The appearances are very similar to those seen in the early stages of a tuberculous lesion, but as there is no progressive collapse, no gross narrowing of the disc space, no paravertebral abscess shadow and no convincing clinical evidence of a tuberculous lesion, the two conditions can usually be distinguished.

Xanthomatous Deposit

Uniform collapse of a vertebral body in a child, and sometimes in an adult, may be due to destruction of the bony elements of the vertebral body by a xanthomatous deposit (*see* page 132). Once collapse has occurred, the area of erosion may be difficult to detect, but there is generally clear radiological evidence of the local bone destruction. It may be an isolated change, when the diagnosis may be difficult without a biopsy, or it may be associated with transradiant areas in other bones, making this diagnosis probable.

Traumatic and Post-traumatic Collapse

The diagnosis of vertebral collapse due to trauma may be obvious from the history, but sometimes the traumatic incident may have been forgotten or may have occurred unknown to the patient, as in electric shock therapy without muscle relaxants. In some cases the spine may not have been radiographed after a known traumatic incident, perhaps because lesions in other parts overshadowed the spinal condition at the time. In yet other cases the spine may have appeared normal in the initial radiographs, whereas radiographs some weeks or months later showed a collapsed vertebra. The reason for this may have been either that the initial radiographs were of poor quality (especially if radiography was difficult because of the state of the patient) or that the trauma resulted in some damage which was invisible at the time but which gave rise some weeks or months later to softening and then collapse of the vertebra.

A traumatic or post-traumatic collapse is generally wedge-shaped. There is a strong tendency for bony lipping to be visible anteriorly, often uniting the collapsed vertebra to the one above it and sometimes to the one below as well. This localized lipping, projecting well forwards, is not seen with collapse due to an untreated secondary deposit.

Vascular Lesion

A local vascular lesion may cause an increase in density of a vertebral body (*see* Fig. 122), and sometimes vertebral collapse may occur later. In such instances the underlying vascular lesion can rarely be proved, but certain cases of late collapse after trauma may fall into this category, and perhaps some cases of osteochondritis in children.

Hydatid Cyst

A hydatid cyst or other non-neoplastic destructive lesion may also result in collapse of a vertebral body.

Neoplastic Secondary Deposit

In an elderly person an even or more rarely a wedge-shaped collapse, with a normal disc space and normal structure of the adjacent vertebrae, will suggest a secondary deposit from a carcinoma, a plasmacytoma or the fully developed phase of a myelomatosis. Owing to the compression associated with the collapse, the erosion of the tumour is often inconspicuous. Quite commonly only a single

21

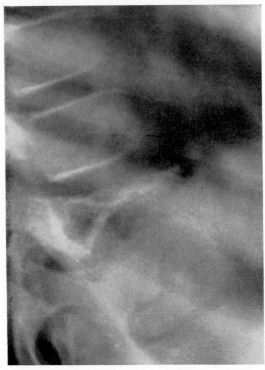

Fig. 37.—Possible osteochondritis (Calvé-type); might be an eosinophil granuloma. Male aged 12 years. Collapse of D. 9 with normal disc space. Slight pain. Ten years later some regeneration.

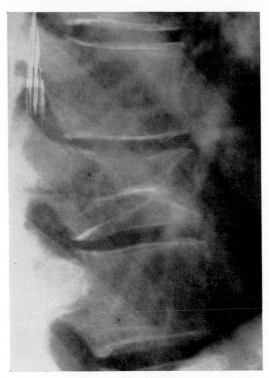

Fig. 38.—Same case as in Fig. 37, 11 years later. Asymptomatic. Plays games. As an adult leads a normal life. Pathology unknown.

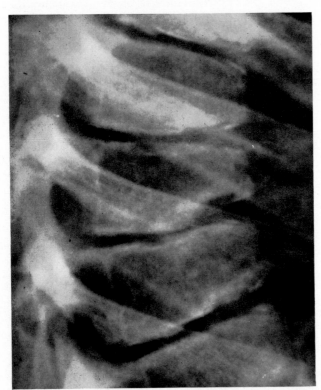

Fig. 39.—Osteochondritis. Male aged 13. Narrow disc spaces with erosion of the anterior-inferior margin and slight wedge shaping of D. 7, 8 and 9. Slight pain after violent exercise, otherwise asymptomatic and no physical signs; E.S.R. 3.

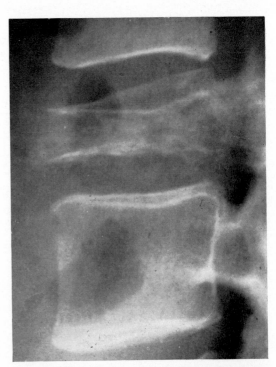

Fig. 40.—Secondary deposit. Female aged 48 years. Even collapse of L. 3 with normal disc space. Carcinoma of the breast. Deposits in other bones some months later. No paravertebral soft tissue shadow.

vertebra is affected (Fig. 40). The primary neoplasm may be known, or may not be detected at first, or there may be evidence of myelomatosis from the electrophoretic pattern or a marrow biopsy. In either case bone erosions may be discovered in other sites by further radiography, or a lung lesion may be found.

NEOPLASTIC SECONDARY DEPOSIT WITH DISC INTRUSION

Occasionally the vertebral erosion by a secondary deposit is so extensive before the vertebra collapses that when this does occur, the disc intrudes into the mass of diseased bone at the same time with consequent narrowing of the disc space. The diagnosis is usually obvious from the presence of a known

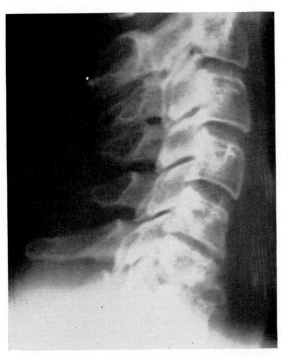

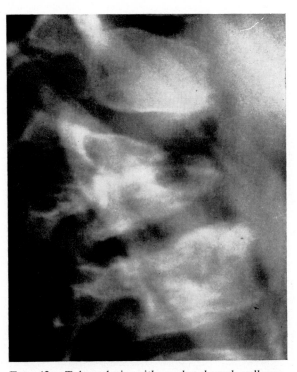

FIG. 41.—Brucellosis. Male aged 40 years with some neck pain. Narrow discs C. 5–7. Erosion of anterior-inferior angle of C. 6 and sclerosis of body. Tests for brucellosis positive.

FIG. 42.—Tuberculosis with wedge-shaped collapse. Female aged 9 years. Complete loss of disc spaces, wedge-shaped collapse of D. 9 and 10, paravertebral and psoas abscess shadow with a little calcium in it.

primary malignant neoplasm, and in such a case there is no paravertebral neoplastic mass. In some cases, particularly in the elderly, disc intrusion, protrusion or regeneration may have preceded the arrival and growth of the secondary deposit, and the narrow disc space would then be unrelated to the vertebral collapse. In such cases there is usually narrowing of several disc spaces.

BENIGN TUMOUR

Vertebral collapse may be due to the extensive erosion of an aneurysmal bone cyst or an osteoclastoma (Fig. 219). Both are rare in a vertebra and may cause erosion without collapse.

DEVELOPMENTAL DEFECT

Occasionally the body of a vertebra is wedge-shaped because it has failed to develop properly. This cannot, strictly speaking, be described as a collapsed vertebra since it has never been normal in shape. It may be an isolated change, but usually some other local developmental abnormality will also be seen, such as non-fusion of the neural arch, and this will make the diagnosis obvious. The height of the vertebra above may be greater anteriorly than posteriorly in compensation for the loss of height anteriorly of the wedge-shaped vertebra. Some cases are the late result of a chondro-osteodystrophy, when the other bone changes, particularly those in the pelvis and femora, will give the diagnosis (*see* page 40). Collapse of a single vertebral body may result from fibrous dysplasia.

INFLAMMATORY LESION (NON-TUBERCULOUS) WITH COLLAPSE

Disc narrowing and a local vertebral body erosion with some collapse may be due to a non-tuberculous inflammatory lesion, either pyogenic or more rarely typhoid or brucellosis (Fig. 41). There is usually some sclerosis as well as the erosion, and after a time secondary lipping is often a conspicuous feature.

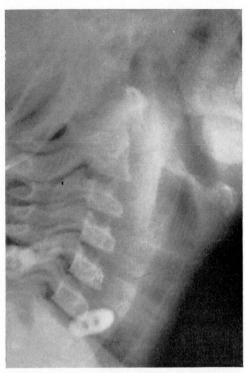

FIG. 43.—Retropharyngeal abscess. Female aged 5 years. Increased width of shadow between lower part of pharyngeal and laryngeal transradiancies and anterior margin of cervical vertebra. Possibly from infected cervical glands. Pus found.

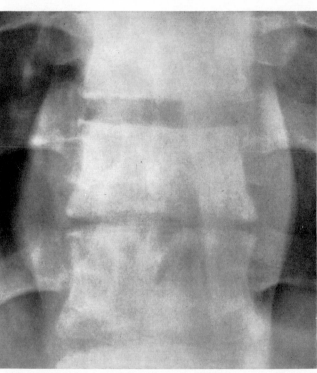

FIG. 44.—Tuberculous paravertebral abscess. Male aged 20 years. Shadow either side of the vertebral bodies in the D. 9–12 region. Lateral view showed narrow disc space and vertebral body erosion. Pain in back 8 weeks.

TUBERCULOUS LESION WITH VERTEBRAL COLLAPSE

A tuberculous lesion will be suggested if a collapsed vertebra is associated with a narrow or absent disc space (Fig. 42). The tuberculous erosion underlying the collapse may be visible if the collapse is relatively slight. Often, however, it is too extensive and the compressed bony debris gives a more or less homogeneous shadow. If one vertebra is collapsed there is generally some erosion of the adjacent surface of the vertebra above or below.

An important feature in the diagnosis is the demonstration of a paravertebral abscess. The appearance of this will depend on its site. In the cervical region an abscess may be presumed if there is forward displacement of the pharyngeal or tracheal transradiancy (Fig. 43). Normally the pharyngeal transradiancy is separated from the vertebrae by a soft tissue shadow some 3 mm. wide, and the tracheal transradiancy by a soft tissue shadow which includes the oesophagus, but which is not as wide as the tracheal transradiancy itself. If an abscess is present, the width of one or both of these soft tissue shadows is considerably increased.

In the dorsal region the shadow of a paravertebral abscess must be distinguished from the shadow caused by the descending aorta and the mediastinal pleural shadow marking the edge of the lung transradiancy medially. If both these normal shadows can be identified, the presence of a third shadow will indicate a pathological lesion, either an abscess (Fig. 44) or a paravertebral neoplastic mass (Fig. 260). In certain anaemias with hyperplasia of ectopic marrow tissue a similar shadow may be seen. All these shadows are shorter than the two normal paravertebral shadows, and tend to show a local lateral convexity, whereas the normal shadows have a straight border. In case of doubt posterior view tomograms may be of value by showing all three shadows at different levels.

In the lumbar region an abscess may cause a prominence of one or both psoas shadows (Fig. 45). Again, whereas the lateral margin of the psoas muscle normally is straight, an abscess tends to show a lateral convex bulge. In the later stages dense spots of calcium may be seen in the abscess. In some cases it is not confined to the psoas sheath, and forms an oval or even reniform shadow in the region below the twelfth rib.

On the whole a collapsed vertebra with a paravertebral shadow will suggest tuberculosis or a pyogenic lesion, while a paravertebral shadow due to a neoplastic mass may be associated with an erosion of the body, but is rarely associated with vertebral collapse.

PAGET'S DISEASE

An even collapse with increased density of the vertebral body and some increase in its width, often combined with marked marginal lipping (Fig. 120), will suggest Paget's disease (*see* page 68). In some cases one vertebra only is affected, though there is often evidence of Paget's disease in some bone other than the spine.

SPINAL OSTEOPOROSIS WITH COLLAPSE OF A SINGLE VERTEBRA

The difficulties of diagnosing spinal osteoporosis are discussed on page 113. The diagnosis is often made on the presence of a vertebral fracture or vertebral compression collapse rather than on the loss of trabecular pattern, the cortical thickness or the clarity with which the lines of the end plates stand out.

The collapse in this condition is commonly confined to the central part of the vertebral body and in a lateral-view radiograph a concave indentation into the upper and lower borders is seen (Figs. 158 and 190). In some cases, however, the collapse is even and the body simply flattened, while in others the body is wedge-shaped. Although a single vertebra may be affected, it is more common for several to be so, and these are not necessarily adjacent or even in the same region.

In an elderly patient the spinal osteoporosis is often simply an age or endocrine change. On the other hand it is possible for an elderly patient to have at the same time a primary neoplasm elsewhere, clinically obvious or latent at the time, with a secondary deposit in the already porotic vertebra precipitating its collapse.

DEFORMITY FROM SOFTENING OF THE BONES

TRIRADIATE PELVIS

Softening of the pelvic bones, whatever the cause, may lead to pressure indentation of the pelvis opposite the hip joints. When this is widespread the pelvis becomes triradiate in shape (Fig. 166). If the softening occurred in childhood and the bones later recalcified, the pelvic bones though deformed will show a normal architecture. If on the other hand widespread under-mineralization is still present, then this will be shown in the pelvic bones too (as described on page 104), osteomalacia being a common cause. Another common cause is Paget's disease, when the typical alteration in bone architecture described on page 178 will be seen.

PROTRUSIO ACETABULAE

In another type of case in which the softening is less general and most marked in the acetabular region, the pressure of the femoral head deepens the acetabular cavity and causes a medial convex bulge of the wall of the pelvic cavity directly opposite, a condition called protrusio acetabulae (Fig. 46). In some cases the bony wall between the articular cortex and the pelvic cavity is much thinned; in others a compensatory boss of cortical bone forms on the medial side.

The condition may be seen with a relatively normal joint interval and relatively normal bone architecture—suggesting a weakening in childhood with normal calcification at a later date or a growth defect of uncertain origin. Often the joint interval is greatly narrowed, possibly due to the mechanical instability of the joint producing a secondary osteoarthritis. In some cases there is a narrow joint interval and lipping, a coarsened irregular trabecular pattern, and an increase in the width of the cortex regionally or throughout the pelvis indicating Paget's disease.

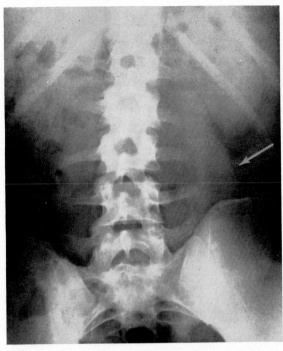

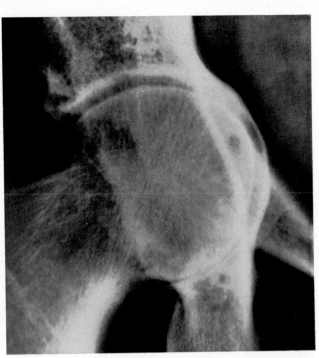

FIG. 45.—Psoas abscess. Male aged 35 years. Bulge left psoas shadow (opposite arrow). Lateral view showed narrow disc space L. 2–3. No bone erosion. Four months' pain in back. Firm mass in loin aspirated and tubercle bacilli found.

FIG. 46.—Protrusio acetabulae. Female aged 47 years. Asymptomatic. Poor calcium content and some trabecular absorption of the femora and pelvis. Looser zone in femur. Condition of protrusio bilateral. Osteomalacia, cause not found.

BOWING OF THE LONG BONES

Softening of the long bones often leads to bending of the bone. Anterior convex bowing of the femora and tibiae is common in osteomalacia, particularly in children, and is usually present in softening due to Paget's disease. In either case the radiograph will often indicate the cause of the deformity.

In young children a minor degree of anterior bowing of the tibiae may be seen without any other radiological or clinical evidence of disease, and is generally of no significance apart from its slight unsightliness.

2—Alterations in the Position of a Bone

A group of bones may lie habitually in a position different from that in which it normally lies when at rest, as in congenital elevation of the shoulder girdles, or there may be a pathological alteration in the position of a single bone in relation to the neighbouring bone or bones with which it normally articulates, as in congenital dislocation of the hip. In the first case it may be possible to reproduce the displacement by an exaggeration of normal movement, while in the second the displacement cannot be attained by normal movement.

In the majority of cases of altered bone position the condition is congenital, but occasionally a non-traumatic dislocation of a joint may arise in the early stages of an acute infective arthritis (*see* page 183) or as a result of a long-standing muscular paralysis. If such a pathological, or for that matter traumatic, dislocation occurred in infancy and cannot be recollected it may not be possible to tell, in the absence of clinical clues, whether the condition is congenital or acquired.

In a congenital dislocation there may be an associated congenital bony abnormality predisposing to the displacement, such as faulty development of the pars interarticularis in spondylolisthesis. Whatever the cause of the displacement, secondary alterations in the shape of the bones in the region of the joint will develop in response to the altered direction of the normal mechanical stresses on the bones. When the deformity is marked, it is sometimes difficult to determine how much of the alteration in shape is a congenital failure of modelling and how much is secondary to the dislocation.

Congenital Elevation of the Scapulae

Elevation of the scapulae (Sprengel's deformity) is the result of the failure of the scapulae to descend from the high position they normally occupy in embryonic life. Not only is the whole shoulder girdle abnormally high, but the scapula is small and short. The condition is usually bilateral, but one side may be higher than the other. The clavicle may lie in a relatively high position on the upper and outer edge of the sternum, and the facet for the joint is shallow and poorly developed.

Depressed Sternum

In patients with a depressed sternum, the whole of the lower anterior thorax is depressed and a deep furrow is very obvious on inspection. The condition is perhaps due to a failure of development of the soft parts, particularly the diaphragm, which prevents the sternum from rising forwards to its normal position.

A lateral-view radiograph or tomograph is of value to show how much space is available between the sternum and the vertebral column for the transit of the aorta. The heart is usually displaced to one side. Operative elevation may be necessary either for aesthetic reasons or to relieve cardio-respiratory insufficiency.

Genu Valgum

Minor degrees of knock knees, in which the ankles are separated from each other when the patient stands with knees together, are normal in growing children, but when the condition is more marked it is pathological. In such cases a radiograph may show the relative overgrowth of the medial condyle of the femur which is responsible for the tilting of the joint and consequent lateral alignment of the tibia (Fig. 47), and if long films are taken the angle of deviation can be measured with considerable accuracy.

Spondylolisthesis

Backward displacement of the sacrum on the fifth lumbar vertebra may be traumatic, but is more often either a developmental condition in itself or the result of a congenital defect in the pars interarticularis which allows the displacement to occur in childhood or adolescence under the normal stresses of the body weight.

Cozens (1961) reported 2 cases in which neither the displacement nor the defect in the pars interarticularis was present in a radiograph soon after birth, but both were visible in a radiograph at the age of 7 years.

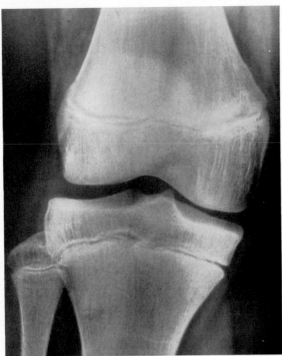

FIG. 47.—Genu valgum. Female aged 11 years. Genu valgum with relative overgrowth of the medial half of the lower femoral epiphysis. Bilaterally symmetrical. Ankle separation when knees touch was 8 cm. at the age of 8 years and is 16 cm. now. Obese but no endocrine defect proved. Correction osteotomy.

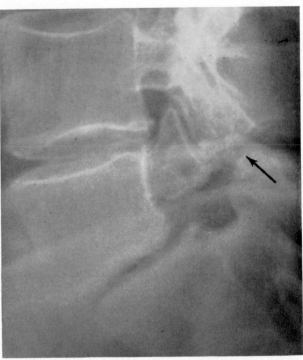

FIG. 48.—Spondylolisthesis. Female aged 59 years, 8 mm. backward displacement of the sacrum on L. 5. Narrow disc space between L. 5 and S. 1. Defect pedicle L. 5 (opposite arrow). No bow-line in posterior view. Slight intermittent backache.

Recorded instances of a late displacement, either traumatic or secondary to a defect in the pars interarticularis, are very rare and so also is the radiological demonstration of any increase in the displacement over the years, though cases are mentioned by Hitchcock (1940). In the vast majority of cases the condition is already established by the time radiographs are taken of the lower spinal region, and, so long as the orientation of the patient and x-ray beam remains constant, the degree of displacement in later radiographs is usually unchanged.

Lateral view

The displacement is best assessed from a lateral-view radiograph by tracing a line downwards along the posterior margin of the body of the fifth lumbar vertebra and continuing it along the posterior rim of the main mass of the body of the sacrum. Normally this line forms a continuous even curve, but it is interrupted at the lumbo-sacral junction in spondylolisthesis. This displacement is usually of several millimetres and quite obvious (Fig. 48). If there is any doubt there is probably no displacement. The degree of displacement may be graded as slight if it is less than a quarter of the width of the sacrum, and moderate if up to half the width; any displacement beyond this can be graded as severe.

The underlying congenital developmental defect is usually clearly seen in the lateral view, when the small spinous process and a transradiant linear defect can be seen in the posterior mass of the bone.

It is probable that this defect is due to the presence of two ossification centres in the neural arch which are joined by cartilage or fibrous tissues instead of bone, thus forming the weak point which predisposes to the displacement. Additional oblique views are therefore rarely necessary to show the defect, nor is there any evidence at present that an exact radiographic study of the site and size of the defect will assist in a decision regarding the line of treatment to be adopted. The relation of the defect and the displacement to the symptoms is also difficult to determine. Some patients are symptom free, others lose their symptoms and yet the defect and displacement remain unchanged.

Posterior view (bow-line shadow)

Spondylolisthesis may also be presumed from a posterior-view radiograph when a continuous bow-line shadow is seen running across the vertebral column near the upper part of the sacrum (Fig. 49). This line shadow will be seen to lie along the inferior margin of the fifth lumbar vertebra and to become continuous at either end, with the cortex forming the inferior margins of the two transverse processes. It is caused by the abnormal forward tilt of the vertebra and is easily distinguished from the oval line shadow seen in cases of gross sacral lordosis, which is formed by the cortex surrounding the upper part of the body of the sacrum when seen almost end-on (Fig. 50).

The bow-line shadow is sometimes of value in that it may be seen in a posterior-view radiograph of a patient's lower abdomen taken for a suspected abdominal condition, and may then be an indication for a lateral-view radiograph of the lumbo-sacral region to confirm or exclude displacement, especially

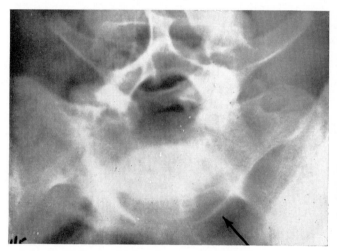

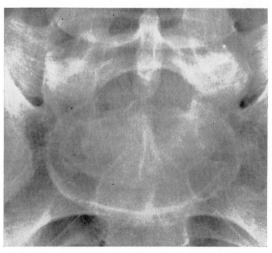

FIG. 49.—Spondylolisthesis. Male aged 19 years. Note bow-line (opposite arrow) joining the transverse processes of L. 5 and passing over the shadow of the sacrum. Lateral view similar to Fig. 48, but whole width of sacrum displaced posteriorly (4 cm.) on L. 5. Pedicle defect.

FIG. 50.—Normal lumbar spine (for comparison with Fig. 49). Male aged 50 years. Note oval line shadow representing the body of the sacrum seen almost end-on in this posterior view. Lateral view normal with moderate lordosis. Radiographed for renal cyst.

in an obese individual when the physical signs of displacement may be indefinite. Spondylolisthesis is often present without this bow-line appearance in a posterior view, and the diagnosis can only be made with certainty from a lateral-view radiograph.

Narrowing of the disc space

Narrowing of the disc space between the fifth lumbar vertebra and the sacrum is common in spondylolisthesis, but is a finding of no great significance since this disc space is frequently narrowed in other lower spinal congenital variations such as a sacralized fifth lumbar vertebra or even as an isolated change (*see* page 205). Unless progressive narrowing is observed, it is impossible to judge whether the narrowing represents a shallow but normal disc, or a degenerated or protruded disc. Secondary bony lipping of the posterior inferior angle of the fifth lumbar vertebra and posterior superior angle of the sacrum is surprisingly uncommon considering the abnormal direction of the stresses. Some sclerosis beneath the end plates may occur in some cases.

Reverse spondylolisthesis

Reverse spondylolisthesis or forward displacement of the sacrum on the fifth lumbar vertebra is sometimes seen. It may be a radiological artefact produced by the diverging rays projecting the lateral part of the sacrum further forward than L. 5 lying closer to the film, or it may be real. It is always slight, often associated with a marked backward tilt of the sacrum, and there is no defect in the pars interarticularis. The relationship of this appearance to symptoms is usually very indefinite. At the most it represents a bad postural habit, or a protective sacral tilt to avoid pain due to some other local cause which cannot be seen in the radiograph.

Displacement of lumbar vertebrae on each other

Forward or backward displacement of a lumbar vertebra on the one above it is not uncommon in elderly persons and is associated with considerable narrowing of that disc space (Fig. 51). The condition

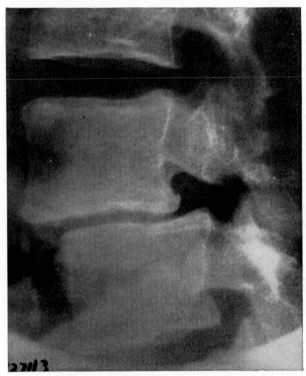
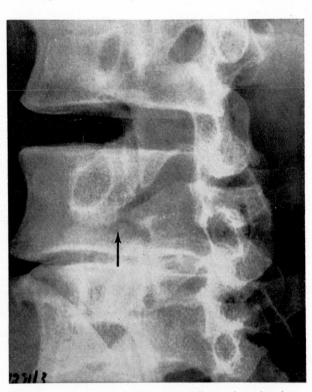

Fig. 51.—Spondylolisthesis L. 4–5. Male aged 49 years. Backward displacement of L. 5 on L. 4 with narrow disc space. Both views showed slight marginal lipping at this site only.

Fig. 52.—Same case as Fig. 51. Oblique view showing defect in the pars interarticularis (opposite arrow). Slight backache following a fall.

appears to be related in some way to the disc degeneration or protrusion, and in some cases, but by no means all, there is an associated defect in the pars interarticularis (Fig. 52). Sometimes several disc spaces are narrowed and more than one vertebra is displaced relative to another. Whether backache is severe or negligible, the prognosis seems to be little different from that seen with a disc protrusion or degeneration without a vertebral displacement.

Congenital Dislocation of the Hip

In an infant

A dislocation of the hip may be present at birth, or may arise soon afterwards because of a congenital shallowness of the acetabulum. The diagnosis will be suspected if the Ortolani "click" is heard on the routine testing of the neonate. The hips are flexed to a right angle, the knees are also flexed and the hips are slowly abducted. If the hip was dislocated, a click is heard when the femoral head goes back into the acetabulum. This sign may be positive and yet no dislocation be present, and a radiograph is therefore necessary in such circumstances to demonstrate or exclude a dislocation and to show whether the acetabulum is well developed or whether there is a shallow acetabular angle. In a baby under the age of 9 months a dislocation may be difficult to demonstrate on a routine radiograph, especially if it is bilateral. Not only is it difficult to assess the position of the femoral head—the epiphysis of which may be unossified or only small and faintly ossified—but it is not always easy or possible to get the patient to lie straight with his legs in the standard position for a radiograph of the hip joint. To overcome this difficulty, a view with both legs adducted 45° and internally rotated is preferable to one with the legs straight (von Rosen, 1962). In a normal baby radiographed in this manner, a line drawn along the long axis of the centre of the shaft of the femur will, if extended, pass through the acetabulum and cross the mid line at the level of L.5–S.1. On the dislocated side a similar line passes above the upper lip of the acetabulum, crosses the mid line at a much higher level, and may pass near the homolateral anterior–superior spine and sacro-iliac joint (Fig. 53).

In some cases a dislocation demonstrated by this method and with the appropriate physical signs on clinical examination may no longer be seen as the child gets older, but in others the dislocation persists. If spontaneous recovery occurs, Leffmann (1959) calls the condition dysplasia of the hip.

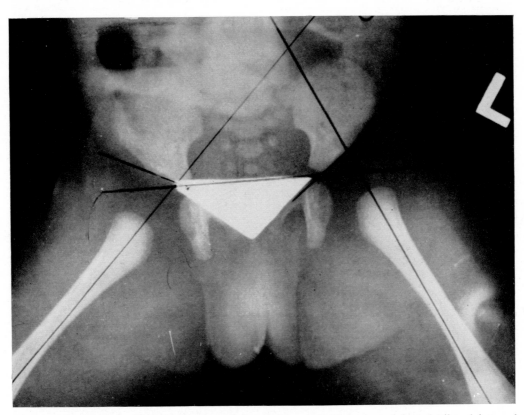

Fig. 53.—Dislocation of left hip (radiograph in von Rosen position—legs abducted 45° and internal rotation). Acetabular angle on left side 45°, on normal right side 28°. Shaft line crosses acetabulum and mid line at L. 5 on right, much higher on left.

The acetabular angle should therefore be measured (line E in Fig. 55). In Fig. 53 the angle is more acute at 28° on the right or normal side, and is shallower at 45° on the dislocated left side. A shallow angle tends to be associated with an unstable hip, and reduction and fixation are then particularly important. A routine radiograph is therefore indicated to see that reduction is complete, and in some cases a further radiograph may be indicated at 1 month and again at 2 months to make sure the reduction is maintained. In a well-developed acetabulum the femoral head is more likely to stay in place after reduction and is unlikely to dislocate if, in spite of a click, it was in place in the initial radiograph.

In young children

In children aged over 9 months the upward and outward displacement of the head of the femur is usually obvious (Fig. 56), but in a doubtful case the diagnosis may be made by certain lines which may be traced on the radiograph, the most useful of which are illustrated in Fig. 55. Shenton's line (A) lies along the upper margin of the obturator foramen and continues outward and downward along the under-surface of the femoral neck and medial aspect of the shaft. A second line (B) goes down the lateral margin of the ilium to the upper and outer edge of the acetabulum and then continues downward and outward along the upper margin of the femoral neck. These two lines form even curves in a normal baby or child, but are interrupted in a dislocation of the hip.

A third line (C) may be drawn across the upper edges of the ischio-pubic bones in the region of the triradiate acetabular cartilage. In a normal child the metaphysis should lie well below this line, and the

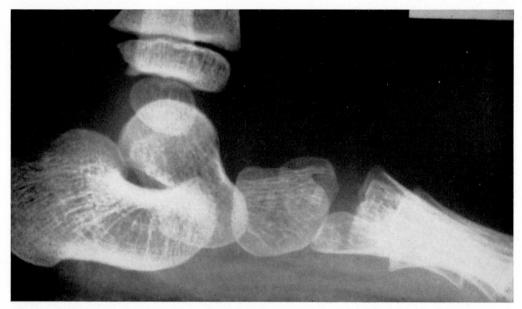

FIG. 54.—Congenital dislocation of the talus. Male aged 4 years. Talus points plantarwards. Symmetrical both feet. Displacement corrected.

epiphysis, while still small as in a baby under the age of 2 years, should only just reach to the line. In a gross congenital dislocation the metaphysis may extend above it. If the displacement is relatively slight, the line may cross the middle or lower third of the epiphysis.

A fourth line (D) marks the lateral distance of the epiphysis, if visible, from some such point as the centre of the triradiate cartilage. A dislocated hip lies more laterally than a normal hip.

A fifth line (E) lies along the angle of the acetabulum, which tends to be relatively obtuse in dislocation of the hip. This line is not always easy to fix since there are no definite points through which to trace it. In addition, asymmetry of the pelvis, due either to faulty positioning or to developmental asymmetry or both, makes it difficult to choose identical anatomical points on the two sides through which to draw the line. If the dislocation is not reduced, the shallowness of the acetabulum becomes very obvious as the child gets older.

Development of the femoral head

The ossified centre of the epiphysis of the femoral head may appear at a later age than normal and may be irregular in shape and abnormally small. This will be particularly noticeable in a unilateral dislocation. If the dislocation is not reduced, the faulty development becomes accentuated in the course of time, and in adult life the head and neck are relatively small and the angle between the neck and shaft is increased so that the neck is almost vertical and in line with the shaft.

When a unilateral dislocation is successfully reduced, the ossification in the abnormal epiphysis may increase more rapidly than that on the normal side until it has reached the same degree of development,

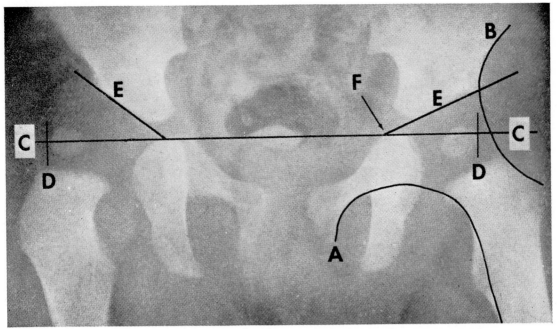

FIG. 55.—Diagram of some lines for use in the diagnosis of displacement of the hip (*see* text). Same case as Fig. 56.

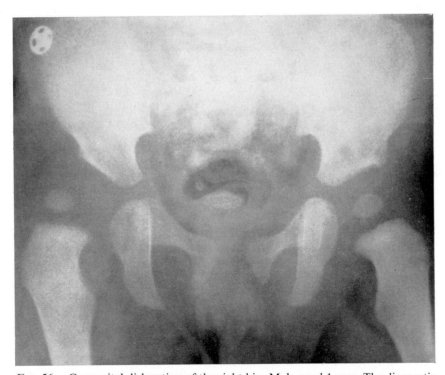

FIG. 56.—Congenital dislocation of the right hip. Male aged 1 year. The diagnostic lines A and B (*see* Fig. 55) cannot be drawn in an even curve on the right side. The epiphysis lies higher above a line C–C, and the distance DF is greater than on the normal left side. The angle CFE is more acute on the normal side and shallower on the side of the dislocation. Radiograph taken because right leg seemed shorter. Manipulative reduction. By age of 8 years virtually normal.

33

thereafter developing in a normal manner so that the two sides are symmetrical. More often in the initial radiograph the epiphysis of the head is smaller than the normal side and remains so for some years. It is often rather fragmented and irregular, thus simulating Perthes' disease, but differing from it in that the head has always been too small and the neck is not widened. In many cases in spite of such an unpropitious start the head may develop and become normal in shape, though frequently a slight shallowness of the acetabulum may persist for life.

More rarely the head develops quite well for a time, but at a later date shows fragmentation and flattening apparently due to osteochondritis. In this case the head may end up rather too large instead of too small.

DISPLACED PATELLA

Congenital displacement of the patella to one side is obvious clinically; radiographs are not needed to show the abnormal position, though they may be of some use in showing the condition of the articular surfaces and any alteration in the shape of the patella.

CONGENITAL VERTICAL TALUS

In congenital dislocation of the talus, the bone lies almost vertically with its distal articular surface facing towards the sole of the foot instead of articulating with the navicular. It is surprising how normal the shape of the displaced bone may be (Fig. 54).

HALLUX VALGUS

In hallux valgus there is lateral deviation of the great toe at the metatarso-phalangeal joint. The aetiology is often obscure, but in the majority of cases the condition seems to be initiated or made worse by badly fitting shoes, and both the displacement and the severity of the symptoms tend to be more marked in women than in men.

In some cases, particularly those appearing in adolescence, it may be the result of faulty development of the head of the first metatarsal, which is narrower and more pointed than normal and thus tilts the proximal phalanx laterally (Fig. 57). In addition, the head of the first metatarsal lies at a greater distance from the second metatarsal than in the normal foot. The degree of deviation can be measured by drawing lines centrally along the shafts of the first and second metatarsals and observing the angle thus formed, which is greater in hallux valgus than in a normal foot. The condition is usually bilateral, but in the case illustrated in Fig. 58 it is much worse in one foot, so that the difference in metatarsal angle is obvious.

In younger persons in the early stages the radiograph is useful to show the exact angle of deviation between the first and second metatarsals and between the first metatarsal and the proximal phalanx, and whether the phalanx is deviated laterally from its normal central position in relation to the articular cortex. Any progression of the lesion can then be observed in serial radiographs, and this may be an indication for surgical intervention.

In older persons the metatarsal head may be enlarged, rather square in shape and with a flat articular surface, while the phalanx may be displaced laterally on the articular cortex (Fig. 58). The degree of displacement of the phalanx on the metatarsal can be graded, being slight when only a few millimetres and gross when the phalanx is hardly in contact with the articular cortex of the metatarsal. In Fig. 58 the displacement is moderate. Bony osteophytic outgrowths are common, as is narrowing of the joint space due to cartilage loss from complicating osteoarthritis (Figs. 58 and 322).

SCOLIOSIS

A scoliosis may be postural, a condition in which the vertebrae are structurally normal, the spine is fully mobile and the curve can be completely corrected by an active effort on the part of the patient; examples are scoliosis secondary to inequality of length of the lower limbs with consequent pelvic tilt, and minor degrees of curvature in adolescents due to faulty posture.

In structural scoliosis the spine may be relatively fixed in the region of the primary defect, but there may be compensatory curves which are mobile; an example is scoliosis secondary to a hemi-vertebra (Fig. 23). Scoliosis secondary to muscular paralysis cannot be corrected by an active effort on the part of the patient, and if the curvature is prolonged and severe, it may itself result in structural changes in the shapes of the vertebrae. Scoliosis may also be secondary to thoracic cage deformities induced by underlying lung conditions, some of which may be obvious on clinical examination, while others are silent. In many cases there is neither an underlying vertebral defect nor muscular paralysis, and the condition is then described as idiopathic scoliosis.

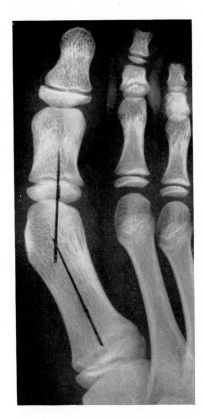
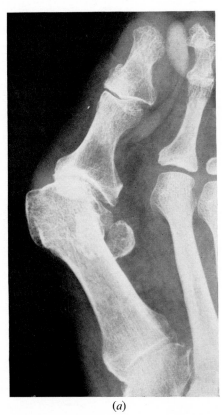
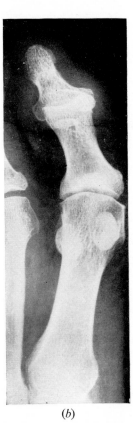

(a) (b)

FIG. 57.—Hallux valgus (developmental). Female aged 9 years. Head of first metatarsal more pointed than normal, and phalanx subluxated somewhat to lateral side. Angle of deviation of phalanx on metatarsal 30°.

FIG. 58.—Hallux valgus (acquired). Female aged 55 years. (a) Angle of deviation of phalanx on metatarsal is 50°, and subluxated laterally. Metatarsal head large, with bony spur below phalanx. Sesamoids enlarged. Deformity for 10 years, pain for 3. (b) Same patient, other foot.

The date of onset is important. If the scoliosis occurs in infancy and is uncorrected, it is likely to be severe and to cause hypoplasia of much of the lung.

Many cases start in adolescence, and if uncorrected these may also become severe.

If there are no clinical clues as to the cause of the curvature, a radiograph may be of value to show or exclude an underlying vertebral lesion. If the lungs are not clearly seen in this, a radiograph of the chest may be indicated if no fairly recent one is available to show or exclude a lung cause.

The most accurate means of recording the degree of spinal curvature and observing any deterioration or improvement is to measure the angles of the vertebrae relative to each other on a radiograph. This is particularly important in growing children, when any deterioration can be detected at an early stage, while the degree of improvement can be factually reported. The severity of a given case can be graded by the angle of curvature, which may form the basis for grouping the cases in order to compare methods of treatment.

Some care should be taken with the technique. In infants the examination is done with the patient supine, but as soon as a child is able to walk, it is best done with the patient standing unless paralytic lesions make this too difficult. If the legs are of unequal length, sufficient blocks can be placed under the foot of the shorter limb to correct the pelvic tilt. The view should as far as possible be antero-posterior, but in severe cases with a rotational curve in addition to the lateral curve, this may not be feasible, and difficulty may be experienced in setting the patient in comparable positions at different examinations. The whole spine below the level of the cervical spine should be included in the radiograph.

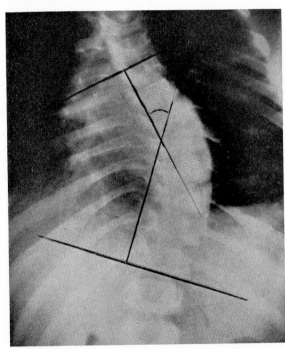 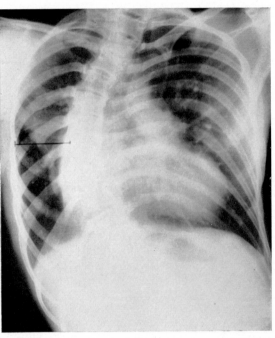

FIG. 59.—Scoliosis. Child aged 9 years. Juvenile idiopathic scoliosis. Angle of curvature 44° and thus moderate.

FIG. 60.—Scoliosis (congenital). Female aged 15 years. Line from vertebra to rib 3·8 cm.; Reid Index therefore grades it as moderate.

Certain lines are then drawn on the radiograph. A line across the iliac crests will be appropriate as a base line provided the pelvic bones are normal, but in severe paralytic disease one ilium may be underdeveloped, and the line is then of no value.

The angle of the appropriate vertebra is then indicated either by a line drawn across from the upper margin of the oval shadow of the pedicle on either side, or by a line along the upper or lower border of the vertebral body (Fig. 59). The pedicle line is easiest to define in some cases and the end plate line in others, depending on how sharply this is projected.

Appropriate vertebrae are chosen for measuring, care being taken that the same ones are chosen when comparative measurements are being made. For convenience, lines are drawn at right angles to the vertebral lines (Fig. 59), and the angle at which they intersect reflects the degree of curvature.

The rotational change cannot be measured from the radiograph, but obvious rotation can be seen and recorded.

A simple means of grading the curve when it is in the mid-thoracic region is to radiograph the chest with both shoulders against the cassette and measure the shortest distance of the vertebrae from the ribs in the axilla (Fig. 60). In an adult a distance of 2–4 cm. would correspond to a curve of 60° by the vertebral lines indicated above, and would be graded as moderate; 0–2 cm. would be severe, while more than 4 cm. would represent a curve of slight grade. In children, moderate would be 1–3 cm.

3—Abnormalities in the Region of the Epiphyses

One group of epiphyseal abnormalities consists of alterations in the rate of maturity of the epiphyses. Centres of ossification may appear earlier or later than normal, or epiphyseal fusion may be premature or delayed, usually as a result of an endocrine disorder.

In the second group there is an alteration in the appearance of the bone in the region of all or nearly all the epiphyses, which may be a congenital developmental defect, the result of an endocrine disorder, or the result of a vitamin D deficiency or of an abnormal dietetic constituent.

In a third group the abnormality is confined to a single epiphysis and consists essentially of fragmentation of the epiphyseal nucleus or of the metaphysis as, for example, in osteochondritis. It is neither inflammatory nor neoplastic, and probably results from a variety of factors leading up to a local vascular disorder with necrosis.

ALTERATION IN THE MATURITY OF THE EPIPHYSES

ACCELERATION OF EPIPHYSEAL MATURITY

General acceleration of epiphyseal ossification in childhood is usually the result of a primary pituitary overaction or a pituitary overaction secondary to adreno-genital virilism. The acceleration of sexual development is obvious clinically, but radiographs are often useful as an index of the patient's precocity. The centres of ossification appear prematurely, sometimes by as much as 5 years or more. In Fig. 61, for example, centres of ossification are present in the trochlea, lateral condyle and pisiform in a child aged 4 years, although not seen normally until the ages of 7 and 11 years respectively.

Since the centre after its premature appearance continues to grow, the epiphyses appear for some time larger than in a normal person of the same age. In Fig. 61 of a child aged 4 years, the capitulum is of much the same size as in a normal child aged 8 years.

In many cases of precocity there is a tendency for epiphyseal fusion and consequent cessation of growth to occur at an earlier age than normal, so that although the patient may be above average height as a child—as was the case with the patient whose elbow is shown in Fig. 61—as a young adult the height may be normal or even less than normal. This is in contrast to the findings in giantism, in which the centres of ossification in the epiphyses may not appear unduly early, but the epiphyses as they grow tend to be larger than normal, and fusion is late so that growth proceeds for a rather longer period than normal.

The parts chosen to demonstrate these changes depend on the age of the patient and the preference of the observer. Under the age of 2 years the lower limbs are most useful for the demonstration of the premature appearance of the centres of ossification. Between the ages of 2 and 11 years there is little to choose between the wrist and the elbow, but the sequence of appearance of the various ossific centres is perhaps rather more regular in the latter, From 11 to 14 years the elbow is the most useful. After the age of 14 years the wrist is again the most useful for demonstrating the dates of fusion of the epiphyses.

Between the ages of about 10 and 16 years, secondary centres of ossification may be expected to appear and persist until fusion takes place between 18 and 24 years. These may be demonstrated in a posterior view of the acromion with the patient reclining slightly backwards, or in a lateral view of the lower thoracic vertebrae. If radiographs of these two parts are inconclusive, a posterior view of the pelvis may be justified, but in view of the inevitable gonadal dose this view for this particular purpose is usually best avoided.

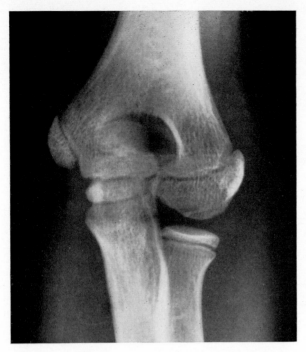 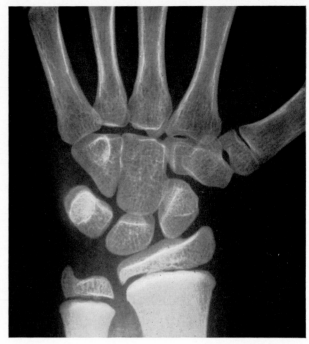

Fig. 61.—Acceleration of epiphyseal maturity. Female aged 4 years. The presence of an ossific centre in the epiphysis of the pisiform and the lateral condyle of the elbow, together with the general appearance of the bones, suggests a child aged 12 years. Child too large and heavy for her age, enlarged clitoris and some pubic hair; 17-ketosteroids 16 mg. per cent (normal 5 mg. per cent).

RETARDATION OF EPIPHYSEAL MATURITY

In cases of stunted growth in which the child is below the average height and size for his age and the cause is not obvious at the initial clinical examination, a radiograph of some of the epiphyseal regions may be of considerable value, especially to show the maturity of epiphyseal development.

A slight retardation with otherwise normal bones, or bones of slightly abnormal shape, will suggest the possibility of pituitary dwarfism. This is in contrast to hereditary dwarfism, in which the epiphyseal maturity is normal, and apart from their small size the structure of the bones is normal.

Rather less marked stunting of growth may be seen with very marked retardation, amounting perhaps to several years, in the appearance of the ossific centres in the epiphyses in hypothyroidism (cretinism). In addition the epiphyses are poorly formed and fragmented, while the metaphyseal line is dense and often a little wider than normal and has a rather wavy contour (Fig. 62). In many cases the cretinoid features will be obvious, though in others the child may merely appear small and rather backward. In a doubtful case the response to thyroid therapy will confirm the diagnosis, since in a cretin the ossification of the epiphyses will then proceed at a very rapid rate, and a response to the hormone will be visible in a radiograph 6 weeks after the commencement of therapy. In a year or less, epiphyseal development may catch up, and the appearances will be those of a normal child (Fig. 63).

These conditions are in contrast to stunted growth with normal epiphyseal maturity but poor epiphyseal disc maturation because of a vitamin D deficiency, whether from an inadequate diet, an alimentary tract disorder, or faulty native vitamin D transformation due to renal disease—*see* pages 92 and 102.

The additional changes in the epiphyseal region—such as the poorly-calcified, irregular, splayed-out metaphyses described in detail on page 44—will indicate the diagnosis. Rickets due to a dietetic vitamin D deficiency is now very uncommon, and when seen is usually in patients under 3 years of age. Renal rickets is seen in rather older children; confirmation of the renal biochemical disorder will either be easy or only be found after full biochemical investigation. In stunting of growth due to a coeliac type of alimentary tract disorder the condition will be clinically obvious.

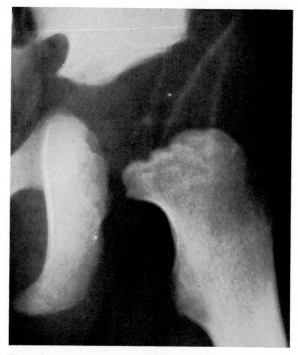

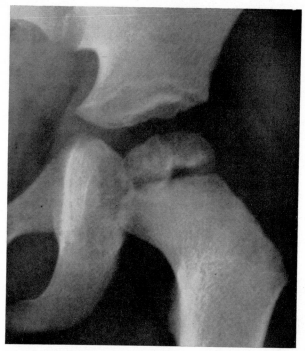

FIG. 62.—Retardation of epiphyseal maturity in hypothyroidism. Male aged 3 years. Very slight ossification of the epiphysis of the femoral head, and wavy metaphysis. Symmetrical on both sides. Similar changes other epiphyseal regions, and no carpal centres visible.

FIG. 63.—Same case 1 year later. Rapid response to thyroid therapy. Centres of ossification appeared within 2 months, growth rapid, mentality improved. The cretinoid features were not very obvious and the x-ray appearances were of diagnostic value.

ACCELERATION OR RETARDATION OF EPIPHYSEAL FUSION

Fusion of the epiphysis to the diaphysis is dependent on the proper functioning of the gonads. If these are secreting in excess at an early age as in virilism, fusion may occur prematurely. If, on the other hand, secretion is minimal or absent, as in hypopituitarism or hypogonadism, then fusion will be greatly delayed (Fig. 64), and may not occur even by middle age.

In hypogonadism there may also be stunted growth and osteoporosis. It may be necessary to give testosterone to accelerate secondary sexual characteristics, but this is unlikely to help the stunted growth since it will probably produce epiphyseal fusion fairly soon, and thus put an end to further growth in length of the major long bones.

Radiography of some of the epiphyseal regions is often of value in these cases, since it will give some indication of the state of the epiphyses and therefore of the overaction or underaction of the gonads.

GENERALIZED ABNORMALITIES IN THE REGION OF THE EPIPHYSES

Certain lesions give rise to an alteration in the x-ray appearances of many or all the epiphyses. A developmental defect, for instance, may be sited in the epiphyseal nucleus, as in epiphyseal dysplasia, and result in fragmentation of the centre with perhaps some alteration of the size. In another type of defect such as chondro-osteodystrophy, the diaphysis may be affected as well as the epiphysis and show some alteration in shape. In a third type such as dyschondroplasia the site is in the epiphyseal plate, which leaves a trail of abnormal tissue as it grows away from the centre of the shaft, resulting in an oval or band-like transradiant zone in the diaphysis.

An endocrine disorder such as hypothyroidism will not only result in the delayed appearance of the ossific centres, but may also cause fragmentation of the developing centre and a wavy metaphyseal line. On the other hand, dietetic deficiencies or abnormal contents will often result in abnormalities of the metaphyseal region such as the irregularity seen in rickets, the submetaphyseal transradiant zone seen in scurvy, and the dense metaphysis seen after the ingestion of certain heavy metals.

DEVELOPMENTAL DEFECTS

Chondro-osteodystrophy (osteochondrodystrophy, chondro-osteo-dysplasia, Morquio–Brailsford disease)

The most severe developmental defect related to the epiphyses is chondro-osteodystrophy, a condition which is often familial. In a severely affected patient the epiphyses are small and fragmented in appearance and are often flattened and of irregular shape. The joint interval appears relatively wide. The metaphyseal line is irregular and rather flattened, and as a result of the abnormal growth the ends of the bones are often wider than normal (Fig. 66). The shaft of a major long bone may be of normal width but will often appear relatively wide in relation to its abnormal shortness. When these changes

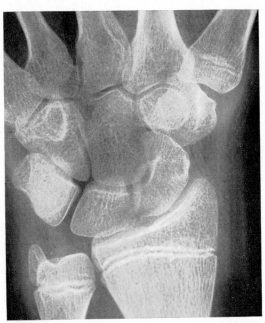

FIG. 64.—Delayed epiphyseal fusion. Male aged 25 years. Epiphyseal discs still wide. Adamantinoma of the pituitary removed. No pubic or facial hair, low metabolic rate.

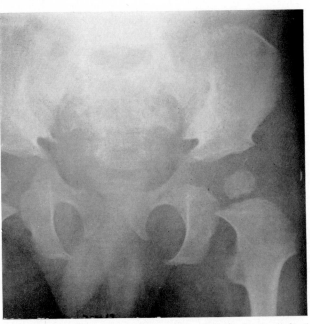

FIG. 65.—Chondro-osteodystrophy (Morquio–Brailsford type). Male aged 3 years. Square-shaped pelvis and femoral neck. Triradiate cartilage near level of sacro-iliac joint. Poor trabecular pattern in epiphysis. Long bones short with splayed-out ends, but not wide.

in shape are associated with gross derangement of the epiphyses, the diagnosis is fairly obvious, but in some cases the change in shape is the most conspicuous feature, the epiphyses showing rather less deformity, and then the changes will approximate to those of a severe case of achondroplasia. However, in most cases of chondro-osteodystrophy the arms are comparatively long in relation to the short trunk, while in achondroplasia they are very short.

The pelvis is rather square in shape (Fig. 65) and the triradiate cartilage lies a shorter distance below the lower margin of the sacro-iliac joint than it does in a normal person. The notch for the gluteal artery is deeper than normal. The acetabular angle may be decreased (Fig. 65) or increased with a shallow acetabulum (Fig. 66). The conspicuous deformity of the femoral head is very characteristic (Fig. 66) but is not found without some changes in other bones.

The vertebral bodies are flat with a tongue-shaped projection anteriorly (Fig. 67). In the lower thoracic or upper lumbar region one vertebra is often particularly poorly developed, wedge-shaped and displaced rather posteriorly. The vertebral changes are best seen in a lateral-view radiograph.

Most of the skeleton except the skull and face may be affected, but the degree of involvement is variable, and in one family some members may have extensive changes and other no more than rather short wide metacarpals of similar length, resulting in a somewhat trident-shaped hand (Fig. 68). In some cases the metacarpals have a thin pointed proximal end; in others, fragmentation of the epiphyses of the fingers is a prominent feature (Fig. 75), the appearances being similar to those of Thiemann's disease (Fig. 76). Anderson and his colleagues (1962) reported a defect in the chondrocytes, which

40

show enlargement and vacuolation and fail to reach the zone of ossification in adequate numbers. The same histological changes were seen in patients with Morquio's disease, dysplasia epiphysialis multiplex and achondroplasia.

The mentality of the patient is usually normal in contrast to the imbecility found in a gargoyle. The x-ray appearances may become less conspicuous as adolescence is approached; on the other hand, the deformities often become relatively worse and very crippling.

The underlying gene defect leads to an enzyme defect, and this is indicated by the presence of an excess of mucopolysaccharide in the urine. In the Morquio–Brailsford type of chondro-osteodystrophy there is an excess of keratosulphate, while in gargoylism (*see* below) the excess is of chondroitin sulphate.

Gargoylism

In gargoylism (Hunter–Hurler syndrome) the bone changes are often very similar to the less severe forms of chondro-osteodystrophy, but the clinical features differentiate the two conditions. Backward displacement of a single wedge-shaped or poorly-developed vertebra in the upper lumbar region is also common in a gargoyle (Fig. 70). The other lumbar vertebral bodies, on the other hand, tend to be square rather than flat with a posterior concavity and without the tongue-like projection anteriorly. The sella is often shaped like a J on its side (Fig. 71). Trident-shaped hands also occur.

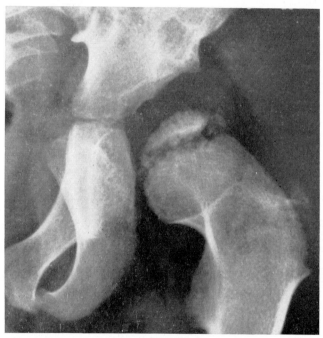

FIG. 66.—Chondro-osteodystrophy. Male aged 5 years. Defective development of the acetabulum, poorly developed and fragmented epiphysis of the head of the femur. Similar defects most other epiphyses. Pointed proximal ends of some metacarpals. Vertebral defects similar to Fig. 70.

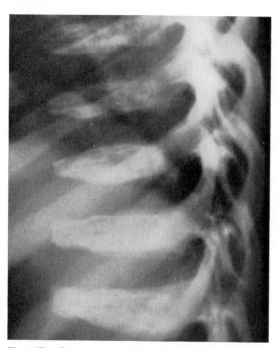

FIG. 67.—Same case as Fig. 65. Flat vertebrae with tongue-shaped anterior border. Boy underdeveloped and weakly. Four years later, practically no change in appearance of the bones. Gross delay in appearance of ossific centres. Father had same disorder.

Dyschondroplasia or chondrodystrophy (Ollier's disease, enchondromatosis)

These terms are generally used to indicate internal chondromas arising from the epiphyseal disc, in contrast to external chondromas or exostoses which may also arise from the epiphyseal disc but presumably from a site nearer the outside edge of the bone.

Internal chondromas frequently fail to ossify or calcify and therefore do not often produce the dense spots so commonly seen in external chondromas or in internal chondromas in specific sites such as the fingers (*see* page 128). Their most usual appearance is that of a vertical band of transradiancy nearly a centimetre wide, extending from the region of the epiphyses towards the centre of the bone for 2 or 3 centimetres and separated from the normal surrounding trabeculae by a narrow rim of dense bone

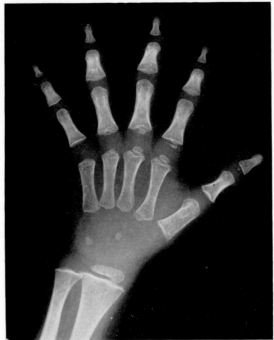

Fig. 68.—Chondro-osteodystrophy. Male aged 3 years. Trident-shaped hand. Metacarpals wide and short and splayed out in position. Epiphyses stunted and deformed. Same case as in Fig. 65.

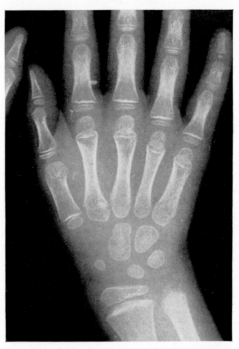

Fig. 69.—Fibrodysplasia ossificans progressiva. Male aged 4 years. Short metacarpals, especially of thumb. Connective tissue ossifications in muscles as in Fig. 382.

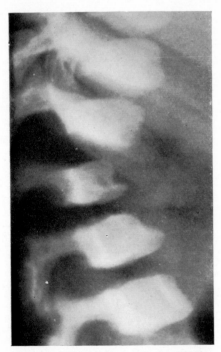

Fig. 70.—Gargoylism (Hunter–Hurler syndrome). Male aged 7 years. Deformed upper lumbar vertebrae with a small L. 2 displaced posteriorly. L. 3 pointed antero-inferiorly. L. 1 square-shaped and narrow disc D. 12. Mental deficiency.

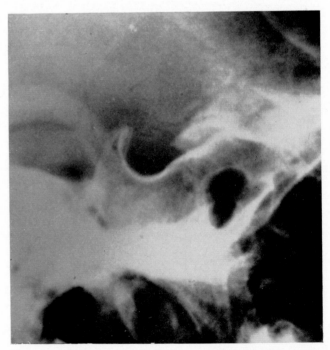

Fig. 71.—Hunter–Hurler syndrome. Male aged 11 years. Lateral view of sella, which is J-shaped with deep recess under anterior clinoid processes.

(Fig. 72). They sometimes lose their connexion with the epiphyseal cartilage and may be seen as oval cyst-like transradiancies a short distance away from the epiphyses which have grown away from them. They no longer grow in size after epiphyseal growth in general has ceased.

Internal chondromas are most conspicuous in the distal thirds of the larger long bones and in the long bones of the hands and feet. They are often associated with external protuberances or exostoses in other sites, either from the same bone or from other bones. They are sometimes confined to the bones of one side of the body, and are sometimes widespread and on both sides.

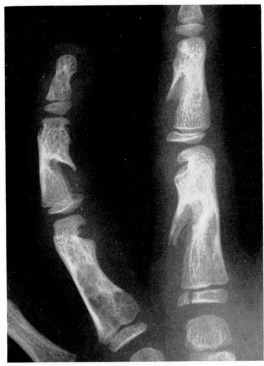

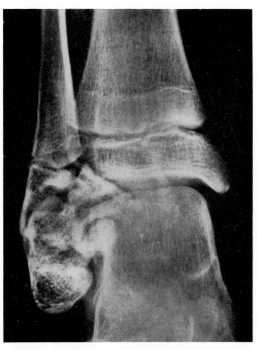

FIG. 72.—Dyschondroplasia (Ollier's disease). Female aged 12 years. Band-like transradiancy middle and proximal phalanx. Biopsy: chondroma. Similar lesion in the ulna.

FIG. 73.—Possible chondrodysplasia. Female aged 12 years. Large fragmented epiphysis at the lower end of the fibula. Asymptomatic.

The cause is unknown, and the appearances are probably due to a failure to transform parts of the epiphyseal cartilage into bone, with later independent proliferation of the cartilaginous islets. McKusick (1966) considers the disease to be a heritable disorder of connective tissue.

Diagnosis

The diagnosis is easy if the typical elongated transradiant bands are seen reaching to or almost to the epiphyses, or if exostoses are present as well. More difficulty will be experienced when this is not the case, or when only a single transradiant zone is seen, perhaps because only a limited area of one bone has been radiographed. If only one transradiant zone is seen and this happens to be oval rather than band-like, it may be mistaken for one of the other types of lesion resulting in a cyst-like transradiant zone described in Chapter 7.

Multiple epiphyseal dysplasia (chondrodysplasia)

Alteration in the structure of many but not all of the growing epiphyses is seen in multiple epiphyseal dysplasia, an apparently developmental and often familial disorder.

The alteration may consist of fragmentation or excessive multinucleation. The affected epiphyses may remain normal in shape and size or there may be flattening of the bony nucleus or, more rarely, a local enlargement or protuberance of the ossific centre (Fig. 73). The epiphyses of the hips and knees are especially affected (Shephard, 1956).

In a variation described by Thiemann (1909) the epiphyses of the phalanges of the hands are particularly affected, being fragmented and flattened (Fig. 76). There may in addition be changes in the hip identical with those seen in Perthes' disease (*see* page 50), or there may be a single localized fragmentation of the lower femoral epiphysis indistinguishable from an osteochondritis dissecans (*see* page 146), but whether these additional changes are part of the epiphyseal disorder or an ordinary osteochondritis developing in an unstable epiphysis is not always obvious. The changes in the hands may become less marked towards the age of 20 years.

Dysplasia epiphysealis punctata

Another alteration in the structure of the epiphyses is seen in dysplasia epiphysealis punctata and consists of small areas of increased density giving a stippled appearance in epiphyses of normal shape and size (Fig. 74).

In the case illustrated, all the epiphyses were affected. There was some interference with the growth in length of the ulna, and the metacarpals were very short. The trabecular pattern was not quite normal, the trabeculae running in the long axis of the bone being thicker and more widely spaced than normal. Cortical development was normal.

ENDOCRINE EPIPHYSEAL DEFECTS

Hypothyroidism (cretinism)

In hypothyroidism the epiphyseal centres of ossification not only make their appearance very late (*see* page 39) but are fragmented or multinucleate with a wavy metaphyseal white line when they do appear (Fig. 62). These changes may not become manifest until the child is nearly a year old. They are most easily seen in the femoral epiphyses up to the age of about 2 years, but may also be seen in the wrists and elsewhere as the child grows older. In some cases the vertebral bodies are irregularly flattened and rather pointed anteriorly in the lumbo-dorsal region (Figs. 28 and 29) (Hubble, 1956).

Whether the disease develops at an early age or in adolescence, the clinical features are frequently indefinite and the radiographic appearances are therefore an important step towards the diagnosis. Successful response to thyroid therapy can be shown more clearly and earlier in the radiograph taken after 6 weeks than clinically. Failure to respond will suggest that the fragmentation is due to some other cause; if the response is good, radiographs have a place in controlling the dosage, which must not be allowed to produce precocious development of the epiphyseal centres.

EPIPHYSEAL DISORDERS AND OSTEOMALACIA

Rickets

Rickets may occur at any time before epiphyseal closure and bone growth are complete. Its presence indicates an underlying mineralization defect or osteomalacia, for which there are several causes (*see* page 94), the underlying pathophysiological events being identical in children and adults. In children, however, rapid bone growth accentuates the mineralization defect, which therefore tends to be clearly seen in the radiographs, particularly at the growing ends of the bones (Fig. 77).

The commonest cause of rickets and adult osteomalacia is vitamin D deficiency. This may be due to nutritional lack, to malabsorption of vitamin D as in steatorrhoea from whatever cause, or to a disturbance of vitamin D metabolism as in renal disease, with a failure to convert native vitamin D to its more active metabolite 1,25-DHCC—*see* page 93. Often there is also renal failure. Rare causes are renal tubular acidosis and familial hypophosphatasia (*see* Fig. 82).

Epiphyseal changes

The early changes are predominantly in the metaphyses. The 1 millimetre wide line of the provisional zone of calcification, which is normally seen at the end of the diaphysis, becomes indistinct or even disappears, while the trabeculae in the bone adjacent to it have a woolly appearance for a depth of 2–3 millimetres instead of the normal fine linear pattern (Fig. 77). The metaphysis becomes concave facing the epiphysis, and the end of the bone is splayed out. The epiphysis itself is usually of normal maturity, but in a severe case it may lose some of its trabecular pattern and the white line normally surrounding it

FIG. 74.—Dysplasia epiphysealis punctata (multiplex). Child aged 7 years. Knee epiphysis shows a spotty appearance; similar appearance in all limb epiphyses. The vertical trabeculae are more widely spaced and thicker than normal and more prominent than the lateral ones.

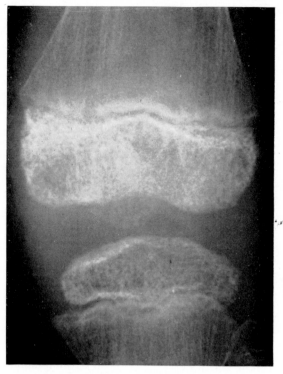

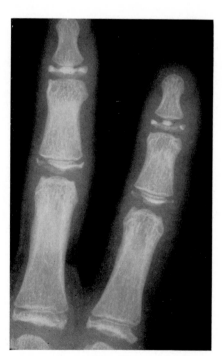

FIG. 75

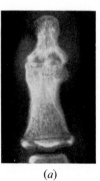

(a)   FIG. 76   (b)

FIG. 75.—Chondro-osteodystrophy. Male aged 14 years. Fragmented phalangeal epiphyses. Other epiphyses similar to Fig. 66.

FIG. 76.—Thiemann's disease. Male aged 12 years. Fragmented phalangeal epiphysis. Also fragmented upper femoral epiphysis like a Perthes' disease, and lower femoral epiphyses like an osteochondritis dissecans. One year later rather nearer to normal.

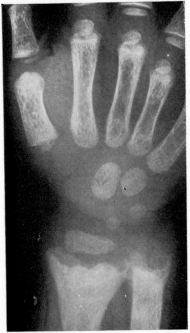 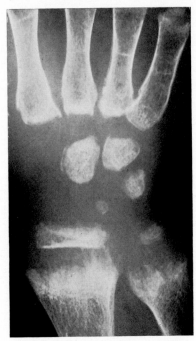 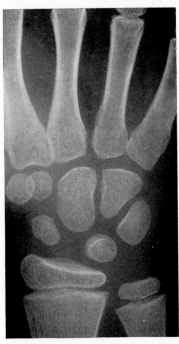

FIG. 77.—Rickets. Female aged 2 years. Metaphysis of the radius concave distally, splayed out and irregular. Deficient trabecular pattern. Fed on boiled milk. Rapid return to normal after vitamin D supplement.

FIG. 78.—Renal rickets in renal tubular acidosis. Male aged 9 years. Widened epiphyseal disc, irregular concave dense metaphyseal region, even loss of density of the diaphysis with trabecular loss. Bright and intelligent but of small stature. Renal calcinosis. Blood urea 32; serum calcium 9·4; phosphorus 3·3; alkali reserve 24·6 CO_2.

FIG. 79.—Same case as in Fig. 78, 3 years later after treatment with large doses vitamin D. Return of epiphyseal regions to normal, trabeculae reformed. Normal centres of ossification. Growth increasing rapidly.

may be broken up or deficient in the region adjacent to the epiphyseal disc. The transradiant zone of the epiphyseal disc becomes widened as the growing cartilage fails to calcify.

These changes are seen in their most marked and easily recognized form in the long bones in the regions of the wrist, and ankle, though most of the epiphyseal regions will show some changes. Splaying out and irregularity of the anterior ends of the ribs may be detected in a routine chest radiograph.

Other bone changes

In severe rickets from any cause there may be widespread loss of bone density. This results from impaired mineralization of newly formed matrix and continuing resorption. Thinning of the trabeculae is seen beneath the epiphysis, and the cortex is poorly formed with narrow transradiant zones within it running parallel to the surface. With a progressive reduction in mineral bone content, softening and consequent deformities occur. The tibiae may bow anteriorly; the pelvis becomes triradiate in shape, with indentation into it of the acetabular regions; the anterior ends of the ribs become bulbous, and the sternum is bowed forwards (pigeon breast). In severe instances, platybasia of the skull may occur, with invagination of the foramen magnum.

Renal rickets

The bone changes produced by renal disease with renal failure are similar to those of other vitamin D deficiency states. However, renal rickets is usually seen in rather older children than dietetic rickets, and the vitamin D deficiency state is more prolonged (though this may also be so in rickets due to malabsorption), so that the transradiant zone of the epiphyseal disc has had time to become unduly wide owing to the continuing growth of uncalcified cartilage cells. The loss of bone density may be

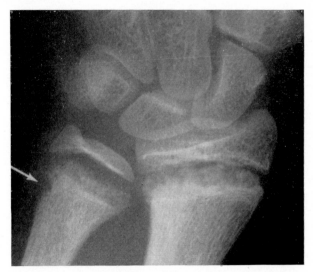

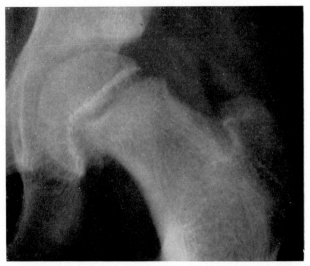

FIG. 80.—Renal rickets with secondary hyperparathyroidism. Female aged 14 years. Widened epiphyseal disc, irregular metaphysis. Cortical erosion of the ulna (opposite arrow). Patchy trabecular loss in the diaphyses of the long bones and vertebrae. Skull normal. Cortical erosions of phalanges similar to Fig. 203a. Severe renal disease.

FIG. 81.—Same case as in Fig. 80. Widened epiphyseal discs. Irregular femoral metaphysis, which is displaced upwards and outwards on the head. Blood urea 230 mg. per cent; serum calcium 7·6; phosphorus 4·9. Bilateral renal hypoplasia. Alkali reserve 4 vols. CO_2 per cent. Alkaline phosphatase 23 K.A. units; urinary calcium output 24 hours 50–70 mg.

more marked, while the changes due to secondary hyperparathyroidism, particularly phalangeal subperiosteal cortical erosions, are also more obvious.

Pathology

Histological examination shows an excess of poorly mineralized bone with much osteoid tissue. At the epiphyseal line the normal orderly pattern is no longer seen. The zone of provisional calcification is virtually absent or very irregular, and the zone of proliferating cartilage accordingly increased. Osteoid tissue is laid down on the cartilage in an irregular manner so that islands of osteoid tissue, blood vessels, osteoblasts, cartilage cells and small foci of calcification all appear in a haphazard and disorganized pattern at the site of the epiphyseal line, which is wider and thicker than normal, with the irregular osteoid tissue and proliferating cartilage cells forming the bulk of the tissue.

Response to treatment

The response to treatment with the vitamin is usually dramatic and rapid, improvements being demonstrable in radiographs after a few weeks and the bones often appearing normal soon after the second month of treatment. Although clinical improvement runs roughly parallel with the radiographic improvement, the latter may be the first evidence that therapy is being effective. In dietetic rickets the ordinary dosage of vitamin D is effective, but in renal rickets, when the conversion of native vitamin D to 1,25-DHCC (*see* page 93) is impaired, either large doses of native vitamin D or the latter metabolite may be needed. Treatment may then be equally effective (Fig. 79).

EPIPHYSEAL DISORDERS DUE TO ENZYME DEFECT

Hypophosphatasia

An appearance similar to dietetic rickets may be seen in hypophophatasia (Fig. 82). The changes may be severe, with bowing of the long bones from softening and, if untreated, pelvic deformity. The metaphyseal white line is absent and the lower radial metaphysis is concave. An associated abnormality is craniostenosis, which may be fatal unless treated by surgical decompression allowing the brain to grow.

The condition is a heritable enzyme defect (an inborn error of metabolism), and the diagnosis can be made if the serum alkaline phosphatase is very low.

DIETETIC EPIPHYSEAL DISORDERS WITH OSTEOPOROSIS

Scurvy

In children, hypertransradiancy of the central part of the epiphysis and a submetaphyseal transradiant zone are typical of scurvy. The centre of the epiphysis is poorly calcified and its trabecular pattern is absent or lost as a result of the depression of osteoblastic activity due to a vitamin C deficient diet. In contrast to the transradiant centre, the surrounding layer of calcified cartilage remains dense and gives the epiphysis a sharply "pencilled" outline (Fig. 144). This surrounding layer is the provisional zone of calcification; it remains dense in spite of the general under-mineralization, and may even appear wider and more dense than normal, because the conversion of calcified cartilage to bone has been arrested without any decrease in the activity of the cartilage cell growth.

The metaphyseal line remains dense and may appear wider than normal for the same reasons. A 1–3 mm. wide transradiant zone may be seen running adjacent and parallel to it (Figs. 83 and 84). This zone may even extend across the cortex so that the edge of the metaphysis is undermined and extends out unsupported by any bone beneath it. This appearance is sometimes known as the corner or angle sign and is occasionally seen in leukaemia in children (*see* page 100). Owing to the weakness caused by such failure of ossification beneath the metaphyseal white line of calcified cartilage, the metaphysis may become separated from the diaphysis and displaced slightly to one side (Fig. 144).

These changes affect all the epiphyses but are most conspicuous and easily demonstrated in the regions of the wrists, knees and ankles. The trabeculae of the shafts are also thinned and indistinct and the cortices are thinner than normal. There may in addition be the shadow of a calcifying subperiosteal haematoma (*see* Fig. 144 and page 80).

Pathology

The presence of vitamin C is necessary for the production of "tissue cement substance" which is essential for the health of blood vessels and for the successful deposition of osteoid tissue. The epiphyseal line in scurvy shows a normal zone of resting and proliferating cartilage and provisional zone of calcification, but the next zone, where osteoid tissue with blood vessels is normally seen, is replaced by a zone of haemorrhagic and gelatinous connective tissue.

Scurvy and rickets

A child may sometimes suffer from rickets and scurvy at the same time, in which case the metaphysis may have the irregular woolly appearance seen in rickets as well as the submetaphyseal transradiant zone seen in scurvy (Fig. 84).

METAPHYSEAL DISORDERS FROM HEAVY METAL DEPOSITION

An increase in the width of the metaphyseal white line shadow is seen if, instead of calcium, certain heavy metals are deposited in this region. A band-like shadow several millimetres wide is then seen (Fig. 85) in place of the normal 1 millimetre-wide line shadow. It is homogeneous and quite well demarcated from the normal trabeculae adjacent to it, and there may be no other radiological abnormalities.

Lead may be ingested in small quantities over a prolonged period if, for instance, a child gnaws a cot bar painted with a lead paint; phosphorus may be ingested in small quantities from sucking matches; fluorine may be present in excess in the water supply; bismuth may be injected medicinally. Each of these heavy metals may produce a similar band-like metaphyseal shadow, though on the whole the increased density in fluorine poisoning is more widespread (*see* page 62).

In chronic lead poisoning the condition may be obvious clinically from the appearance of the gums or from the punctate basophilia of the red cells, but occasionally attention may first be drawn to the possibility by the widened metaphyseal line seen in a radiograph taken for some other purpose such as the exclusion of a fracture. The diagnosis may be confirmed by the detection of lead in abnormal quantities in the serum or urine. In bismuth poisoning the history will indicate the cause, and opacities of bismuth from previous injections may also be visible in the gluteal regions.

DELAYED GROWTH

A slight widening of the metaphyseal lines may be seen as a temporary phenomenon during periods when growth is slowed down for one reason or another.

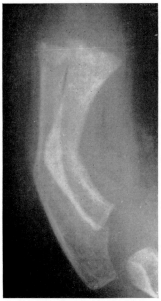

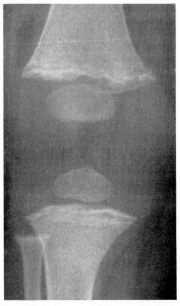

FIG. 82.—Hypophosphatasia in child aged 9 months. Metaphyseal line radius is concave distally and indistinct. Bones are soft and bowed. Reconstitution after vitamin D therapy. Patient also had craniostenosis. Alkaline phosphatase 7·6 K.A. units.

FIG. 83.—Scurvy. Male aged 1 year. Dense metaphyseal line, submetaphyseal transradiant zone extending across cortex on medial side of femur to give corner sign. Pencilled outline to epiphysis with trabecular resorption of the interior. Given vitamin C; rapid recovery and return of bones to normal.

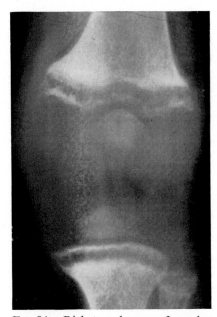

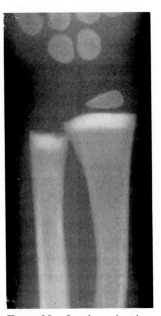

FIG. 84.—Rickets and scurvy. Irregular lower femoral metaphysis, wide submetaphyseal transradiant zone, poorly developed ossific centres with incomplete rim of dense bone. Rapid recovery following treatment with vitamins C and D.

FIG. 85.—Lead poisoning. Female aged 2 years. Metaphyseal dense line 5 mm. wide. Anorexia, loss of weight and constipation. Chewed paint off newly-painted cot. Punctate basophilia, serum lead 4 µg. per ml. (normal less than 0·5). Urine lead slightly above 0·1 mg. per litre.

ABNORMALITY OF A SINGLE EPIPHYSEAL REGION

Fragmentation or deformity of a single epiphysis, with neither diminution of the joint space nor nearby loss of density, is usually due to osteochondritis or osteochondrosis (Williams, 1959). Although the aetiology of the various types of osteochondritis is not definitely known, it appears that a local failure of the blood supply to the epiphyseal bone is an important factor. It is often assumed that there is occlusion of a small end artery, but in some cases a venous occlusion may initiate the local bone necrosis. A vascular lesion may disturb the action of "organizer" locally, so that another mechanism might be added to the circulatory factor, and this would make it easier to understand the distribution of the changes seen for instance in Perthes' disease. In some cases the precipitating cause of the vascular disturbance appears to be swelling and distintegration of the cartilage cells in the region of the metaphysis, as in Perthes' disease, while in others, especially in adults, trauma seems to set off the vascular disturbance, as in a march fracture of a metatarsal or the disintegration of a lunate bone following gross trauma.

The few histological studies available have shown the changes of an aseptic necrosis of the bone with areas of haemorrhage and sequestrum formation. There follows a reparative process with formation of callus which is subsequently converted into normal bone.

An abnormality of a single epiphyseal disc, also of uncertain aetiology, will occasionally lead to a loss of the adhesive properties of the cells and therefore to epiphyseal displacement, as in coxa vara.

Osteochondritis of the Femoral Head (Perthes' Disease)

Fragmentation of the epiphysis

Fragmentation and flattening of the epiphysis of the femoral head is characteristic of Perthes' disease, and usually by the time the first radiograph is taken the changes are well developed and obvious in the radiograph, as in Figs. 86 and 87. The fragmentation may affect the whole of the epiphysis or it may be relatively localized.

Occasionally the radiograph is taken at an earlier stage when the changes are comparatively slight and may amount to no more than a small erosion of the articular cortex and the bone beneath. Such a change may be invisible or difficult to see with certainty in the standard posterior view, but can be clearly seen in a posterior view taken with the leg abducted and everted—the so-called "frog" position (Fig. 88)—or in a view with the patient rotated some 60° towards the affected side so that the epiphysis is seen almost as in a lateral view. These early erosions usually lie in the anterior third of the epiphysis. In other cases the earliest change is an area of erosion near the metaphyseal aspect (Fig. 89) or near the centre of the epiphysis, but wherever the initial erosion, multiple erosions may appear later to give the appearance of widespread fragmentation and flattening.

The fragmentation is the result of localized areas of bone resorption in a previously normal epiphysis, and is to be distinguished from the multinucleate centres of ossification which may be seen in hypothyroidism or congenital dislocation of the hip (see page 32).

Flattening of the epiphysis

Some flattening of the ossific centre of the epiphysis often follows the fragmentation. In the early stages this is the result of resorption rather than collapse, since the joint interval or distance between the white rim of bone forming the under-surface of the acetabular rim and the upper surface of the ossific centre of the femoral head is wider than on the normal side. This joint interval is always either normal or wider than normal and never narrower. In the later stages, pressure collapse may result from the stress of normal weight-bearing, thus adding to the flattening and deformity of the epiphysis. In the early stages the distance from the acetabular cortex to the metaphyseal white line of the neck of the femur is increased relative to the normal side, but is reduced or the same in spite of the widened joint interval if flattening of the head is appreciable.

The uneroded bone fragments in the flattened epiphysis may become relatively dense or sclerotic due either to compression or to excessive calcification resulting from the altered blood supply.

Other bone changes

The architecture of the trabeculae and the cortex of the neck and shaft is normal, and there is no evidence of any local loss of bone density near the affected epiphysis.

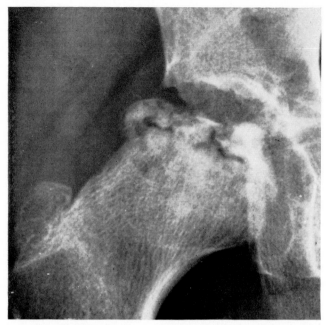

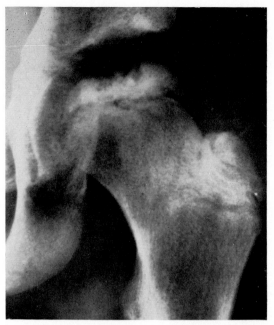

FIG. 86.—Osteochondritis hip (Perthes' disease). Male aged 8 years. The joint interval is slightly wider than the normal side, but the distance from the acetabular rim to the metaphysis is less. In initial radiograph both distances were slightly increased. Acetabular, femoral epiphyseal and metaphyseal erosions. Epiphysis flat and fragmented, neck wide and short. Initial lesion was deep in the epiphysis with deep sclerosis.

FIG. 87.—Osteochondritis hip (Perthes' disease). Male aged 9 years. Localized erosion of articular aspect of epiphysis and bone beneath. Joint interval 3 mm. wider than on the normal side, but distance between acetabular rim and metaphysis is 3 mm. less. Limp 5 weeks. Took usual course with fair recovery.

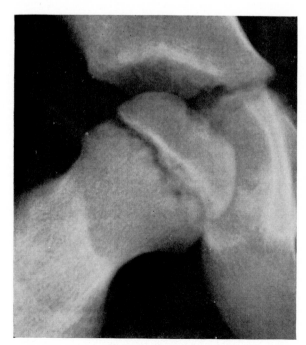

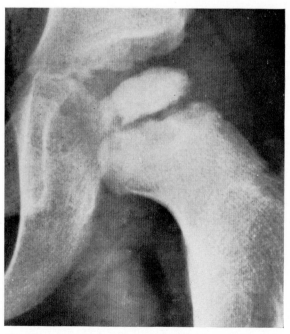

FIG. 88.—Osteochondritis hip (Perthes' disease). Male aged 10 years. Radiograph taken with leg in "frog" position; small erosion of articular aspect of epiphysis near fovea capitis, not visible in routine posterior view. Metaphyseal line pitted. Joint space widened. Pain and limitation movement. Good reconstitution.

FIG. 89.—Osteochondritis hip (Perthes' disease). Female aged 8 years. Early erosion metaphyseal aspect of epiphysis and obvious erosion of metaphysis. Slight pain knee, limitation movement hip.

The femoral neck often appears to be wider than normal, and the metaphysis is often slightly irregular with some widening of the epiphyseal line. These features cannot be easily explained on the theory of a vascular disorder of the epiphysis. The acetabulum may be normal in shape and structure, or there may be small areas of erosion and fragmentation in the region of the articular cortex due to an apparently similar lesion at this site.

Incidence and course

The incidence is higher in children with an endocrine disorder than in normal children. The disease is most commonly seen between the ages of 3 and 10 years and there is usually no history of trauma. It is more often unilateral than bilateral and is often the only abnormality. The symptoms are usually slight, so that it is unusual to see the patient until a relatively late stage of the disease.

The course is slow once a moderate degree of fragmentation and flattening has occurred and there may be no change in the x-ray appearances for many months. Serial radiographs should therefore be widely spaced, since even with suitable shielding some rays will reach the gonads and may do permanent damage. Eventually the epiphysis starts to grow again and the fragmentation disappears, so that the final appearance is that of a flattened epiphysis which is wider than normal and fitting on a definitely widened femoral neck. The trabecular structure becomes normal.

The late results of 52 cases of Perthes' disease were reviewed by Evans (1958). Judged radiographically, one-third showed a good femoral head and one-third a poor one, and the whole of the latter group showed evidence of secondary osteoarthritis. Evans and Lloyd-Roberts (1958) found no difference in the late radiological appearances between those treated as in-patients and those as out-patients.

SLIPPED UPPER FEMORAL EPIPHYSIS (ADOLESCENT COXA VARA)

A slipped upper femoral epiphysis (adolescent coxa vara) is seen in children aged between 10 and 14 years, and the symptoms may be relatively slight and easily mistaken for "rheumatism" at first. The only physical sign may be slight limitation of movement; the condition is more often unilateral than bilateral, and the radiographic appearances may give the most important evidence on which to make the diagnosis.

Posterior view of the hip

In a posterior-view radiograph a slipped upper femoral epiphysis may be diagnosed if the femoral neck is displaced upwards and outwards in relation to the epiphysis of the femoral head. The displacement may be a slight one of no more than 2–3 millimetres.

More often, however, especially in the early stages, the posterior-view radiograph may appear almost normal, in which case certain tests for the abnormality may be useful. One is to look for a slight widening of the transradiant zone of the epiphyseal disc relative to the normal side and a slight irregularity of the metaphysis, which also appears slightly widened since the angle of the ray does not pass through it quite tangentially (Fig. 90). Another test is to see whether the inferior media angle of the metaphysis fails to overlap the shadow of the acetabulum as in a normal hip at this age.

A third test is to draw a line along the lateral margins of the epiphysis of the head and the femoral neck. In a normal hip this line will run in an even curve with a lateral concavity. In a slipped epiphysis the line may be uneven at the point where the neck is displaced 2–3 millimetres laterally on the epiphysis; in addition, because of rotation of the neck, the line along it will be straight or show a slight lateral convexity (Fig. 90).

Lateral view of femur

In a lateral view the forward and upward displacement of the neck relative to the epiphysis will often be quite obvious (Fig. 91), so that this view ought to be taken if the condition is suspected clinically or if the line of the metaphysis appears abnormal in any way in the posterior view.

A final test is to draw a line on the lateral-view radiograph from the anterior to the posterior inferior angles of the epiphysis of the femoral head, and another centrally along the neck, as illustrated in the diagram (Fig. 94). In a normal hip these two lines meet almost at right angles. In a slipped epiphysis the forward displacement of the neck rotates the epiphysis posteriorly so that the angle will be 70° or less. In a long-standing case the line of the metaphysis itself becomes tilted, so that in a lateral view it forms an angle of about 30° with the shaft instead of 10° as in a normal person.

Aetiology

The condition appears to be due to the development of a weakness in the adhesive power of the epiphyseal disc, and as a rule trauma beyond the normal stress of standing plays no part. The underlying irregularity of the metaphysis is the only indication of an abnormality in the region of the epiphyseal disc, and the cause of this is unknown. The child is often rather overweight, but beyond this there may be no evidence of an endocrine disorder.

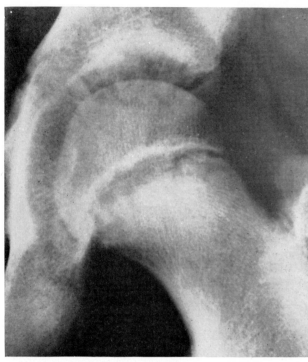

FIG. 90.—Slipped upper femoral epiphysis. Male aged 11 years. Epiphyseal transradiant zone wider than normal side, and slight irregularity of metaphysis. Fat boy, with 1 month's pain in the hip when walking.

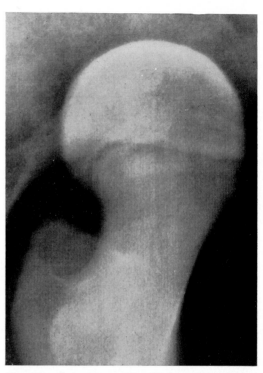

FIG. 91.—Same case as Fig. 90; lateral view showing forward and upward displacement of the neck in relation to the head. Treated first as rheumatism, then radiographed, then reduced and pinned.

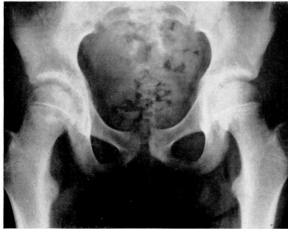

FIG. 92.—Slipped upper femoral epiphysis; almost normal in standard A.P. view.

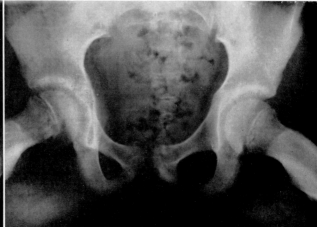

FIG. 93.—Same case with legs in frog position. Forward displacement of neck on head is clearly shown on right side; left side normal.

In a few cases material has been available for pathological study and a disease of the cartilage plate has been revealed.

Displacement of the epiphysis on the femoral neck is also seen in younger children with a generalized epiphyseal disorder such as renal rickets (Fig. 81) or osteopetrosis. It may also occur in Gaucher's disease.

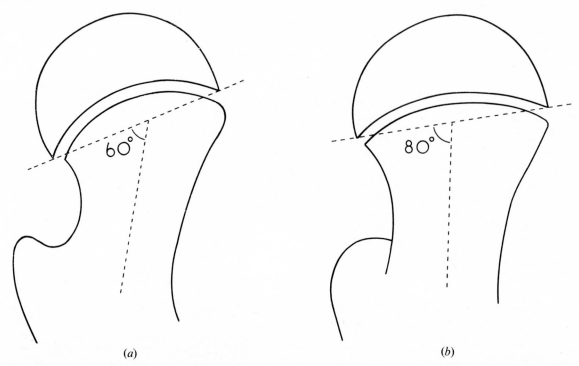

(a)   (b)

Fig. 94.—(a) Tracing from the radiograph of Fig. 91. Head–neck angle 60°. (b) Same patient—opposite normal hip. Head–neck angle 80°.

Serial radiographs to assess position and union

Because of the inevitable gonadal dose of radiation even with suitable shielding, the number of radiographs taken should be as small as possible. A posterior-view and a lateral-view radiograph will be required after reduction to ensure this has been achieved. Thereafter there is no urgency for further radiographs except perhaps to check that the position has been maintained, although this can be assumed without radiology if an effective form of fixation is being employed, such as a graft or nail, or if there has been no weight-bearing.

Since the slip occurs in the region of the epiphyseal cartilage, there will be no calcified callus formation to show whether the cartilage has united firmly, so that radiographs for this purpose should not be taken in the first few weeks. Whatever method of treatment is adopted, after some months the epiphysis usually shows premature union, and the disappearance of the transradiant zone of cartilage can be demonstrated in a radiograph. Thus in a straightforward case, two sets of radiographs are enough, one immediately after reduction and one some 3 months later.

Premature union will limit the growth in length of that limb and cause some shortening. However, satisfactory reduction will result in less shortening than if the neck remains up relative to the head, and will ensure that the lines of stress pass through the hip joint in a normal direction, so that secondary osteoarthritis will be less likely to develop some years later.

OSTEOCHONDRITIS OF THE TIBIAL TUBEROSITY (OSGOOD–SCHLATTER DISEASE)

Fragmentation and elevation anteriorly of the tongue-like projection of the upper tibial epiphysis in the region of the tibial tuberosity is seen particularly in boys between the ages of 11 and 15 years (Fig. 95). A return to an almost normal appearance in a few months is the usual outcome, and epiphyseal fusion occurs in a normal manner. The condition seems to be due to a vascular disturbance the cause of which is unknown. Minor trauma, such as may be incurred when simply running about, seems to be a precipitating factor in many cases. Quite often the opposite painless knee shows similar but less marked fragmentation of the epiphysis. The lesion seems to be of the type known as osteochondritis, though the exact pathology is not known. There is often slight pain and tenderness.

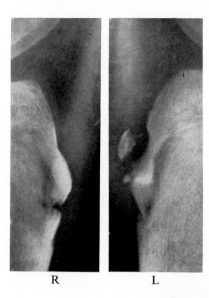

R   L

FIG. 95.—Osteochondritis of tibial tuberosity (Schlatter's disease). Female aged 12 years. Left knee epiphysis displaced forwards and fragmented, right normal. Slight pain on the left; rapid recovery.

FIG. 96.—Osteochondritis second metatarsal. Female aged 13 years. Wide joint space, flat fragmented epiphysis, wide neck. Eight months' pain in the region of the second toe. Recovery.

FIG. 97.—Osteochondritis navicular (Köhler's disease). Male aged 5 years. Fragmentation and flattening both navicular bones with wide joint spaces. Very slight pain in both feet.

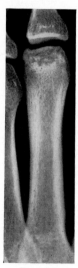

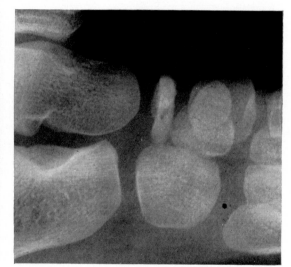

FIG. 96   FIG. 97

OSTEOCHONDRITIS OF A METATARSAL EPIPHYSIS

Fragmentation and flattening of the epiphysis of the second metatarsal is usually seen at a rather later age than Perthes' disease, but is associated with a similar widening of the neck of the bone (Fig. 96). The joint space tends to be widened, and there is no local loss of bone density. After some months the epiphysis itself becomes more normal in appearance, but the flattening of the head and widening of the neck may remain as permanent changes.

Some pain in the foot is commonly present during the initial phases of the lesion, but some cases are asymptomatic throughout.

Fragmentation and flattening of the epiphysis of the first metatarsal is seen more rarely but takes a similar course. Again, the cause and exact pathology of the condition are unknown, though they seem to be similar to those of lesions referred to as osteochondritis or epiphysitis in other sites.

OSTEOCHONDRITIS OF THE NAVICULAR (KÖHLER'S DISEASE)

Fragmentation and flattening of the navicular (Fig. 97) can be considered an epiphyseal lesion during the age of active growth of the bone. The lesion is usually seen early, that is, from about the age of 4 to 8 years. The joint space is normal or wide, the fragmentation and flattening last only a few months, and the bone eventually becomes normal in appearance: a sequence suggesting a lesion of the osteochondritis type. It is presumably due to a local vascular disorder, but the cause of this is unknown. Many fewer cases have been observed by the author during the last 20 years than in the 20 years before that.

Clinically there may be slight pain in the foot, but some cases are virtually asymptomatic, being discovered during an x-ray examination of the foot for some other purpose.

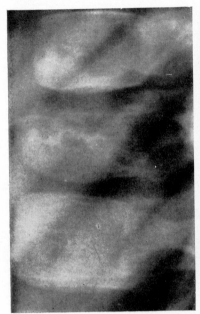

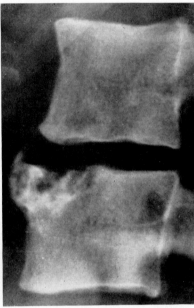

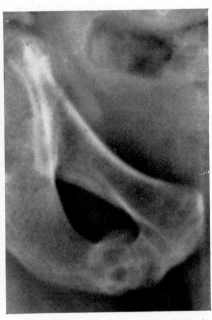

FIG. 98.—Possible osteochondritis vertebral body. Male aged 5 years. D. 11 fragmented and a little flat, with some narrowing of the disc space between it and D. 12. Asymptomatic. E.S.R. 7. Normal radiograph previous to this and some resolution later.

FIG. 99.—Possible late local osteochondritis vertebra. Male aged 25 years. Erosion and separated fragment anterior superior angle L. 3, with slight narrowing of the disc space above. Increasing backache over 18 months. Slight limitation of movement. Improved with plaster and bed rest.

FIG. 100.—Possible osteochondritis ischio-pubic ramus. Male aged 14 years. Widening and erosion in the region of the uniting epiphysis, which is firmly united on the other side. Lasted 9 months, then bone became normal.

OSTEOCHONDRITIS OF THE PRIMARY CENTRE OF A VERTEBRAL BODY

Fragmentation of a vertebral body, usually in the lower dorsal region, with a narrow disc space in a child aged 10–15 years will suggest an aseptic necrosis of the osteochondritis type (Fig. 98), especially if the symptoms are slight and the other bones are normal. A more limited erosion or fragmentation of the anterior third of an end plate of the upper or lower surface together with a limited area of the bone beneath, with narrowing of the disc space (Figs. 39 and 99), may be due to a similar type of lesion.

The limited or the more extensive type of lesion is usually associated with some prolapse of the nucleus pulposus into the affected bone, but whether this is the cause or the result of the bone lesion is often uncertain.

In both of these forms, distinction must be made from a similar appearance caused by a tuberculous infection, but the latter is commonly associated with a paravertebral abscess (*see* page 24), a raised E.S.R. and constitutional disturbances.

Pathological proof of the nature of these appearances is rarely forthcoming, and the cause can therefore only be surmised. Clinically the symptoms are trivial and soon disappear; radiologically the lesions tend to resolve without specific treatment, but some residual wedge-shaped deformity is common.

OSTEOCHONDRITIS OF THE SECONDARY CENTRE OF A VERTEBRAL BODY (SCHEUERMANN'S DISEASE)

In Scheuermann's disease (if there is such an entity), fragmentation of some of the secondary centres of ossification is most clearly seen near the anterior angles of the vertebral body. It is not always possible to distinguish the fragmented appearance due to normal multinucleate centres of ossification from pathological fragmentation. A pathological lesion will be probable if the fragmentation is more marked in a single epiphyseal region or is confined entirely to one site, and if there is an abnormality in the shape of the antero-inferior or antero-superior corner of the body itself. The antero-superior corner is most commonly affected. The centre may never unite to the body, persisting as a single 5 millimetre triangular fragment of bone adjacent to the corner. The condition is probably a normal variant like a bipartite patella.

It is doubtful whether such lesions really account for any pain which may be present, or for any residual spinal curvature. Often the vertebral body becomes rather wedge-shaped, and this is probably a secondary effect of the curvature and not the cause of it. Pathological examination of cases with adolescent kyphosis usually shows a series of vertical prolapses of the nucleus pulposus (Schmorl's nodes) which appear to have affected the normal growth of the vertebra leading to wedge-shaped deformities, and there is no evidence of epiphyseal osteochondritis.

UNCOMMON SITES OF EPIPHYSEAL FRAGMENTATION (OSTEOCHONDRITIS, EPIPHYSITIS)

Fragmentation with or without flattening may occur in almost any epiphysis, but is relatively uncommon apart from the sites mentioned above. The lesion may be asymptomatic, or associated with slight pain; complete resolution is the usual outcome.

Four other sites require special mention—namely the calcaneum, lower dorsal spine, patella and ischio-pubic ramus—in that it may be hard to distinguish a pathological fragmentation in these parts from a fragmented appearance due to multinucleate centres of ossification.

The calcaneum

A fragmented appearance of the epiphysis of the calcaneum around the ages of 8 to 14 years is quite common, but in the majority of cases this is not a pathological change. When present with some pain and tenderness at that site, it may be difficult not to attribute the fragmentation to osteochondritis, but similar appearances can frequently be seen without any symptoms, so that it is impossible to be dogmatic from the radiographic appearances. Quite commonly the appearances are more or less symmetrical in the two feet, though sometimes more marked on the side of the painful heel, the other side being without symptoms. Whether pain is present or not, the epiphysis develops normally and finally fuses to the metaphysis, which then appears quite normal, while pain, if present, rarely persists for any length of time.

Lower dorsal spine

Multinucleate centres for the secondary centres of ossification are common in the lower dorsal spine between the ages of 12 and 20 years. The rim of epiphyseal bone appears broken up into several pieces instead of appearing as a single white line of bone. There may be no other changes, and the end plates are normal. As in Scheuermann's disease (see above), it is very doubtful whether the term "disease" or osteochondritis should be applied to these x-ray appearances. Fusion of these epiphyses to the vertebral body occurs in a normal manner. The vertebral body may be normal or may show some slight wedge-shaped deformity. The relation of this deformity to the abnormal appearance of the secondary centres is unknown and it may even be the cause and not the effect of the latter.

The patella

Multinucleation of the patella is normal in the early stages around the ages of 4 to 6 years, but uncommon after this, except for the occasional non-fusion of one or two pieces near the upper and outer margins. Any fragmentation beyond this may represent a pathological lesion of the osteochondritic type. If the lesion is of this type, resolution will occur and the patella will be seen as a single bone shadow, whereas in anatomical multinucleation in an older child, a small separate fragment will never unite to the main mass of bone.

The ischio-pubic ramus

Just before union of the ischio-pubic rami at the age of 7 to 8 years, there may be a bulbous expansion and some irregularity of the adjacent surfaces of the two bones. This is usually normal, and only lasts a few months. If much exaggerated, this too may represent a pathological lesion of the osteochondritic type (Fig. 100).

4—Increases in Bone Density

A generalized increase in bone density may be the result of a developmental defect in which the calcified cartilage either fails to be converted into bone or is converted into primitive or cortical instead of cancellous bone, as in osteopetrosis; or the bone histology is normal but the bones are abnormally thick; or the normal trabeculae become thickened in response to widespread secondary deposits or myelofibrosis. An increase in density may be due to the ingestion of fluorine or an excess of vitamin A. A localized increase in density in the submetaphyseal region of many bones is seen after the ingestion of substances of high atomic weight such as lead or the absorption of injected bismuth, and is present in some cases of hyperparathyroidism—*see* page 108.

A localized increase in the density of a single bone may be due to a local developmental defect, a vascular lesion, a local osteoblastic response to a neoplasm or infection, an alteration in the bone architecture as in Paget's disease or hyperparathyroidism, or a local increase in width due to added periosteal new bone.

GENERALIZED INCREASE IN BONE DENSITY

DEVELOPMENTAL OSTEOPETROSIS

A generalized increase in density affecting all or most of the bones may be seen in osteopetrosis (Albers–Schönberg disease or marble bones), a rather uncommon and often familial developmental defect. The increased density, which may be even in some bones and patchy in others, is usually quite obvious in the radiographs either from the abnormally marked contrast between the whiteness of the bones and the blackness of the surrounding soft tissues or from comparison of the affected parts with the more normal parts of the bones should these be present. In addition to their great density, the opaque areas appear structureless without a visible trabecular pattern (Fig. 101).

There may also be changes in the shape of the major long bones with a flask-like expansion (Fig. 101) similar to that seen in many cases of Gaucher's disease (*see* page 16).

Patterns of increased density

Various patterns of increased density are found. In classical Albers–Schönberg disease (osteopetrosis) there is a homogeneous increase in the density of the proximal and distal thirds of the major long bones of the limbs, the middle third being relatively unaffected and almost normal in appearance (Fig. 103). The vault and base of the skull, all the ribs and the ischio-pubic rami show a homogeneous increase in density throughout. The vertebrae show the increase in density along the upper and lower thirds of the bodies, the middle third again being relatively transradiant (Fig. 102). A similar "rugger jersey" appearance, though with much less dense transverse bands, may be seen in secondary hyperparathyroidism (*see* page 108 and Fig. 180).

Variations of these patterns are seen in some of the bones. In the bones of the hands and feet the increased density may be confined to the middle third of the long bones (Fig. 105), the ends being of normal density with normal trabecular structure. In the carpals and tarsals the increase in density may be evenly distributed or may be confined to the peripheral part leaving a relatively transradiant central zone. In the long bones of the hands and feet and in the ilia there may be transverse bands of transradiancy across the dense areas, 2–3 millimetres wide and spaced a few millimetres apart (Figs. 104, 106 and 107); in the ilia these alternating dense and transradiant bands run either parallel or at right angles to the iliac crests (Fig. 107). All these changes may be present in the different bones of a single patient and are, as a rule, roughly symmetrical on the two sides.

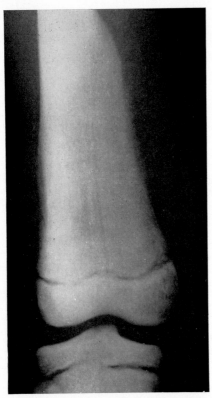

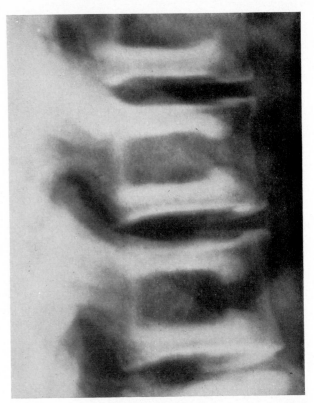

FIG. 101.—Osteopetrosis (marble bones, Albers–Schönberg disease). Male aged 10 years. Dense epiphysis and lower third of shaft (middle third normal). Flask-like expansion lower third. Middle third phalanges and carpals as Fig. 105.

FIG. 102.—Osteopetrosis dorsal vertebrae. Female aged 33 years. Dense upper and lower thirds of vertebral bodies with transradiant central zone. Major long bones as Fig. 101. Ilia show dense 5 mm. wide bands parallel to the crests.

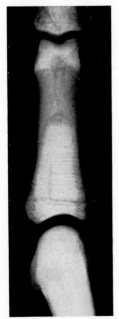
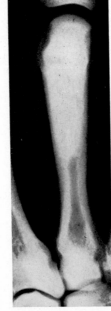

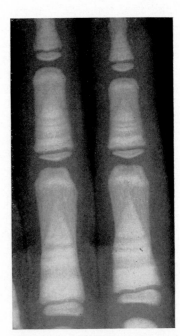

FIG. 103.—Osteopetrosis finger. Female aged 27 years. Transverse bands of dense bone in phalanx. Ends of metacarpal dense. Other bones similar to Figs. 101 and 102.

FIG. 104.—Osteopetrosis of fingers. Transverse bands of dense bone with more normal bone between them.

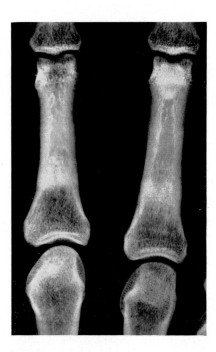

Fig. 105.—Same case as Fig. 102. Phalanges dense in middle thirds with a normal trabecular pattern at both ends.

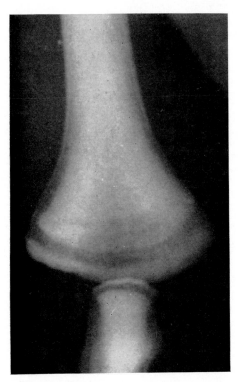

Fig. 106.—Osteopetrosis of humerus. Male aged 2 years. The transradiant band is normal bone with the dense bone on either side.

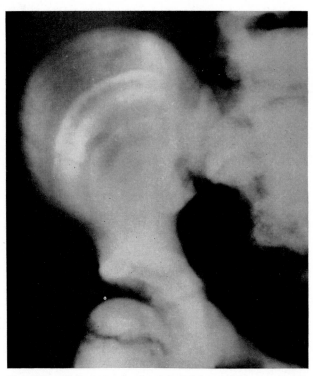

Fig. 107.—Osteopetrosis of pelvis. Male aged 9 years. Bands of dense and more normal bone, some parallel and some at right angles to the iliac crest. Femoral epiphysis dense.

In a variation known as Voorhoeve's disease, the pattern is quite different, the dense regions consisting of vertical bands some 2–3 millimetres wide mainly in the major long bones near their ends (Fig. 108).

Pathology

Osteopetrosis is a hereditary disorder of the skeleton which is transmitted as a Mendelian recessive character. The symptoms are the result of the pathological changes; for instance, the bones are brittle, so that transverse fractures of the long bones are common. They usually unite well, but residual deformities such as coxa vara are sometimes seen. Anaemia is a direct result of encroachment of bone on the marrow spaces, while narrowing of the cranial foramina may cause deafness or defects of vision.

The bones formed in cartilage are extremely hard and dense, and can be cut only with difficulty. A cross-section shows no demarcation between the dense cortical bone and deeper bone which shows no evidence of a trabecular structure, while this homogeneous dense bone encroaches on or may completely occupy the marrow cavity. There is therefore no cancellous bone.

Microscopically the abnormality starts at the epiphyseal plate, where the zone of calcified cartilage is a prominent feature. Instead of being absorbed, this calcified cartilage persists throughout the shaft of the long bone and becomes surrounded by dense bone. There is thus a defect of bone remodelling with a failure of bone resorption, so that dense calcified bone occurs in all the affected areas.

DEVELOPMENTAL OSTEOPOIKILOSIS

Localized dense areas of bone, circular or oval in shape, well demarcated and some 3–5 millimetres in size, may be seen widely distributed throughout most of the skeleton in developmental osteopoikilosis (Fig. 109). In each bone there may be a large number of such dense areas or only a few, and in either case they tend to lie within a few centimetres of the metaphysis.

The condition is asymptomatic and without clinical significance. The areas do not enlarge when general cessation of growth has occurred.

McKusick (1966) considers osteopoikilosis to be a heritable disorder of connective tissue because there are often associated but inconspicuous skin lesions showing collagen fibrosis yet with preservation of elastic tissue elements. Histologically one bone lesion examined showed clumps of thickened trabeculae, probably from a local hyperplasia of collagen in the bone matrix.

MYELOSCLEROSIS

A fairly generalized increase in bone density may be seen as a result of a myeloproliferative disease of unknown aetiology, first inducing fibrosis of the marrow which in turn results in a secondary bone sclerosis. There is thus an inevitable anaemia, and in some patients there is also a myeloid type of leukaemic response, an example being seen in the case illustrated in Fig. 110. The increased density is often rather less marked than that seen in osteopetrosis or secondary deposits, but there is a similar loss of the trabecular pattern and of the clear distinction between cortical and cancellous bone (Fig. 110).

In the ribs, pelvis and vertebral column the increase in density is usually quite even, giving the bones a rather grey, homogeneous appearance (Fig. 111). In the shafts of the major long bones it may be uneven and in the form of a linear criss-cross pattern of the cancellous bone. In the skull any increase in density due to myelosclerosis cannot usually be demonstrated since the patients are elderly and prone to have a rather dense structureless vault in any case.

FLUOROSIS

A generalized even increase in bone density is seen following the accidental ingestion of small quantities of fluorine over a prolonged period due to a fault in the water supply to a district. In its lesser manifestations the appearances are similar to those of myelosclerosis, but in severer cases the increase in density is greater (Fig. 113). The characteristic mottled discoloration of the teeth which is usually present will indicate the diagnosis. The bones in this condition become twice as heavy as normal, but the exact histological appearances are not recorded, nor is the mechanism known by which these changes are produced. There may be calcifications in the region of tendon insertions or periosteal shadows.

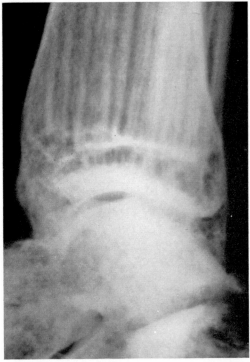

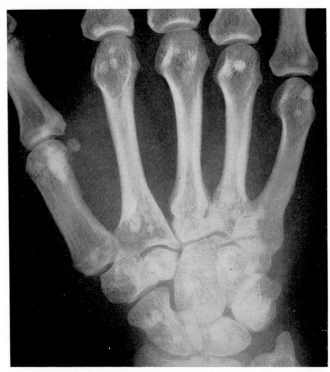

FIG. 108.—Osteopathia striata (Voorhoeve's disease). Vertical coarse linear dense pattern affecting the lower third of the tibia. Also in all limb bones. Each vertebral body has a 1 cm. wide dense horizontal band across the middle third. Ribs homogeneous density. Asymptomatic. Normal blood chemistry and Hb. level.

FIG. 109.—Osteopoikilia. Female aged 25 years. Circular well-demarcated 3 mm. areas of increased density towards ends of all the long bones of the arms and of the carpals. Asymptomatic. X-ray taken for possible fracture.

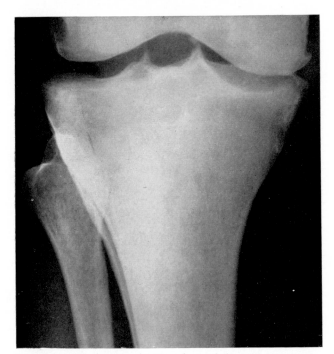

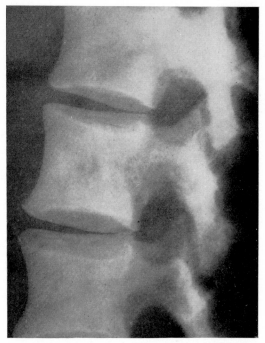

FIG. 110.—Myelosclerosis. Female aged 61 years. Structureless dense area upper third tibia. Similar areas in other major long bones of limbs and ribs. Hepato-splenomegaly. W.b.c. 80,000. Rib biopsy showed myelosclerosis.

FIG. 111.—Myelosclerosis. Female aged 71 years. Dense structureless vertebrae. Also ribs, pelvis and to a lesser extent femora. Splenomegaly. Hb. 46 per cent. W.b.c. 54,000. Mainly metamyelocytes.

HYPERVITAMINOSIS

A generalized increase in the bone density in the submetaphyseal region may be seen in children treated with a considerable excess of vitamin A.

SECONDARY DEPOSITS

An even or patchy increase in density throughout much of the skeleton may be the result of an osteoblastic sclerosis in response to and starting from multifocal widespread secondary deposits. The changes are generally most marked in the vertebral column, pelvis and ribs, but sometimes the major long bones of the limbs are also involved. The skull and the distal bones of the limbs are rarely affected.

Even increase in density

The whole of a bone may appear uniformly grey and structureless without any clear distinction between the cortical layer and the bone beneath (Figs. 116 and 117). The increase in density is not as marked as in developmental osteopetrosis, though there is a similar loss of the trabecular pattern, nor is there any increase in the width or alteration in the shape of the bone, in contrast to Paget's disease (see page 178). In Hodgkin's disease the sclerotic reaction often results in a similarly even, structureless appearance of a number of vertebral bodies, but unlike secondary deposits from a carcinoma of the prostate, it rarely affects the whole of the vertebral column or all the ribs.

Patchy increase in density

In the early stages before the foci coalesce, and even in the later stages if the deposits are more widely spaced, the increase in density is often patchy. The dense areas may be about 3–8 millimetres in size, oval or circular in shape and well demarcated (Fig. 118), or they may be much smaller, giving a granular appearance to the bone (Fig. 116). In some forms the sclerosis is more linear and the appearance is that of a coarse linear pattern throughout the bone, a change seen only in the vertebrae or pelvis (Fig. 119).

These more patchy forms of sclerosing secondary deposits must also be distinguished from Paget's disease. In the latter the cortex is thickened and there is a disorientation of the nearby trabecular pattern in addition to the coarse linear or granular pattern, features which are not seen in secondary deposits. In addition, biochemical tests may show a raised alkaline phosphatase in Paget's disease and a raised acid phosphatase in secondary deposits from the prostate, though not in other types of secondary deposit.

Pathology

The most common cause of sclerosing secondary deposits is a carcinoma of the prostate. Similar bone changes may be seen in carcinomatous deposits from other primary sites such as the breast, or more rarely in secondary deposits from a primary osteogenic sarcoma or in one of the reticuloses, particularly Hodgkin's disease. Histologically the site of the osteosclerosis will reveal tumour cells, often but not invariably in a fibrous stroma. In the stroma of the tumour tissue, osteoblastic activity is visible with new bone formation showing irregular and prominent cement lines.

PAGET'S DISEASE

In one of the many manifestations of Paget's disease, the vertebral column and pelvis in particular may show a more or less uniform increase in density rather similar to that seen in sclerosing secondary deposits. Other features are usually present to indicate the diagnosis, particularly softening of the bones with flattening and widening of the vertebrae, the characteristic alteration of the trabecular pattern (see Chapter 9, page 178) and an increase in width of many of the bones, particularly the pelvis. The increased width is most easily seen in the ischio-pubic rami.

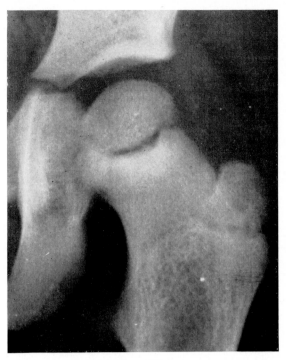

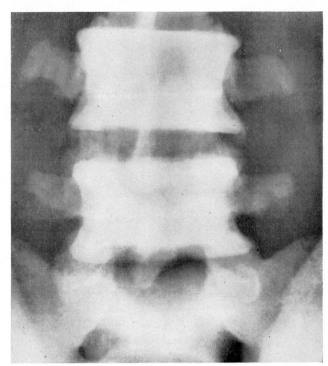

Fig. 112   Fig. 113

Fig. 112.—Renal osteosclerosis. Female aged 6 years. Submetaphyseal zone of dense bone in femur. Fanconi's syndrome. Serum Ca. 9·4 mg. per cent; P. 4·5 mg. per cent. Amino aciduria. Initially appearance of rickets; improved on high dose of vitamin D, so was really healing rickets.

Fig. 113.—Fluorosis. Adult. Dense homogeneous appearance of lumbar vertebral bodies. Similar appearance pelvis and upper femora. Aden area where fluorosis endemic. Sodium fluoride 6 parts per million in local well water.

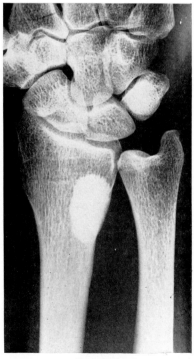

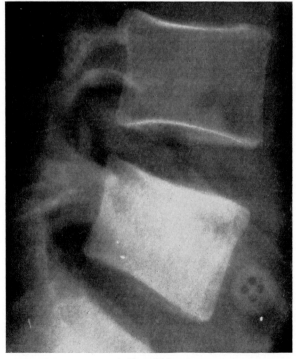

Fig. 114   Fig. 115

Fig. 114.—Ex-hyperparathyroidism. Female aged 32 years. Two years previously typical hyperparathyroidism, and adenoma removed. Cystic area lower end of radius now seen as dense oval shadow. Some of cystic areas healed in a similar manner, others showed reconstitution of normal bone architecture.

Fig. 115.—Hodgkin's disease. Male aged 48 years. Single dense fifth lumbar vertebra with normal disc space. Biopsy of lymph gland: Hodgkin's disease.

INCREASE IN BONE DENSITY CONFINED TO METAPHYSEAL REGION

HEAVY METAL DEPOSITION

An increase in bone density of the submetaphyseal region of the long bones may occur after the intake of heavy metals such as lead or bismuth—*see* page 48.

RENAL OSTEOSCLEROSIS AND HYPERPARATHYROIDISM

Submetaphyseal sclerosis is seen in some cases of hyperparathyroidism, particularly in hyperparathyroidism secondary to renal disease, as in the "rugger jersey" appearance of the vertebral bodies with sclerosis beneath the end plates (*see* Fig. 180) or a relative increase in density of the submetaphyseal region of the major long bones. Though the increase in density is not as marked as in heavy metal poisoning, it can often be seen if carefully looked for, and can be confirmed by densitometry by comparing the ratio of a point 1 cm. and 8 cm. from the lower end of the ulna as described by Doyle (1966). For mechanism *see* page 108.

INCREASE IN DENSITY OF A SINGLE VERTEBRA

SECONDARY DEPOSIT OF CARCINOMA

A fairly even increase in density throughout the body of a single vertebra, with no change in its shape and no alteration in the transverse processes or in the width of the intervertebral disc, is often seen with a secondary deposit, particularly from a carcinoma in the breast or prostate, though sometimes from a carcinoma in some other site. The presence of the primary neoplasm may already be known from the clinical examination, or the dense vertebra may be discovered incidentally in, for example, a lateral-view chest radiograph, or a radiograph of the spine taken for the exclusion of a fracture or of a lesion causing backache.

The finding of a single dense vertebra may present considerable difficulty in diagnosis. Sometimes a more thorough clinical examination will reveal the primary neoplasm which was not detected at the initial examination. Sometimes a careful inspection of the initial radiographs or of additional radiographs taken to include more of the spinal column, the whole pelvis and the ribs, may show another area or several areas of increased bone density or of erosion, thus suggesting widespread secondary deposits. On the other hand a single dense vertebra may be the only bony abnormality.

In some elderly patients there may be a rather misleading narrowing of the adjacent disc space. This is simply the result of disc degeneration or protrusion, very common in normal persons over the age of 50, and has no connexion with the secondary deposit which it may well have preceded by a number of years. In such cases other disc spaces will also be narrowed.

HODGKIN'S DISEASE

An increase in the density of a single vertebra may be due to the sclerotic bone reaction to intra-osseous deposits of Hodgkin's tissue. Histologically this tissue is composed of a polymorphic mixture of large mononuclear tumour cells, giant cells containing two or more nuclei, eosinophils and lymphocytes in a fibrous stroma of varying maturity and cellularity. For mechanism of erosion or sclerosis, *see* page 150. The vertebral body tends to have a very even, rather grey, ground-glass appearance (Fig. 115).

The diagnosis will usually be known from glandular enlargements with biopsy proof or presumed from a large mediastinal shadow, but occasionally it is unsuspected until the vertebral density is observed in a radiograph taken perhaps because of persistent spinal pain.

Often two or three adjacent vertebrae are affected as well as the vertebral end of one or two adjacent ribs, which may show an even or a patchy sclerosis, or a mixture of erosion and sclerosis. There may be a paravertebral shadow about 1 centimetre wide and several centimetres long due to paravertebral deposits, which will have an appearance similar to that of an abscess (*see* Fig. 44) but with a straighter and therefore less obviously convex lateral margin (*see also* Fig. 260, a secondary deposit of carcinoma).

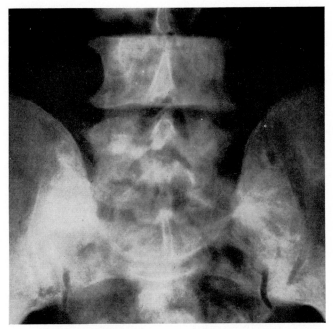

FIG. 116.—Sclerosing secondary deposits from the prostate. Male aged 64 years. Rather granular increase in density lumbar vertebrae and even increase near sacro-iliac joints. Sternal biopsy: sclerosis from secondary carcinoma of the prostate. Some backache.

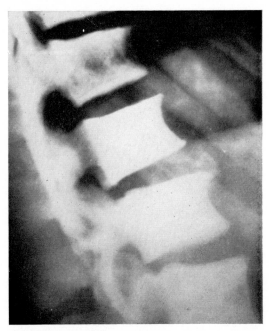

FIG. 117.—Sclerosing secondary deposits from prostate. Male aged 81 years. Even increase in density of lumbar vertebrae, also of the pelvis and the upper femora. Serum alkaline phosphatase 5 K.A. units; serum acid phosphatase 7 K.A. units; P.M. sclerosing secondaries vertebrae, etc., from carcinoma of prostate.

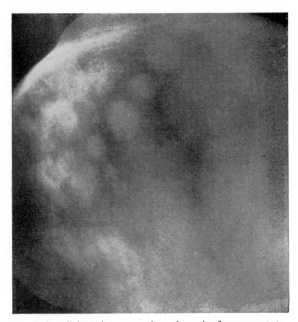

FIG. 118.—Sclerosing secondary deposits from prostate. Male aged 71 years with 5–8 mm. circular shadows in the ilia, also in the lumbar vertebrae. Femora more even density and periosteal new bone. Proved carcinoma of the prostate. Later severe lower back pain. Some control by stilboestrol.

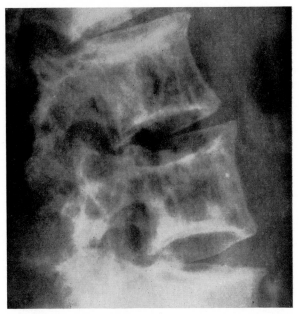

FIG. 119.—Sclerosing secondary deposits. Female aged 52 years. Carcinoma of breast. Vertical striate bands in vertebrae. Also erosions and striate bands in pelvis and femora.

PAGET'S DISEASE

Paget's disease may affect a single vertebra, and the resulting increase in density is usually striate with a particularly coarse and rather irregular trabecular pattern. More rarely it is confined to a marginal band some 5–8 millimetres wide running parallel to the upper, lower and posterior margins, while the anterior margin and central portion of the body are of more or less normal density. This latter appearance differs from a secondary deposit, in which any uneven increase in density tends to be discrete with a few small circular or oval areas scattered throughout the body.

On the other hand, the increase in density may be even throughout the body, in which case it may simulate a secondary deposit.

In Paget's disease the affected body tends to be not only flattened, a feature common in both conditions, but also widened (Figs. 120 and 121), a change which is not seen in secondary deposits. Since this change in shape gives rise to unusual stresses over a long period, it is often associated with gross bony marginal lipping, which is either confined to the region of the deformed vertebra or more marked there than elsewhere.

Evidence of Paget's disease in some other bones such as the skull, pelvis or major long bone of a limb does not necessarily point to this diagnosis of the dense vertebra, since a secondary deposit may be present as well as Paget's disease.

LOCAL VASCULAR DISORDER

More difficult to distinguish from a secondary deposit is the late sclerosis of a single vertebra due to a local vascular disorder with secondary osteochondritis or aseptic necrosis. There is generally no history indicating the cause or date of onset of the lesion and no clinical clues after the lesion has been seen in radiographs. Even if pathological material becomes available, it is not always possible to be certain of the cause of the dense sclerosis (Fig. 122).

LOW-GRADE CHRONIC OSTEOMYELITIS

Another cause of a dense vertebra with few signs or symptoms is a low-grade chronic sclerosing osteomyelitis. There is usually some diminution of the disc space between it and the vertebra above or below, but this may be inconspicuous. On the other hand, local secondary marginal lipping is both usual and conspicuous (Fig. 41).

BENIGN TUMOUR OR DEVELOPMENTAL DEFECT

A diagnosis of haemangioma is frequently made when a dense vertebra is seen, especially in a young adult. The density is often not quite homogeneous and the vertebral body has a coarse striated pattern which extends into the transverse processes on either side (Fig. 123). It must be admitted that in the majority of cases the diagnosis is not proved by histological examination and it is possible that other benign lesions such as a fibrous dysplasia may be responsible for the x-ray appearances. In either case the lesion is without symptoms and rarely shows progression in serial radiographs. In fibrous dysplasia there may be some flattening of the affected vertebra.

A case of osteoid osteoma of a vertebra with an increased density of most of the vertebral body is reported by Mustard and Duval (1959) and Fett and Russo (1959).

PRIMARY BONE SARCOMA

A very rare cause of increased density of a vertebra is a primary sarcoma, either an osteogenic sarcoma or a chondrosarcoma. There may be a slight increase in the size of the vertebra, but apart from this a chondrosarcoma may closely simulate an osteochondritis with little diminution of the disc space and a rather mottled increase in density of the vertebral body (Fig. 124).

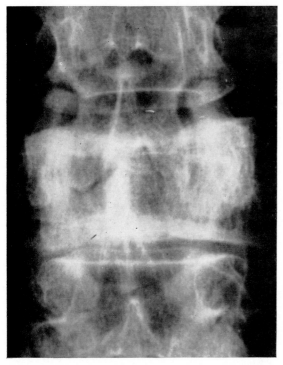

FIG. 120.—Paget's disease. Male aged 78 years; asymptomatic. L. 3 dense with coarse trabeculae; height less and width greater than adjacent vertebrae.

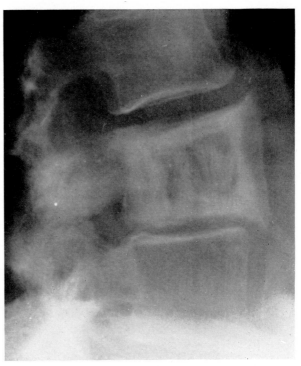

FIG. 121.—Male aged 76 years; same case as in Fig. 120. Lateral view. A.P. diameter increased. Alkaline phosphatase 46 K.A. units.

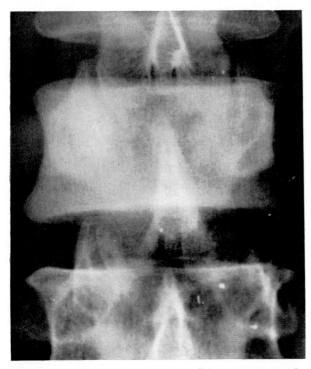

FIG. 122.—Dense vertebra, possibly post-traumatic. Elderly male. P.M. Marrow fibrotic and bone sclerosis, presumably the result of old trauma. No evidence of neoplasm or Paget's disease.

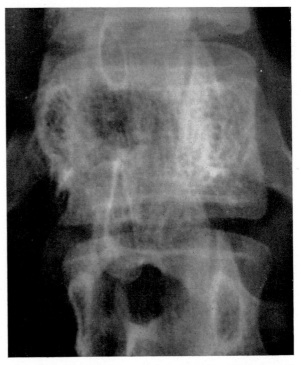

FIG. 123.—Possible haemangioma vertebra. Female aged 29 years. Striated pattern D. 12. Asymptomatic, no pathology available.

ISOLATED INCREASE IN BONE DENSITY IN A LIMB BONE, RIB OR PELVIS

DEVELOPMENTAL DEFECT

An increase in density of part of a limb bone or rib, without any periosteal new bone, is often due to a developmental defect in which dense cortical bone has been laid down in an area normally occupied by cancellous bone. The defect is longer (sometimes several centimetres long) and relatively narrower than in osteopoikilosis. It lies against the cortex on one or other side and is well demarcated on its inner side from the adjacent cancellous bone (Fig. 125). It is often widest near the middle and tapering to a thin line at each end. When the lesions are confined to some of the limb bones on one side of the body only, it might be termed melorheostosis.

A single well-demarcated 1 centimetre circular or oval shadow deep in a bone some distance from the metaphysis is a common finding. It remains stationary after adolescence and is often called a bone island.

DEEP BONE INFARCT

A band-like increase in bone density about 1–2 centimetres wide and several centimetres in length, lying deep in the medullary part of the bone, is seen as the result of a bone infarct (Fig. 126). A common site is the lower third of a femur or upper third of a tibia. This lesion was first detected in caisson workers and was thought to be due to a too rapid decompression resulting in bubbles of gas in the blood stream which presumably caused the infarct. A similar shadow is sometimes seen when no such occupational risk exists and can only be presumed to be an infarct because no precipitating incident can be recollected. A similar appearance may be seen in sickle cell anaemia, presumably due to intra-vascular clotting.

Pathology

The avascular bone at the site of the infarct retains its calcium although the bone is dead and all the osteocytes have disappeared leaving ghost-like spaces in the bone trabeculae. A vascular fibrous reaction frequently occurs at the margin of the dead area and this produces a degree of mineral loss of the surrounding living bone, so that the area of the aseptic necrosis with its full calcium content is clearly contrasted against the nearby living bone.

ENCHONDROMA

A band-like increase in bone density in the medulla with an appearance similar to a bone infarct may be due to a calcifying enchondroma (*see* Fig. 127).

HEALING CYST

Following treatment of hyperparathyroidism, a cyst-like area in a bone may become reconstituted with dense calcified material instead of being filled in with normal cancellous bone with a trabecular structure, or perhaps remaining unchanged. In such a case a well demarcated 1–2 centimetres dense oval shadow will be seen deep in the bone (Fig. 114).

AVASCULAR NECROSIS OR OSTEOCHONDRITIS

Dense lunate

An even or a patchy increase in density throughout the whole of a semilunar bone in the wrist is usually due to a local vascular accident of the type producing an avascular necrosis or osteochondritis (Fig. 128). It may follow some weeks after severe trauma or there may be no known preceding incident. In some cases the bone disintegrates and collapses, but in others the trabecular pattern eventually reforms and the bone, after being dense for perhaps some months, becomes normal in appearance.

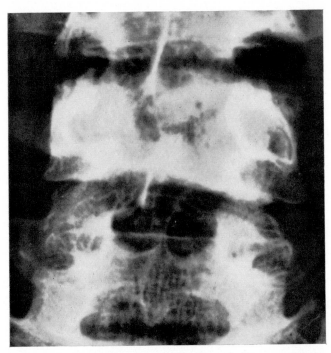

FIG. 124.—Chondrosarcoma. Female aged 13 years. Dense fourth lumbar vertebra. Unchanged for 4 years. More pain, so biopsy which showed a chondrosarcoma. Radiotherapy; 10-year survival.

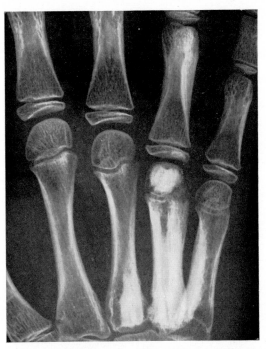

FIG. 125.—Developmental defect (melhorheostosis type). Female aged 13 years. Dense areas centre of carpals, external cortical thickening fourth and fifth metacarpals and phalanx, internal thickening third. Unchanged 5 years later.

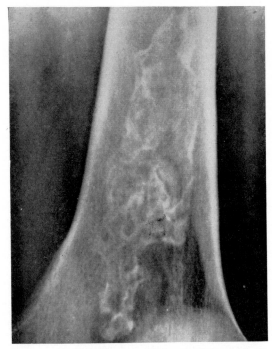

FIG. 126.—Possible bone infarct. Male aged 54 years. Slight pain in the knee. Band-like dense area in medulla might be an infarct. No clinical or pathological proof as yet. No transradiant zone; longer and less spotty than a chondroma.

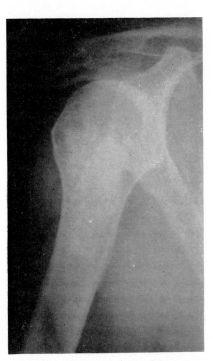

FIG. 127.—Enchondroma of humerus. Female aged 71 years. Asymptomatic. Post-mortem examination showed deep calcifying chondroma.

Dense talus or scaphoid

A similar even increase in density of one fragment of a fractured scaphoid (Fig. 129) or talus is often seen and usually lasts some months. In some cases bone union occurs and the bone returns to a normal appearance, but in many bone union never occurs.

Dense patella

In a patella there may also be an even increase in density of one fragment after a fracture, or a patchy increase in density with perhaps some loss of density in the areas between may occur without a history of trauma. The benign course with eventual resolution suggests an avascular necrosis. It is quite different from a necrosis of a part of the patellar articular cartilage, a condition known as chondromalacia patellae, in which there are often no changes visible in the radiograph.

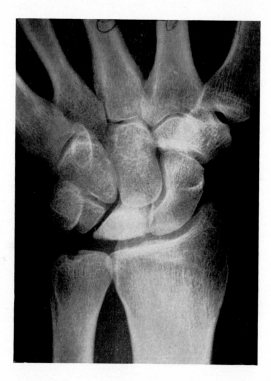

FIG. 128.—Aseptic necrosis of lunate. Male aged 30 years. Dense lunate. Twisted wrist 1 year ago, with pain since.

Dense femoral head

An increase in density of the head of the femur may be seen some weeks after a fracture of the femoral neck, and may be the first radiological evidence of avascular necrosis of the head (Fig. 130). The head tends to become flattened and may totally disappear.

Aseptic necrosis of a femoral head may also occur in cases of renal failure treated with a renal transplant and steroids (Fig. 131). It is probable that the subcapsular end arteries are blocked by fatty myxoedematous tissue. Aseptic necrosis may also occur in a patient with severe thalassaemia.

Dense terminal phalanx

An increase in density of one or several terminal phalanges is sometimes seen as a result of a vascular disorder. The presence of Raynaud's phenomena makes the diagnosis obvious (*see also* page 145 describing absorption of the tip of the phalanx). The change may affect the whole of each phalanx or only the distal or middle third (Fig. 132). A similar radiological appearance may be seen without any obvious cause, when it probably represents a developmental defect with an excess of dense bone at the expense of the cancellous bone (Fig. 133).

Secondary Deposit

One or several dense areas in a pelvic bone, a rib or a major limb bone may be the result of secondary deposits, particularly from the prostate or breast. In some cases the shadow is circular and quite well demarcated, and about ½–1 centimetre in size (*see* Figs. 118 and 134). Rather less commonly there is a larger, rather poorly demarcated area of increased density, sometimes seen in an ilium adjacent to the sacro-iliac joint (*see* Fig. 116). Such an area is usually due to Hodgkin's disease rather than to a carcinoma.

Sclerosing Osteitis and Sarcoma

An even increase in density of a metacarpal or metatarsal is sometimes seen with a sclerosing osteitis but may also be seen with a bone sarcoma. The early diagnosis of a sclerosing osteitis or sarcoma of a vertebra may be possible only by a bone biopsy. The increase in density is of the deeper parts and the distinction between cortical and cancellous bone is lost. There may be a little periosteal new bone or a small area of erosion, but these are often very inconspicuous.

In a rib an even structureless increase in density, usually in only a part of the bone, may also be due to a chronic sclerosing osteitis. It is generally secondary to an underlying pleural condition which will be obvious in a chest radiograph.

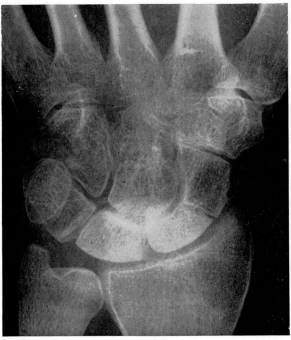

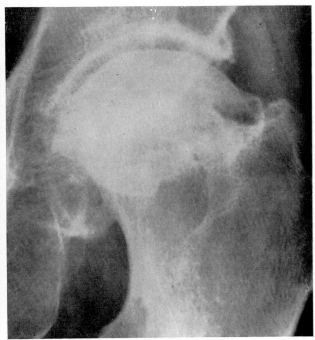

Fig. 129.—Aseptic necrosis. Male aged 34 years. Dense medial fragment of scaphoid; presumed avascularity of medial fragment, with loss of bone density from immobilization of lateral fragment and surrounding bones.

Fig. 130.—Aseptic necrosis. Female aged 85 years. Dense deformed femoral head; 3 years ago transcervical fracture following fall. Pain started 1 year later and persisted.

Condensans Ilii

A localized area of increased bone density is occasionally seen in women of the child-bearing age in the ilium adjacent to the sacro-iliac joints. It is situated towards the lower third of the joint and is 2–3 centimetres long and roughly triangular in shape, with its base against the joint and its apex pointing downwards and outwards (Fig. 135). It is well demarcated from the surrounding normal bone, and the joint space and articular cortex are quite normal, thus differing from sacro-iliitis (*see* Chapter 10, page 197). It is usually bilateral and almost symmetrical.

There are often no symptoms, though some patients experience a transient low back pain which is difficult to relate to the x-ray appearances. The disease is not progressive, though occasionally regressive. Such histology as has been reported is rather indefinite and has failed to indicate the aetiology.

OSTEOID OSTEOMA

An osteoid osteoma (*see* page 176) may appear as a roughly circular 1 centimetre well-demarcated shadow deep in a bone. More commonly it is diffuse and associated with periosteal new bone and a small erosion.

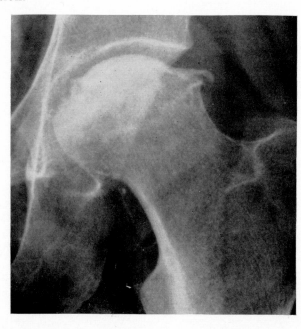

Fig. 131.—Dense femoral head. Female aged 26 years. Chronic renal failure; renal transplant and on steroids. Hip normal 2 years previously.

ISOLATED INCREASE IN DENSITY IN THE SKULL OR FACIAL BONES

ANATOMICAL VARIATIONS

The bone density in the vault varies considerably between different normal persons and between the different bones in a single normal person. The frontal bone may be thicker and denser than the parietal or occipital bones.

Occasionally a band of denser bone runs parallel with the transradiant lines of the sutures, extending out for a few millimetres. In the case of the lambdoid suture a similar increase in density may be caused by an overlap of the bones (bathrocephaly).

A 1–2 centimetre circular shadow may be seen in the mid line of the occipital bone in a posterior (Towne's) view, representing a large external occipital protuberance seen end on. The cause of the increase in density will be visible in a lateral view if it is not overexposed.

HYPEROSTOSIS FRONTALIS

An increase in the density and width of the anterior part of the frontal bone is seen in hyperostosis frontalis. There is a loss of diploic structure in the affected area which ends sharply posteriorly, often with a knobbled contour.

The changes are usually bilateral but not quite symmetrical. Many cases are asymptomatic, but in some cases there is a complaint of headache which is probably not directly related to the bone changes.

MENINGIOMA

In the vault or base of the skull a localized increase in bone density is often the first radiographic evidence of an underlying meningioma (Fig. 136). There may be clinical evidence of an intracranial

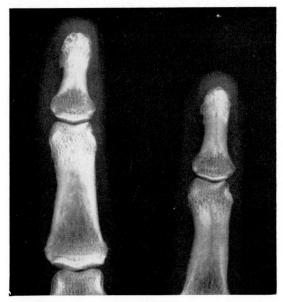

FIG. 132.—Vascular disorder. Female aged 35 years. Increased density of terminal phalanges. Raynaud phenomena many years with tendency for hands and feet to go cold and blue. Improved after ganglionectomy.

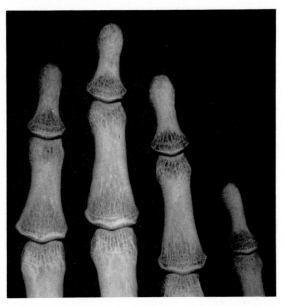

FIG. 133.—Developmental defect. Female aged 20 years. Dense terminal phalanges. Asymptomatic. Active nurse.

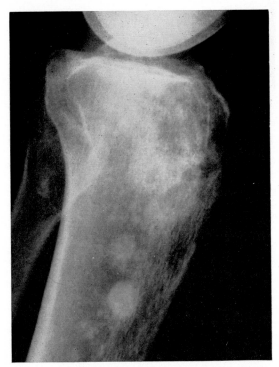

FIG. 134.—Secondary deposit. Female aged 55 years. Circular dense areas in the upper tibia, also in the pelvis and spine, and erosive lesion of the femur. Carcinoma breast. Recent pain over tibia.

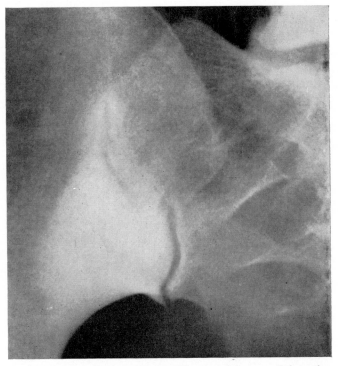

FIG. 135.—Condensans ilii. Female aged 25 years. Triangular dense area in ilium adjacent to sacro-iliac joint. Articular cortex normal. Same on other side. Asymptomatic.

lesion, or this may not be obvious at the initial clinical examination. The increase in density is generally associated with some thickening of the bone, often with an increase in the depth of the vascular grooves, and in some cases with erosion nearby. Calcification in the tumour itself may reinforce the shadow of the increased bone density.

INFLAMMATORY LESION

A long-standing localized osteomyelitis or syphilitic lesion may result in an area of bone thickening and increased density with a poorly demarcated edge, and some erosions nearby.

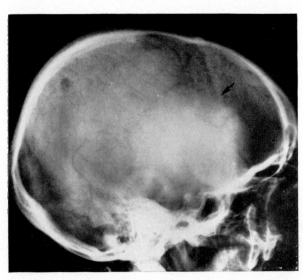

FIG. 136.—Meningioma. Male aged 46 years. Sclerotic area right temporo-parietal area. Complaining of lump on head. Nil else found. Dense bone and underlying meningioma excised.

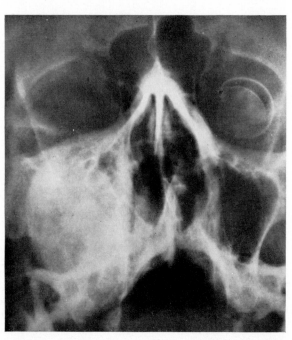

FIG. 137.—Leontiasis ossea. Male aged 75 years. Almost homogeneous opacity obliterating outline of the right antrum. Twenty years' painless swelling of the right cheek.

SECONDARY DEPOSIT

A sclerosing secondary deposit may result in a localized increase in density of the vault. Generally there are several such areas.

FIBROUS DYSPLASIA AND OSSIFYING FIBROMA

An increase in the thickness and therefore the density of the facial bones, and in some cases the anterior part of the base of the skull, is seen in fibrous dysplasia and in an ossifying fibroma. Distinction between these two conditions can be made only by a histological examination of a piece of the bone. The condition may be confined to one side but is sometimes bilateral. It is generally painless, reaches a certain degree of development and then becomes stationary. In some cases the patient may record that there has been some swelling of the face for 20 years or more.

LEONTIASIS OSSEA

A gross increase in the density of the facial bones on one or both sides, with slight or considerable increase in size, is called leontiasis ossea. This may be the result of a chronic low-grade osteitis of bacterial origin, or more commonly of a developmental defect such as a fibrous dysplasia or an ossifying fibroma (Fig. 137).

PAGET'S DISEASE

An increase in density of the facial bones on one side may be due to Paget's disease. Superficially the lesion may simulate fibrous dysplasia, but the later age of onset and the presence of the changes of Paget's disease in other bones will usually suffice to differentiate the two conditions. In Paget's disease the increase in density is less homogeneous and more striated.

5—New Bone and Calcification Outside the Cortex (Periosteal Shadow or Periostitis)

Three types of extracortical (periosteal) shadow are seen in radiographs. The first is the so-called "onion-skin appearance" in which periosteal new bone has been formed in layers with transradiant tissue between them (Fig. 283), and the second is the "sun-ray appearance" in which subperiosteal calcifications have been formed at right angles to the shaft of the bone (Fig. 281). These two types are nearly always associated with erosion or sclerosis and are therefore described in detail in Chapter 8.

The third and most common type is a relatively narrow linear shadow running parallel to the cortex which strongly suggests periosteal new bone formation, although it can equally well represent calcification in a haematoma or in neoplastic tissue. Like the onion-skin and sun-ray appearances, it is often referred to in x-ray reports as "periostitis". This is an unsuitable term since it can properly apply only when the cause of the shadow is inflammatory; it is inappropriate when, as is often the case, the cause is traumatic, neoplastic or circulatory.

The shadow varies in width from a hair line so thin that it can be seen only with the aid of a magnifying glass or by radiographic or photographic enlargement techniques (Fig. 138) to a band as wide as, or even wider than, the diaphysis adjacent to it (Fig. 143). Very wide shadows are generally seen with a subperiosteal haematoma resulting from trauma or from a haemorrhagic state such as scurvy (Fig. 144).

The length of the shadow varies from a few millimetres to the whole length of the diaphysis. A very short shadow will suggest a traumatic lesion or an underlying stress fracture.

The periosteal shadow may occur adjacent to the diaphysis of any of the long bones or large flat bones such as the scapula (where it is most common in the subglenoid region) or the pelvis. It is uncommon in the vault of the skull and often less in extent than in a similar type of lesion elsewhere (see Chapter 7). In the mandible it is often most conspicuous on the inferior aspect, though it is also seen on the lingual or labial aspect in an occlusal vertical view. It is occasionally seen on the lateral or anterior margin of a vertebra. Since there is no periosteum round the epiphyses or articular surface of a bone, it is unusual to see a periosteal shadow in a carpal or tarsal bone, although it is sometimes seen on the undersurface of the calcaneum.

In the early acute stage of the lesion the periosteal shadow is often separated from the outer edge of the cortex by a 1–3 millimetre transradiant zone (Fig. 138). At this stage the periosteum has become separated from the cortex by inflammatory products such as pus or oedema, by a subperiosteal haemorrhage or by neoplastic cells, and the new bone or calcified tissue has begun to arise from the elevated periosteum but has not yet completely replaced this relatively transradiant material. The transradiant zone may persist for some time, but will eventually disappear as the periosteal new bone or calcification spreads right back to the cortex. At this middle stage the periosteal new bone is still distinguishable from the adjacent cortical bone, because it is rather less radio-opaque and the clear-cut outer margin of the cortex demarcates the two shadows (Fig. 145). Finally, as healing proceeds, the periosteal new bone becomes denser and fuses with the cortical bone (Fig. 149), and the x-ray appearances become indistinguishable from those of an area of primary cortical hyperostosis. In some cases the periosteal new bone may eventually disappear completely, leaving the bone with a normal x-ray appearance.

POST-TRAUMATIC PERIOSTEAL SHADOW

Trauma without a local wound may result in a subperiosteal haematoma even in the absence of a fracture. Calcification in the haematoma, or a periosteal response to the presence of the blood, may be apparent 7–14 days after the incident (Fig. 140). In some cases the history of a recent traumatic incident may make the diagnosis reasonably certain. In others there is no such history, the precipitating blow or stress having passed unnoticed by the patient, and the localized area of periosteal new bone may be discovered either accidentally during radiography for some other purpose or when investigating slight pain in the area. In either case the traumatic cause may not at first be apparent. If the lesion remains stationary for some weeks and then slowly resolves, it is almost certainly a post-traumatic subperiosteal haematoma (Fig. 141). In an adult a post-traumatic haematoma after a minor injury is usually localized, the periosteal new bone being seen only along a small length of the shaft of a long bone, perhaps only for $\frac{1}{2}$–2 centimetres (Fig. 141).

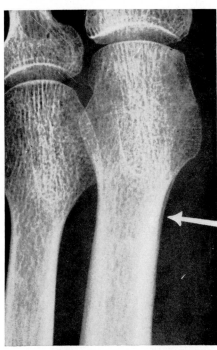

FIG. 138.—Periosteal new bone. Male aged 40 years. Hair-line shadow adjacent to the shaft of the second metatarsal (opposite arrow), visible only with a magnifying glass; 4 weeks' pain and swelling of the left foot, and local tenderness (magnification, × 2).

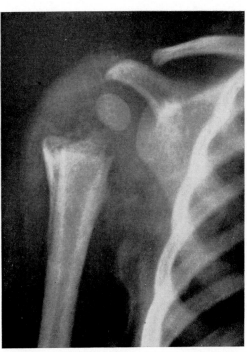

FIG. 139.—Caffey's or "battered baby" syndrome. Male aged 9 months. Periosteal new bone round upper third of shaft of humerus. Shaft lateral on epiphysis. Said to have been accidentally bumped while shopping. Other arm similar.

On the other hand, in infants the periosteal shadow may be very extensive and as long as, and often wider than, the diaphysis (Fig. 143). Several bones may be affected. After a few weeks the subperiosteal calcifying haematoma may be converted into bone which fuses with the cortex, and the condition may then be described as infantile cortical hyperostosis.

In some cases the periosteal shadow is the only feature; in others there is some separation of the epiphysis in addition (Fig. 139), suggesting that trauma is indeed the cause. There may also be some erosion of the metaphysis, probably secondary to the epiphyseal separation with haemorrhage.

Although trauma is the cause in most cases, it may be impossible or very difficult in an infant to elicit a history of injury (Caffey, 1957). This difficulty was also found in a series of cases of the "battered baby" syndrome reported in England by Griffiths and Moynihan (1963).

Infantile Non-traumatic Cortical Hyperostosis

In some babies with similar radiological features (Fig. 142), trauma can actually be excluded with reasonable certainty, the bacteriological examination is negative and a mild inflammatory reaction may be seen in a biopsy; the aetiology of this pseudo-traumatic lesion is obscure.

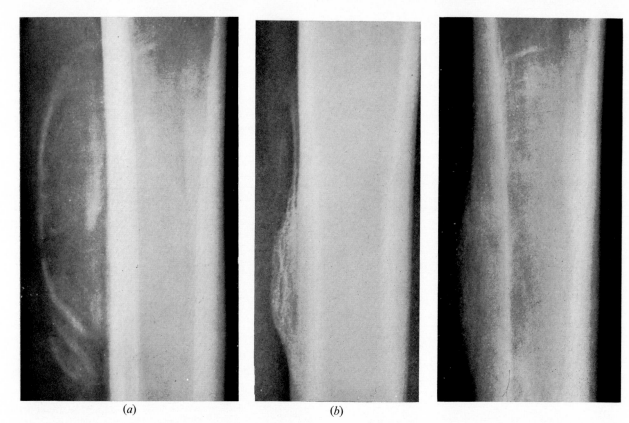

(a) (b)

FIG. 140.—(a) Subperiosteal haematoma. Male aged 25 years. Linear shadow 2 centimetres from cortex of lateral aspect of femur. Kicked on thigh 16 days before. (b) Four months later. Shadow denser and smaller and closer to cortex. Narrow transradiant zone between it and the cortex.

FIG. 141.—Same case as in Fig. 140 (a) and (b) 8 months later. Periosteal shadow fused with the cortex.

NON-TRAUMATIC HAEMATOMA

In an infant a subperiosteal haematoma with an extensive periosteal shadow may be due to scurvy (Fig. 144), the haemorrhage resulting from some day-to-day stress, and may sometimes be the first indication of this condition. The periosteum is generally much raised and the calcification beneath it 1–2 centimetres wide. There may be other radiological changes of scurvy such as osteoporosis and submetaphyseal transradiant zones (described on page 48).

STRESS, FATIGUE AND PSEUDO-FRACTURE

STRESS FRACTURE OF A METATARSAL (MARCH FRACTURE)

A short localized periosteal shadow separated from the cortex of the shaft of the second or, less commonly, the third or fourth metatarsal will suggest a periosteal reaction occurring with a stress or "march" fracture. The lesion may be seen in the middle third of the shaft or may be just below the neck. It may be either a fine hair-line shadow, visible only with the aid of a magnification technique (Fig. 138), or an obvious shadow about 1 centimetre long and 2–3 millimetres wide (Fig. 145) with a lateral convex prominence (Fig. 145). It is separated from the cortex by a narrow transradiant zone in the early stages, but soon extends right up to the cortex.

The lesion may be asymptomatic, especially in the early stages, or there may be some localized pain in the foot. In some cases there is a history of much walking a week or two before the radiograph shows any changes; in others there is no significant antecedent history of stress. Sometimes no abnormality is visible in the initial radiograph, the periosteal shadow appearing only a week or two later.

The actual fracture may be visible as a transverse or oblique hair-line transradiancy across the shaft. This sometimes precedes and sometimes succeeds the appearance of the periosteal shadow. In asymptomatic cases the fracture line may have filled up with calcified callus and therefore be invisible by the time the first radiograph is taken. The periosteal shadow, on the other hand, remains visible for some months, first fusing with the cortex and finally becoming indistinguishable from it as the new bone becomes absorbed.

The aetiology of the condition is uncertain. It may well be due to a local vascular incident with increased brittleness of the shaft, and thus be allied to a local necrosis.

Stress or Fatigue (Pseudo-fracture) of the Tibia in Children and Athletes

In older children a small periosteal linear shadow on the lateral aspect of the upper third of the tibia may be the only evidence of a stress or fatigue pseudo-fracture (Fig. 147). There may be a history of minor trauma, or no relevant history apart from some slight pain, and there may be some tenderness but no other sign of disease. Eventually the tell-tale 2–3 millimetre wide transradiant zone of bone resorption may be seen running horizontally to indicate the diagnosis, or resolution of the periosteal new bone may occur without the transradiant zone being seen. Similar cases are reported by Devas (1963).

Fatigue pseudo-fractures of the tibia are reported in athletes by Devas (1958). The majority of these were found in the lower third of the tibia, and a periosteal shadow was the only change in 6, while the narrow horizontal transradiant zone was visible in 11.

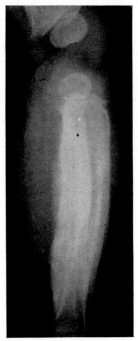 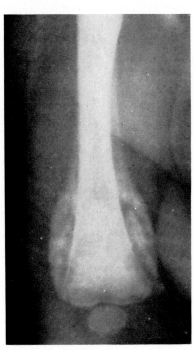 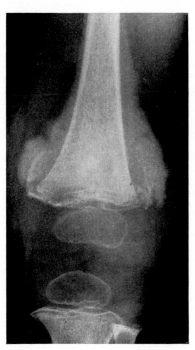

| Fig. 142 | Fig. 143 | Fig. 144 |

Fig. 142.—Infantile cortical hyperostosis. Female aged 1 year with fever and bone pain. Periosteal new bone round tibia. Most major long bones similar, and symmetrical deposits round ribs.

Fig. 143.—Subperiosteal haematoma. Male aged 5 weeks. Birth injury with subperiosteal haematoma of the femur. Structureless shadow either side of the shaft separated from the cortex by a narrow transradiant zone.

Fig. 144.—Subperiosteal haematoma in scurvy. Male aged 3 years. Homogeneous shadow almost the width of the femoral shaft on either side of the cortex. Note submetaphyseal transradiant zone in the femur and tibia and relative absence of the trabeculae in both epiphyses.

STRESS FRACTURE OF A RIB

A rather similar condition is sometimes seen in the middle or anterior third of the first rib. The fracture line and the periosteal new bone are usually quite obvious, but in contrast to the metatarsal lesion the fracture line persists for a year or more. The condition is usually asymptomatic and may be bilateral.

A localized periosteal shadow is sometimes seen in some other rib (Fig. 146), usually the seventh, eighth or ninth, on one side only. This may be on one or both sides of the shaft and is usually in the middle or anterior third. The fracture line in this site may be visible only if a localized coned-down beam is used or if a tomogram is taken. The condition may also be asymptomatic.

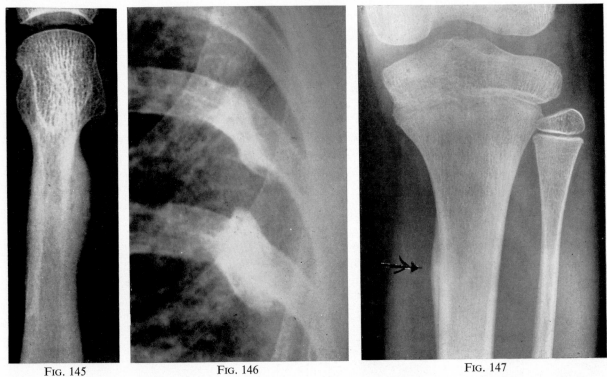

FIG. 145   FIG. 146   FIG. 147

FIG. 145.—Periosteal new bone in march fracture. Homogeneous shadow with convex outer margin distinct from but touching the cortex of the second metatarsal. Asymptomatic.

FIG. 146.—Periosteal shadow or calcifying callus round united fractures of the left sixth and seventh ribs. Male aged 51 years. Chronic cough with sputum.

FIG. 147.—Stress fracture of the tibia. Male aged 11 years. Periosteal new bone (opposite arrow). In original radiograph, faint dense horizontal line for short distance beneath periostitis. Two months' ache in tibia. Resolution.

In these rib lesions it is not always possible to say whether a stress fracture was in fact the precipitating cause or whether there had really been quite severe trauma unnoticed by the patient, as during severe coughing or in the course of surgery. This is especially true when the periosteal shadow is only discovered long after the incident, perhaps in a routine chest radiograph, and the fracture line has filled with calcified callus and is invisible.

PSEUDO-FRACTURE (LOOSER ZONE)

A small 3–5 millimetre periosteal shadow with a convex outer border may be the most conspicuous radiological evidence of a pseudo-fracture (Looser zone). The short transradiant zone of resorption extending into the bone beneath the periosteal shadow is sometimes quite inconspicuous, although it may become more obvious at a later stage (*see* Chapter 6, page 104).

Generalized trabecular thinning or absorption indicating the underlying osteomalacia may give the diagnosis in some cases, but may be too slight to be appreciated in others.

POST-IRRADATION FRACTURES

Following therapeutic irradiation, a bone may become unduly brittle so that a spontaneous fracture may occur. This type of lesion is sometimes seen in the anterior ends of the third, fourth and fifth ribs after treatment of a carcinoma of the breast by a field glancing this part of the thorax. Pain is often absent or slight. A similar fracture may occur in the pubic bone following pelvic irradiation. In either site there may be some sclerosis along the fracture line, suggesting in some cases that it represents a pseudo-fracture.

INFLAMMATORY CONDITIONS

PYOGENIC OR TYPHOID BONE INFECTIONS

In acute pyogenic or typhoid inflammatory lesions of the bone there is a latent period of from 10 to 14 days between the onset of pain and fever and the appearance of bone and periosteal changes in the radiograph. Nevertheless a radiograph may be justified, since it is sometimes possible to see a slight increase in the radio-opacity and width of the surrounding soft tissues. With present day antibiotic therapy the latent period may be even longer. After it has elapsed, a narrow linear periosteal shadow often precedes other bone changes by a few days (see Chapter 8, page 158). If the acute infection is overcome at an early stage, erosive or deep sclerotic bone changes may never develop and the periosteal shadow may then remain the sole radiographic change of an acute osteomyelitis.

In a less acute infection the changes may be virtually confined to the periosteum, often in a limited area of the shaft, and on one side only. The clinical diagnosis may at first be uncertain, and the demonstration of a periosteal shadow in a radiograph may be of considerable diagnostic value.

In a secondary infection of the periosteum from an adjacent local inflammatory lesion in the soft tissues, a narrow linear shadow of periosteal new bone may be seen. Such a linear shadow, for instance, close to the deep aspect of the pelvic brim near the ischial spine may be the first evidence of a deep pelvic inflammation. Periostitis of a rib is not uncommon secondary to an inflammatory condition of the underlying lung and pleura, particularly in a chronic empyema.

SYPHILITIC BONE LESIONS

Periosteal new bone adjacent to the cortex of a single bone or several bones may be the presenting sign of a syphilitic bone lesion. The periosteal new bone deposits vary in quantity, sometimes giving no more than a hair-line shadow and sometimes giving a shadow several millimetres wide. The major long bones of a limb are often affected and the changes may be almost symmetrical on both sides. A syphilitic periostitis may occur at any age but is now uncommon.

In babies the sole osseous manifestation of syphilis may be a dactylitis with fairly abundant periosteal new bone around the cortex of a phalanx. This may mask any underlying bone erosion in some cases, while in others both changes may be seen.

TUBERCULOUS BONE LESIONS

In tuberculosis of a long bone of a hand or foot, periosteal new bone may be the only radiological change for a time (Schintz and his colleagues, 1951) and the condition may therefore simulate a syphilitic lesion. A rib is another site for a tuberculous lesion. More commonly some erosion of the bone is present as well (see Chapter 8, page 162).

FUNGUS INFECTIONS OF BONE

Periosteal new bone formation may be the result of a fungoid infection and is usually secondary to a lesion adjacent to rather than in the bone. For instance, periostitis of one or more ribs may be the result of a spread from an intrathoracic actinomycosis.

Haematogenous bone infection is seen with blastomycosis and coccidioidomycosis.

BENIGN NEOPLASM

OSTEOID OSTEOMA

A small localized area of periosteal new bone may be the sole x-ray change in an osteoid osteoma (Fig. 148), neither the small deep erosion nor the surrounding cortical sclerosis being visible in such a case (*see* Chapter 8, page 176). The patient is usually over the age of 15 years; pain is often a conspicuous feature and the lesion is only slowly progressive.

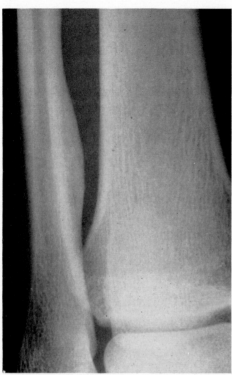

FIG. 148.—Osteoid osteoma. Male aged 19 years. Homogeneous shadow with convex medial margin on the inner aspect of the fibula, touching but distinct from the cortex. Pain for 6 months in the ankle region, gradually getting worse. Removal of nidus (which is invisible in the radiograph); histology—osteoid osteoma.

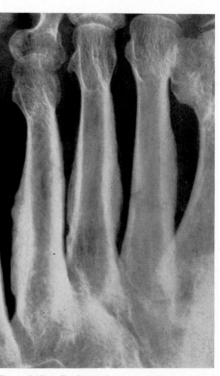

FIG. 149.—Periosteal new bone around metatarsals. Female aged 67 years. Shadow around the shaft of the second indistinguishable from the cortex, that around the third separated from the cortex on one side by a narrow transradiant zone. Diabetic, peripheral vascular disease, ulcer under great toe.

MALIGNANT NEOPLASM

A periosteal shadow without other x-ray changes is an uncommon manifestation of a bone neoplasm, but may be seen with a Ewing's type of tumour or a secondary deposit from a neuroblastoma. In some cases the periosteal shadow is narrow, linear and rather wavy in contour, extending almost the whole length of the shaft of a long bone such as the fibula, and separated from the cortex by a narrow transradiant zone. In other cases the periosteal shadow is in linear layers with transradiant zones between them, giving an "onion-skin" appearance.

Rather different is a more localized dense shadow protruding from the cortex for 1–2 centimetres and showing its periosteal connexion at one or other end, where it tapers down parallel to the shaft. Such an appearance may be caused by a so-called "parosteal" sarcoma. Both at operation and on superficial examination of an often inadequate biopsy specimen this lesion is sometimes misdiagnosed as myositis ossificans, a mistake which is unlikely to occur if the pathological findings are interpreted in relation to the x-ray appearances.

Finally, a rather thin periosteal shadow may be the only x-ray evidence of a nearby fibrosarcoma in a muscle or of a synovioma arising from an adjacent tendon sheath.

VASCULAR DISORDERS

VARICOSE VEINS AND ARTERIAL OCCLUSION

Extensive periosteal deposits are seen quite commonly on the tibia and fibula in severe cases of varicose veins with venous capillary stasis and oedema of the leg.

Extensive periosteal deposits are also seen, though less commonly, on the tibia and fibula following femoral or popliteal artery occlusion without gangrene. In diabetic patients with associated occlusive arterial disease and a poor circulation to the foot, such deposits may be seen around the metatarsals and are often the result of infection as well as the arterial occlusion (Fig. 149).

PULMONARY OSTEOARTHROPATHY

Narrow linear shadows of periosteal new bone adjacent to the cortex of many long bones are characteristic of pulmonary osteoarthrophy (Fig. 151). Common sites are the lower end of the radius and ulna just proximal to the wrist joint, the lower end of the femur just above the condyles, and the tibia

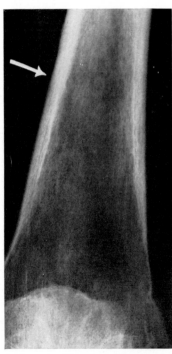

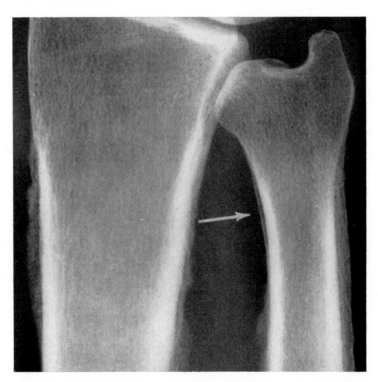

FIG. 150.—Pachydermo-periostosis. Male aged 42 years. Extensive periosteal new bone shadows adjacent to the cortex of the femur (opposite arrow). All major long bones and some metacarpals. Large hands and feet with soft tissue overgrowth. No acromegaly. Bone pain at times.

FIG. 151.—Periosteal new bone in pulmonary osteoarthropathy. (Magnification × 2). Male aged 42 years. Line shadow adjacent to cortex of the radius and ulna, the latter separated from it by a transradiant zone (opposite arrow). Complained of swelling of the ankles and knees. Treated as rheumatism, then wrist radiographed; so chest radiographed and large shadow seen. Pneumonectomy proved it to be a carcinoma.

and fibula just above the malleoli. In severe cases periosteal new bone may be seen around the shafts of the metacarpals and metatarsals and occasionally around the proximal and middle phalanges. There is usually a narrow transradiant zone between the periosteal new bone and the cortex even when the condition is of relatively long standing. The bones of both sides of the body are affected in a roughly symmetrical manner.

In some cases the causative underlying pulmonary lesion has already been recognized, but in others the condition may be found accidentally when a bone or joint is radiographed for some other purpose such as exclusion of a fracture, or arthritis because the patient complains of some pain and swelling as a result of the arthropathy.

When bone changes have been seen, a radiograph of the chest should be taken if this has not already been done. This will probably show an abnormal shadow suggesting a bronchial carcinoma or, more rarely, a pleural fibroma, or it may show small nodular shadows and a ground-glass haze suggesting a fibrosing alveolitis (diffuse idiopathic interstitial pulmonary fibrosis). Nowadays rarely, it may follow

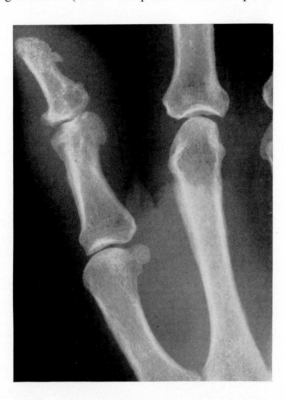

FIG. 152.—Thyroid acropachy. Female aged 56 years. Periosteal shadow adjacent to cortex of proximal phalanx of thumb and second metacarpal. None in lower forearm. Hyperthyroidism 30 years ago; now myxoedematous, with pre-tibial myxoedema and swollen thumbs.

a chronic abscess or empyema. Occasionally a routine anterior-view chest radiograph is normal but the shadow of a bronchial carcinoma is seen in a lateral view or in tomograms of the regions obscured by the upper ribs or hilar vessels, or the carcinoma is found on bronchoscopy. In fact, with perseverance the lung cause can nearly always be found.

Should the lung tumour be removed or the hilar nerves cut, symptoms may be relieved at once. The periosteal new bone usually disappears some months after removal of the tumour.

An increased blood flow to the limb has been demonstrated in this condition, which is therefore probably the result of a vascular disorder secondary to the pulmonary condition.

ASSOCIATED WITH GENERAL DISEASES

Periosteal new bone may be seen associated with thyroid acropachy. The patient is usually known to have had hyperparathyroidism in the past, and later to have become myxoedematous. In thyroid acropachy (Fig. 152) the distribution of the periosteal line shadows is round the shafts of the meta-carpals including the thumb, without involvement of the forearm bones, which also serves to distinguish it from pulmonary osteoarthropathy. The great toe may be involved.

Periosteal new bone formation with a distribution similar to pulmonary osteoarthropathy is some-times seen in association with severe liver disease (biliary cirrhosis).

Periosteal new bone may also be seen in a patient treated with a large excess of vitamin A and occa-sionally in the familial type of hypophosphatasia—see page 47.

IDIOPATHIC HYPERTROPHIC OSTEOARTHROPATHY

Occasionally periosteal linear shadows are seen along the shafts of many of the long bones which look the same as in hypertrophic pulmonary osteoarthropathy but for which, however, no precipitating intrathoracic or other lesion can be demonstrated either by clinical examination or by full-scale radiological examination of the chest including bronchography.

PACHYDERMO-PERIOSTOSIS

Extensive periosteal new bone deposits are seen in pachydermo-periostosis (Fig. 150), an idiopathic condition in which the hands and feet are very large. In this respect but in no other it resembles acromegaly. The sella is normal and there is thickening of the skin.

Because the condition is long-standing, the periosteal new bone reaches the cortex, and in some of the bones it may fuse to it so completely as to become cortical thickening.

DEVELOPMENTAL PERIOSTEAL BONE THICKENING

MELORHEOSTOSIS (LERI)

A peculiar increase in the density of the middle third of the shaft of several long bones of one limb only, with irregular wavy deposits of periosteal new bone fused with the cortex, the x-ray appearance of the bone resembling dripping candle wax, will suggest melorheostosis as described by Leri and Joanny (1922). A variant of this appearance is for the cortical bone thickening to be mainly internal and at the expense of the cancellous bone. Both forms are shown in Fig. 125. The condition may be asymptomatic or there may be some pain at times.

The causation of this disease is unknown, but some of the bony outgrowths have cartilaginous caps and it is possible that their formation is analogous to exostoses in these instances.

6—Widespread and Regional Reduction in Bone Density

Written in collaboration with

N. J. Y. Woodhouse

DIAGNOSTIC CRITERIA AND TECHNIQUES

When widespread and severe, a reduction in bone density can be deduced without doubt from the appearances of the bone in a radiograph. When the reduction is less severe, subjective assessment becomes uncertain and therefore strict criteria must be observed in making the x-ray diagnosis, or else special techniques must be used for confirming a reduction in bone mineral content. Some of these techniques are described below.

With all simple radiological methods, a general loss of bone mineral content can be detected only when it is severe and between 30 and 40 per cent of the calcium has been lost. The various methods available are perhaps more useful in revealing progressive loss in serial radiographs than in detecting slight or moderate loss in the initial radiographs. Finally, the loss may be regional, and vertebral compression may occur before any changes can be detected in, for instance, the bones of the hand.

Visual quality of the image

If a bone is absorbing most of the incident radiation, it tends to give a white image in a properly developed radiograph. If only a small proportion is absorbed, there is a relatively grey image compared with the surrounding soft tissues, especially if the kVP used was below 80. A generally grey image of the bones may be an indication of their poor mineral content, or it may be due to purely technical factors producing a radiograph with poor contrast. Overall greyness of the bone images in the presence of severe and widespread loss of density is of little value for diagnosis, since other and more objective criteria for the specific diagnosis will then invariably be present.

Comparative image

Abnormal greyness of the bone image is fairly easy to detect if it is localized and the loss of bone density can thus be compared with the whiter image of nearby bones or, in a limb, with equivalent bones on the opposite side (*see* Fig. 298), but a general greyness throughout the skeleton presents more difficulty in diagnosis. In one technique the patient's hand, for instance, can be radiographed with the same x-ray beam and on the same film as the hand of a normal person placed adjacent to it, as in Fig. 157. Owing to the difficulties of matching the patient with a normal person of similar age, sex and body build and the theoretical dangers of the examination to the normal person, this method is little used.

Using a dried metacarpal bone mounted on a 4 mm. thick block of aluminium or an aluminium step wedge alongside as a control is one alternative, but this, although traditional, rarely gives information of value.

The cortical–cancellous bone index

Another technique is to measure the combined width of the cortex on each side of the second metacarpal at its mid point (Fig. 153) and the total width of the shaft at the same level. The metacarpal index is then calculated:

$$\frac{\text{Combined width of layers of cortex on each side} \times 100}{\text{Total width of shaft}}$$

The normal cortical index in men aged 40–50 years ranges from 55 to 58. Since the mineral content decreases with age, in women more rapidly than in men, the result in any case should be assessed in relation to this factor, which is shown in the graphs prepared from presumed normal persons by Morgan and his colleagues (1967) (Fig. 154*a*) and by Doyle (1966) (Fig. 154*b*).

Accuracy can be increased by measuring the cortical width on a slightly enlarged image using a magnifying glass.

If the cortex appears abnormal in the second metacarpal, the index can be calculated from measurements of the third metacarpal. The humerus is another bone that lends itself to this technique, but no figures for decrease with age are available as yet. The proximal phalanx of the third finger, the mid humerus and the mid femur have also been used to obtain an index.

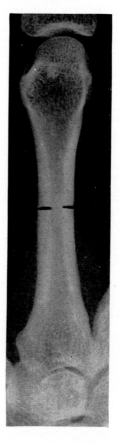

FIG. 153.—Radiograph of second metacarpal of a normal male adult aged 40 years. Anterior view. Lines show how width of cortex is measured.

Light densitometry method

By using a pin-point spotlight and a selenium cell detector and scanning across the mid point of the second metacarpal, the difference in density between the cortical and the cancellous bone can be measured, or the metacarpal index can be calculated as mentioned above.

By means of a similar technique, the density of the mid point of the shaft of the ulna 1 centimetre and 8 centimetres from its distal end can be compared. An increase or loss of bone density in hyperparathyroidism in particular can be detected with some assurance by this method as described by Doyle (1966).

Radiation absorption methods

The quality of the x-ray beam emitted from a conventional x-ray tube is so heterogeneous that the results of absorption of such a beam by a bone are difficult to interpret. However, by using an isotope source of radiation with a monochromatic beam and measuring the incident and emergent beam, the degree of absorption by a piece of bone can be found, and this can be related to the mineral content with considerable accuracy. The patient's hand is immersed in a water bath to give a constant thickness of the soft tissue component.

Such methods are rather too elaborate for routine clinical use.

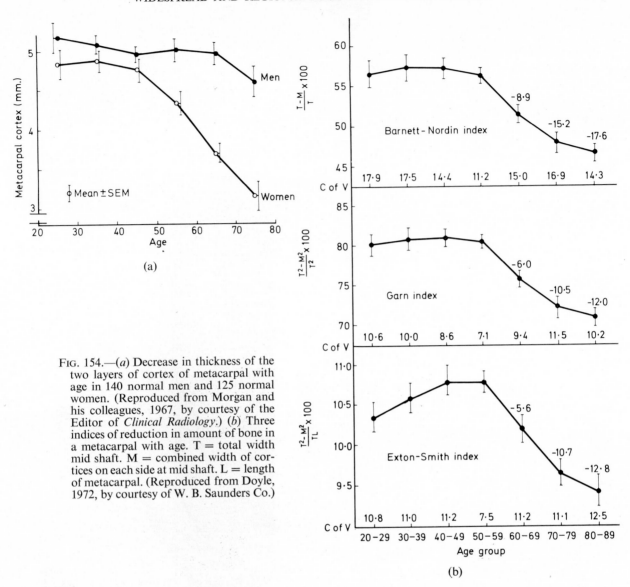

FIG. 154.—(*a*) Decrease in thickness of the two layers of cortex of metacarpal with age in 140 normal men and 125 normal women. (Reproduced from Morgan and his colleagues, 1967, by courtesy of the Editor of *Clinical Radiology*.) (*b*) Three indices of reduction in amount of bone in a metacarpal with age. T = total width mid shaft. M = combined width of cortices on each side at mid shaft. L = length of metacarpal. (Reproduced from Doyle, 1972, by courtesy of W. B. Saunders Co.)

Visual analysis of bone architecture

Somewhat less sensitive for the detection of loss of bone density than densitometry methods is a study of the bone architecture together with the metacarpal cortical index in a borderline case. This method is adequate in some clinical situations when applied to the limb bones. In the vertebral column, particularly in persons over 45 years old, the visibility of the trabecular pattern is very variable, as is the width of the cortex and therefore the cortical–cancellous bone index. Loss of bone density can thus often be inferred only when a vertebral compression fracture or collapse can be seen. Sometimes the vertebral end plates show a relative increase in density and cast a prominent white line shadow, so drawing attention to the poor mineral content of the bone beneath (*see* Fig. 168).

Radiologically, changes in the trabecular pattern due to a loss of bone density are of three types.

(1) The even changes in which all the trabeculae are affected and the pattern is thin and widely spaced (*see* Fig. 157). Since the trabecular pattern varies somewhat from person to person, a slight pathological thinning may be difficult to recognize, but a more marked thinning will be obvious and the trabecular pattern will appear as though sketched with a very fine-pointed pencil. The thinner trabeculae will inevitably look more widely spaced than in a normal pattern, but when the loss of bone density is advanced they may be even more widely spaced, since some trabeculae lose so much mineral that they become invisible (*see* Figs. 157 and 162).

In very severe loss of bone density, the whole trabecular pattern disappears as if erased by a brush and the bone between the still visible cortical layers has a homogeneous grey appearance (*see* Fig. 300). There is nearly always an even thinning of the cortex which gives the appearance of a thinly pencilled outline to the hazy grey interior of the bone. When this degree of extreme mineral loss is present, the bones are exceedingly transradiant, so that where they overlie other structures such as the lungs or abdominal viscera or the thicker muscles they may be quite difficult to see. This state of affairs may even suggest a poor quality radiograph when in fact the fault lies with the bones.

(2) The coarsened pattern in which some trabeculae are so thinned as to be invisible while the remaining ones are widely spaced and broadened by compensatory hypertrophy (Fig. 162).

(3) The patchy change in which small groups of trabeculae here and there lose their mineral content, the bone between them being less affected (*see* Fig. 188).

Somewhat analogous radiological changes may be present in the cortical bone at the same time. For instance, with even trabecular absorption the cortex is often reduced in width to an even thin line (*see* Fig. 300); with a coarsened trabecular pattern the cortex may be split up into a coarse lace-like pattern (*see* Fig. 203*a*); and with patchy trabecular loss the cortex may show similar erosions (*see* Fig. 177).

This distinction between an even loss of bone density (*see* Fig. 157), a coarsened trabecular pattern (*see* Fig. 203) and patchy loss of bone density (*see* Fig. 187) is often very obvious in the radiograph and is frequently of some importance in diagnosis. Such changes may be widespread throughout the skeleton or may be confined to one region or to one group of bones.

WIDESPREAD REDUCTION IN BONE DENSITY

The aim of this section is to describe those diseases and, where possible, the underlying pathophysiological mechanisms which can produce a widespread loss of bone density. A brief account of the physiology of bone and the major calcium-regulating hormones, parathyroid hormone, calcitonin and vitamin D is also included.

It should be remembered that a radiological loss of bone density is common to many diseases and implies a considerable reduction in skeletal mineral content. Furthermore, although the radiological features may provide clues to the underlying disease process, in isolation they are seldom diagnostic.

Normal bone

Bone is a connective tissue the matrix of which consists of collagen fibres set in an amorphous mucopolysaccharide gel or ground substance. Its rigidity is derived from the orderly deposition of crystals of a complex calcium phosphate salt. Two types of bone are seen, cortical and cancellous. Cortical bone is structurally designed to withstand stress and everywhere surrounds cancellous bone. Both types have the same lamellar structure and differ only in their arrangement. Cortical bone is compact and made up in concentric lamellae, each unit being referred to as an osteon. Cancellous bone has a sponge-like morphology, the trabeculae of which are surrounded by marrow spaces. Bone is constantly being destroyed and reformed, a process referred to as remodelling. This occurs at different rates within a single bone and between different bones. Cancellous bone remodels faster than cortical bone, and the vertebrae, ilia and ribs remodel faster than the long bones. This may explain why in some diseases a reduction in bone density is more readily apparent in trabecular than in cortical bone, and more easily seen in the vertebrae and ribs than in the peripheral bones.

Bone cells

Osteoprogenitor cells differentiate into two cell types, the osteoblast and the osteoclast. Osteoblasts are responsible for bone matrix formation and line almost the total surface of bone. During bone matrix mineralization, osteoblasts gradually become surrounded by mineralized bone tissue and are then referred to as osteocytes. These cells are present throughout the bone and are linked to each other and to osteoblasts on the surface of the bone by cytoplasmic processes. They can remove surrounding bone mineral (osteocytic osteolysis) and may form new bone. Osteoclasts are multinucleated, unlike the other bone cells, and are responsible for the removal of mineral and the underlying matrix from the bone surface (osteoclastic resorption). In health these cells are relatively few in number.

Parathyroid hormone

Human parathyroid hormone is a polypeptide with a molecular weight of approximately 9,000. It has not yet been synthesized. Parathyroid hormone secretion is controlled by the ionized serum calcium level; a fall in this level will increase the secretion and a rise will diminish it.

The hormone acts on three major target organs—the bone, the gut and the kidney (Figs. 155 and 156). At the bone level, osteoclastic resorption and osteocytic osteolysis are increased. Bone formation may also increase. Parathyroid hormone has two major actions on the kidney: tubular reabsorption of phosphate is reduced and tubular reabsorption of calcium is increased. Normal subjects whose serum calcium levels are raised artificially to those of patients with hyperparathyroidism will consequently

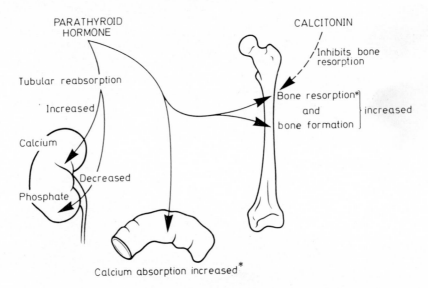

FIG. 155.—Diagram showing action of parathyroid hormone and calcitonin.

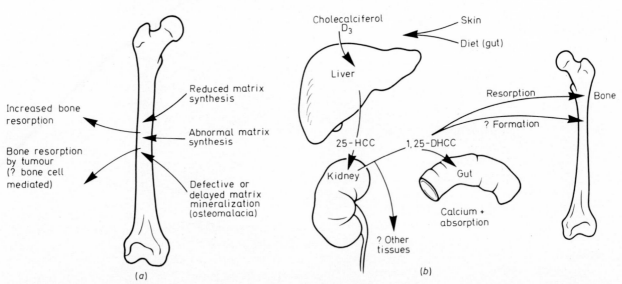

FIG. 156.—(a) A simplified scheme illustrating the mechanisms by which a loss of bone density can occur. In most diseases more than one of these is involved. (b) Diagram illustrating the metabolism of vitamin D₃ in simplified form. The production of the active metabolite 1,25-DHCC is controlled by a complex feedback system involving calcium, parathyroid hormone and calcitonin. 1,25-DHCC promotes bone resorption and intestinal absorption of calcium. There may also be an effect on bone mineralization and on skeletal muscle (*see* page 93).

have a decreased secretion of parathyroid hormone and will therefore excrete a much greater quantity of calcium in the urine. Parathyroid hormone also stimulates the intestinal absorption of calcium and phosphate. All these actions are reversed in hypoparathyroidism.

It may now be seen that there are three mechanisms which produce hypercalcaemia in primary hyperparathyroidism: (1) increased tubular reabsorption of calcium by the kidney; (2) increased intestinal absorption of calcium; and (3) increased removal of calcium from bone. The last effect will contribute to the hypercalcaemia only when there is a relative reduction in the rate of bone formation.

Calcitonin

This polypeptide hormone has a molecular weight of 3,500 and is produced by the "C" cells which, in man, are found in the thyroid and sometimes in the parathyroid glands and thymus. Its secretion is also controlled by the serum calcium level, a rise in the latter increasing and a fall reducing calcitonin secretion, the opposite to the case with parathyroid hormone. Calcitonin assays are available, but these are not yet sensitive enough to measure normal blood levels. Nevertheless, there is good indirect evidence that calcitonin circulates normally in man.

The major target organ is bone, calcitonin inhibiting osteoclastic bone resorption. This hormone is probably important in regulating the differentiation of osteoprogenitor cells and thus controlling the normal bone remodelling process. It may also serve to protect the bone in hyperparathyroidism and during pregnancy. Human calcitonin has been synthesized, and its long-term administration will produce a progressive and sustained reduction of bone turnover in some patients with Paget's disease, with relief of bone pain and radiological healing of bone.

Vitamin D

Cholecalciferol or native vitamin D_3 is probably inert, and further transformation to one or more active metabolites is required for biological activity. Some of the metabolic pathways are illustrated diagrammatically in Fig. 156b.

Cholecalciferol, synthesized by the skin or absorbed by the gut, is converted by the liver to 25-hydroxycholecalciferol (25-HCC) and hydroxylated further by the kidney to 1,25-dihydroxycholecalciferol (1,25-DHCC). This is the most active metabolite yet discovered, and its secretion is regulated by the serum and probably the intracellular calcium level. When this level falls, the conversion of 25-HCC to 1,25-DHCC is enhanced. Conversely, when the serum (or cell) calcium rises, the secretion of 1,25-DHCC is reduced. The major target organs for 1,25-DHCC appear to be gut and bone, although other tissues such as striated muscle may also be important. The metabolite rapidly induces intestinal calcium transport and stimulates bone resorption, and there is some evidence that vitamin D is responsible for the initiation of normal bone mineralization as well (see page 104). The secretion of 1,25-DHCC by the kidney and its accumulation in target tissues now means that this substance should be regarded as a calcium metabolite.

Interrelationship between parathyroid hormone, calcitonin and 1,25-DHCC

The secretion of all three hormones is regulated by the level of ionized calcium. Hypocalcaemia induces a rise in circulating parathyroid hormone and 1,25-DHCC levels and a fall in calcitonin levels. This results in an increased rate of bone resorption, intestinal absorption and tubular reabsorption of calcium, with a consequent rise in serum calcium. Hypercalcaemia has the opposite effect: calcitonin levels rise, and parathyroid hormone and 1,25-DHCC levels fall. Bone resorption is inhibited, less calcium is absorbed, and tubular reabsorption of calcium is diminished. It should be noted that the bone and gut actions of parathyroid hormone require the presence of 1,25-DHCC.

Recently a direct link between these hormones has been demonstrated. In the absence of a change in serum calcium, calcitonin enhances the conversion of 25-HCC to 1,25-DHCC. Parathyroid hormone has the opposite effect and inhibits the production of 1,25-DHCC when the serum calcium is elevated. This observation might explain the occurrence of osteomalacia in primary hyperparathyroidism, as both the serum calcium and the parathyroid hormone levels are high and presumably 1,25-DHCC production is low (see page 106).

MECHANISMS LEADING TO REDUCTION IN BONE DENSITY

The relevant pathophysiological events are shown in Fig. 156a. A reduction in bone density will occur when the rate of bone removal exceeds that of formation, that is, when more calcium leaves bone than goes in.

Bone formation is determined by (1) the ability to synthesize normal matrix and (2) the effectiveness of matrix mineralization. Mineralization can be normal when the rate of matrix synthesis is reduced, or, conversely, defective or delayed when matrix formation is normal. Alone or in combination, either situation will result in a reduced bone density even if the rate of bone removal is not increased. When abnormal matrix is synthesized, bone mineralization is defective.

DISEASES CAUSING WIDESPREAD REDUCTION IN BONE DENSITY

The diseases causing a widespread reduction in bone density are listed below.

Osteoporosis

Endocrine disorders

Cushing's syndrome
Thyrotoxicosis
Hypogonadism

Dietary deficiencies

Famine
Vitamin C deficiency
Calcium deprivation

Drug-induced osteoporosis

Steroids
Heparin

Metabolic osteoporosis

Homocystinuria
Mucopolysaccharidoses

Idiopathic osteoporosis

Under 65 years of age
Over 65 years of age

Marrow diseases

Childhood leukaemia
Histiocytosis (Gaucher's disease)
Neoplastic disease (myelomatosis, lymphosarcoma, anaplastic carcinoma secondaries)

Osteomalacia

Nutritional vitamin D deficiency
Malabsorption of vitamin D
Disturbed vitamin D metabolism

Rare causes

Phosphorus deficiency; familial or acquired hypophosphataemia
Hypophosphatasia
Fibrogenesis imperfecta ossium
Renal tubular acidosis
Uretero-colic anastomosis

Hyperparathyroidism

Primary hyperparathyroidism
Secondary hyperparathyroidism

In most diseases associated with an increase in the rate of bone removal (osteoclastic resorption and osteocytic osteolysis) there is a compensatory increase in the rate of bone formation. In Paget's disease or acromegaly the latter may be adequate to prevent net loss of bone, but in other diseases this is not usually the case.

These mechanisms are discussed more fully under the individual disease headings.

OSTEOPOROSIS

Osteoporosis can be defined as a reduction in the amount of normally mineralized bone. It may occur in various situations as discussed below, and these should be excluded before a patient is labelled as having "idiopathic" osteoporosis.

Endocrine disorders

Cushing's syndrome

Cushing's syndrome may be diagnosed from the clinical and biochemical findings. The former include adiposity (though this is not invariable), a moon-shaped face, skin striae, hypertension and, in women, hirsutism and amenorrhoea.

In approximately 30 per cent of such patients there will be evidence of bone disease in the radiographs. There may be fractures (compression collapse) of one or more vertebrae or multiple rib fractures. In severe cases, the decrease in bone density may be so great that the shadows of the vertebrae are difficult to see and the trabecular pattern is absent even in a young adult (Fig. 158). In some cases the callus round a uniting fractured rib may be more conspicuous than the undermineralized rib which it surrounds and can be mistaken for an intrapulmonary lesion. Similar changes in several scattered ribs may be mistaken for multiple intrapulmonary secondary deposits.

In the early stages of Cushing's syndrome the visible bone lesions may be limited to the vertebral column. In the later stages there may be thinning of the cortex and trabecular thinning and loss throughout most of the skeleton, including the bones of the hands. A fifth of all clinical cases have features indicating a pituitary tumour, and a radiograph of the sella is therefore indicated as a routine.

The bone disease results from impaired matrix synthesis and probably excessive resorption as well. Thinning of the skin points to a general disturbance of collagen metabolism.

Most cases of Cushing's syndrome are due to increased ACTH secretion by the pituitary. The remainder are associated with ectopic ACTH production by a neoplasm in some other site or with an adrenal adenoma or carcinoma. In some patients a radiological examination of the suprarenal regions is therefore indicated to exclude a tumour of this gland. On the whole an aortogram is more reliable than the outlining of the glands by gas after a pre-sacral injection. Hyperplasia or a small tumour may pass undetected by either method.

Thyrotoxicosis

Usually thyrotoxicosis is promptly diagnosed and treated and osteoporosis is consequently uncommon. In subclinical cases, however, a considerable reduction in bone density may occur before the condition is recognized and treated. The decreased bone density is due to an increased rate of bone resorption produced by elevated thyroxine and tri-iodothyronine levels. Bone formation also increases but fails to keep pace with resorption, and bone loss occurs. There is widespread and even thinning of the trabeculae and cortical bone, and unlike most other forms of osteoporosis, the peripheral skeleton is involved early in the disease and vertebral compression is less common. The reason for this is not clear.

Hypogonadism

Low or absent circulating levels of androgen or oestrogen occur with pituitary gonadotrophin deficiency and bilateral disease of the gonads. In young persons, sexual development is retarded and epiphyseal closure delayed (see Fig. 64). When hypogonadism is acquired in adult life, regression of the secondary sex characters is seen and skin thickness decreases. The osteoporosis is due to a reduction in bone matrix synthesis and possibly to an increase in the rate of bone resorption. In adults the axial skeleton is predominantly involved and there may be vertebral body compression.

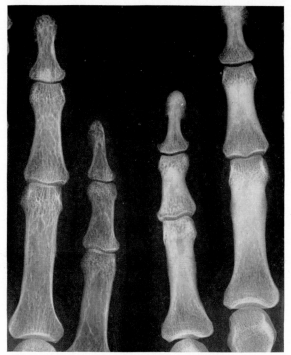

FIG. 157

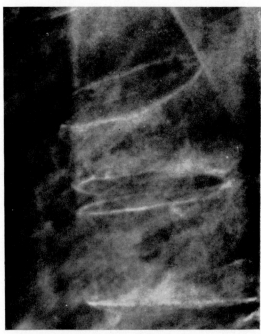

FIG. 158

FIG. 157.—Osteomalacia. Female aged 30 years. Widespread loss of bone density. Widely spaced and thin trabecular pattern. Thin cortex. (Control of same age on right.) Steatorrhoea many years.

FIG. 158.—Cushing's syndrome with spinal osteoporosis. Female aged 25 years. Even loss of density of lower thoracic vertebrae with even and wedge-shaped collapse. Normal disc spaces in some areas, biconcave indentation into vertebral bodies in other areas (*see* bottom of Fig.). Hands and skull normal. Amenorrhoea, adiposity, skin rash on face, thirst and polyuria. One suprarenal removed. Periods returned, all symptoms lost.

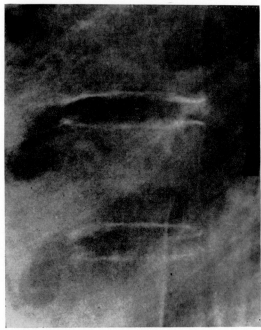

FIG. 159

FIG. 160

FIG. 159.—Rheumatoid arthritis. Male aged 53. Lateral view of dorsal spine before steroid therapy. No vertebral collapse.

FIG. 160.—Steroid therapy. Same patient as Fig. 159 six months after prednisolone 15 mg. 8-hourly. Collapse D. 7 and trabecular loss D. 8.

Treatment

Successful treatment of these endocrine diseases is associated with an increase in bone mineral content. The degree of improvement is greatest when the skeleton has a capacity for further growth as in children and young adults, and is less obvious with advancing age.

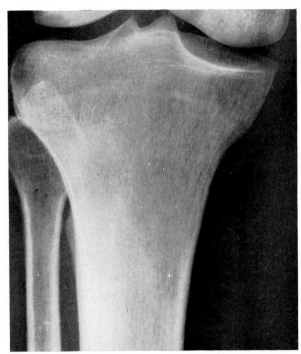

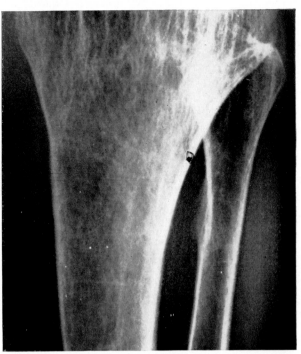

FIG. 161.—Senile osteoporosis. Male aged 86 years. Some trabecular loss with thinning of the trabeculae still seen.

FIG. 162.—Osteomalacia. Female aged 42 years. Even trabecular loss, middle third tibia; compensatory thickening with coarse striate pattern at upper end. Thin cortex. Other bones the same. Steatorrhoea of unknown cause (probable gluten metabolic defect). Bulky yellow stools.

Dietary deficiencies

Famine

Famine conditions involve multiple deficiencies including protein, carbohydrate, fat, minerals and vitamins. In this situation a reduction in bone density may result from a combination of reduced matrix synthesis, mineralization and excessive resorption.

Vitamin C deficiency

A deficiency of vitamin C may occur in isolation and cause impaired bone matrix synthesis. In children the trabeculae throughout the shaft and in the epiphyseal nuclei are thin and indistinct, those in the submetaphyseal region being particularly affected and often forming a transradiant band across the bone (see Fig. 83). The cortex is often thin, but the metaphyseal white line is never thinned and may even be wider than normal. A periosteal shadow from a subperiosteal haemorrhage is common (see Fig. 144).

Calcium deprivation

In the experimental animal, dietary calcium deprivation causes osteoporosis as the rate of bone resorption exceeds that of bone formation. If this ever occurs in man, it must be uncommon, since the South African Bantu have apparently normal skeletons with dietary calcium intakes of 200 mg. a day compared with a daily intake of 600–1,000 mg. in Western Europe.

Drug-induced osteoporosis

Steroids

The bone changes resulting from an excess of steroids given for therapeutic reasons are identical with those seen in Cushing's syndrome (*see* above) except that avascular necrosis of the femoral head (*see* Fig. 131) seems to be more common. Compression collapse of one or more vertebral bodies is often the first radiological abnormality to be seen (*see* Fig. 160). In other cases an apparently spontaneous fracture of one or more ribs—often a mid rib in the axillary region—may be the only abnormality visible. Sometimes several ribs are fractured, but without radiological evidence of a loss of bone density. Bone changes are not usually seen unless therapy has been given for at least 6–12 months and the dosage has been maintained at a relatively high level. In elderly patients it may be difficult to determine whether vertebral compression is due to age, to the disease for which the steroids are being given, or to the steroid therapy itself. It is therefore useful before embarking on long-term, relatively high dosage steroid therapy to take an initial lateral view radiograph of the lower half of the dorsal spine (*see* Fig. 159).

Heparin

Treatment with heparin in some way results in structural damage to collagen, and if given for long periods may produce osteoporosis.

Metabolic osteoporosis

Homocystinuria

Homocystinuria may result in a loss of bone density. McKusick (1966) considers that it may affect the metabolism of mucopolysaccharide and thus bone matrix synthesis. The deficiency of bone mineral may be very gross and all the vertebrae may show compression collapse (Fig. 163). The vertebral bodies are enlarged antero-posteriorly.

Mucopolysaccharidoses

Chondro-osteodystrophy, Hunter–Hurler syndrome (*see* pages 40 and 41).

Idiopathic osteoporosis

Albright and Reifenstein (1948) defined osteoporosis as "too little bone, but what there is, is normal", and suggested that the disorder resulted from a failure of bone matrix synthesis. Although having the merit of simplicity, this definition has two drawbacks. First, it implies that osteoporosis has a single cause when in fact there may be several, and secondly, "too little bone" is not quantitatively defined. For the purpose of this section it may be simpler to think of osteoporosis in clinical terms, that is, as the occurrence of vertebral or other fractures, the specific morbid event being the fracture. When other causes of osteoporosis have been excluded, such patients may be divided arbitrarily into two groups, (1) those under 65 and (2) those over 65 years of age, the latter group being referred to by Albright as "senile osteoporosis".

Osteoporosis of unknown cause in persons under 65 years of age

This group includes juvenile, post-pregnancy and post-menopausal osteoporosis. The presence of compression of some of the vertebral bodies may be the predominant radiographic finding (*see also* page 113). In some cases the whole skeleton is involved.

The occurrence of vertebral compression (fractures) and loss of bone density is clearly abnormal in young persons. An endocrine disorder is postulated in juvenile osteoporosis, as the disease usually remits during puberty. In some young male patients and some females in the post-menopausal group there is histological evidence suggesting the presence of hyperparathyroidism, but the basic abnormality in these variants of idiopathic osteoporosis is as yet unknown.

Osteoporosis of unknown cause in patients over 65 years old (senile osteoporosis)

Whereas the presence of vertebral compression fractures and a loss of bone density is clearly abnormal in young persons, in older persons these appearances may be just due to their age. In the words of Adams, Davies and Sweetnam (1970), "the main difficulty lies in finding diagnostic criteria which will

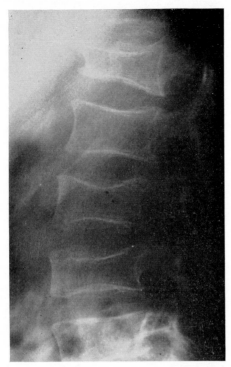

Fig. 163.—Homocystinuria. Male aged 12 years. Lumbar vertebrae flattened. End plates relatively dense. Lens dislocation. Plasma methionine twice normal. Plasma homocystine 2·8–3·1 mg. per 100 ml.

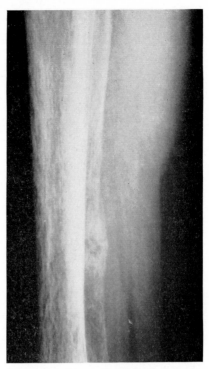

Fig. 164.—Hypophosphatasia of tibia and fibula. Female aged 53 years. Cortex indistinct with vertical linear pattern. Trabeculae widened and widely spaced. Transradiant Looser zone across fibula. Serum alkaline phosphatase 3 K.A. units; Ca. 9·7 mg. per cent; P. 4·8 mg. per cent.

afford a means of separating out patients with osteoporosis from normal persons of the same age. In the case of senile osteoporosis none may exist".

Diagnostic difficulties apart, there are a fairly large number of old people with compression fractures of several vertebrae not due to trauma. How might these have occurred? After a certain age all persons begin to lose bone, and women start to lose bone somewhat younger than men. If a person initially had too little bone, a normal rate of bone loss as they grew older might produce osteoporosis. However, measurement of the mineral content of peripheral bone does not separate normal women from women with unexplained vertebral compression fractures. It has therefore been suggested that the fault may lie in (1) the axial skeleton having too little bone to begin with; (2) a selective loss of bone from the vertebrae; or (3) a normal amount of bone with reduced strength (Doyle, 1972).

Gonadectomy in women increases bone resorption, possibly by increasing the sensitivity of the osteoclast to parathyroid hormone. By increasing bone resorption and diminishing bone formation, oestrogen withdrawal may thus be an important factor in the genesis of osteoporosis in patients with "too little bone to begin with". A further important factor is muscular development. Bone and muscle mass correlate well, and the incidence of hip fractures in the elderly is lower in those countries where hard physical work is common than in more "developed" western societies. The pathogenesis of "senile osteoporosis" is clearly complex and at present is poorly understood.

Whatever the cause, there is eventually an even thinning of the trabeculae and the cortex (*see* Fig. 161). In many regions the trabecular pattern may disappear completely, while in others a few thin trabeculae may still be seen. All the bones tend to be affected to much the same extent except in some cases where the spine is more affected (*see* section on spinal osteoporosis, page 113).

The progression of the changes is slow, usually extending over many years. In the skull the dorsum sellae is often less dense than the surrounding bone, so that the appearances may be confused with a similar loss of density sometimes occurring in response to a raised intracranial pressure. However, in old age the cortical line or lamina dura lining the floor and clinoid processes is always intact, while in raised intracranial pressure and in some cases of hypertension it may be eroded.

Osteoporosis in marrow diseases

Childhood leukaemia

A widespread loss of bone density is sometimes seen in children with leukaemia. Usually the diagnosis will be established from the clinical and laboratory investigations, but in rare instances the peripheral blood film is normal, the radiological features resemble those of juvenile idiopathic osteoporosis, and the diagnosis can be made only on examination of a bone marrow smear. The whole skeleton may be affected, including even the bones of the hands and feet. In the vertebral column the absence of trabeculae may be noticed and may stand out clearly against the dense white lines of the end plates. Compression collapse may occur (Fig. 168), and if this involves only one vertebral body, the appearances may be mistaken for those of tuberculosis, although the disc space will not be narrowed. In some cases the presenting symptom is backache, and a radiograph taken to investigate the cause of this may give valuable evidence which will lead to the diagnosis.

In the long bones there is often a submetaphyseal transradiant zone (Fig. 167) which is similar to that seen in scurvy (*see* Fig. 83). As in scurvy, it may extend across the cortex to give a "corner sign" just below the metaphysis (Fig. 166).

In some cases there is a small linear shadow of periosteal new bone which may be due either to a minor trauma with subperiosteal haemorrhage or to subperiosteal deposits of leukaemic cells. Sometimes the loss of bone density is patchy (*see* pages 109 and 113).

Histiocytosis (Gaucher's disease)

A very even trabecular absorption with cortical thinning is seen in the long bones in Gaucher's disease (Fig. 169). In addition there is a flask-shaped expansion of the ends of the major long bones, particularly of the lower third of the femora (*see* page 16 and Fig. 169). In some cases localized cyst-like transradiant areas may also be visible (*see* page 133 and Fig. 223).

In most instances, radiographs of the major long bones are taken because the condition is suspected clinically. An enlarged spleen is found either during routine clinical examination or because the patient complained of swelling of the stomach. There may be pigmentation and eye changes (pingueculae), and the diagnosis is usually confirmed by the finding of Gaucher cells on histological examination of the marrow or spleen after marrow biopsy or splenectomy. These Gaucher cells are large with darkly staining nuclei and an abundant hyaline or reticulated cytoplasm containing the lipoid cerebroside. The accumulation of these cells causes bone resorption.

Neoplastic disease

Diffuse loss of bone density, although uncommon with tumours, may be seen in multiple myelomatosis, lymphosarcoma or diffuse secondary deposits from an anaplastic carcinoma infiltrating the bone. One mechanism for the reduced density is increased bone resorption by osteoclasts which are stimulated in some way by the tumour cells. Compensatory new bone formation is unusual, and bone mineral loss may be rapid. When the amount of calcium liberated by the bone exceeds the capacity of the kidneys to excrete it, hypercalcaemia and a rising blood urea rapidly follow.

OSTEOMALACIA

Osteomalacia is a disorder of bone as a tissue in which newly formed bone matrix fails to mineralize normally and promptly. Although several diseases cause osteomalacia, three major factors seem to be important in its development: (1) the absence of vitamin D or one of its metabolites; (2) low serum phosphate levels; and (3) the production of abnormal bone matrix.

The development of a mineralization defect is reflected by a progressive accumulation of unmineralized bone matrix or osteoid which results in an increase in both the extent and the thickness of the osteoid surface covering the bone. The ability to cut thin undercalcified bone sections and the use of quantitative histological techniques have allowed progressively earlier diagnosis of this disorder.

The commonest cause of osteomalacia is vitamin D "deficiency", which may occur in three situations.

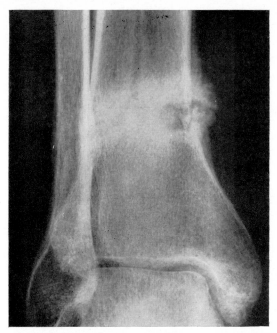

FIG. 165.—Possible stress fracture simulating Looser zone in Paget's disease. Male aged 64 years. Fracture line, sclerosis around, and some periosteal new bone; 18 months some local pain. Other bones showed typical Paget's disease. Serum alkaline phosphatase 15 K.A. units. Pain-free after short period of rest.

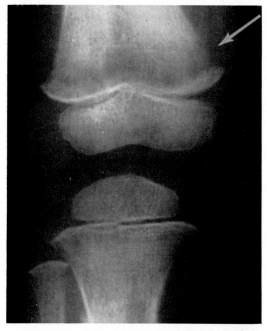

FIG. 166.—Leukaemia. Female aged 2 years. Sub-metaphyseal transradiant line of decalcification in femur and tibia, extending across cortex opposite arrow to give "corner sign". Periosteal shadow on tibia. Bleeding from gums and lumps on skin; biopsy of one of these showed leukaemic deposit. W.b.c. 110,000 per c.mm. (85 per cent blast cells).

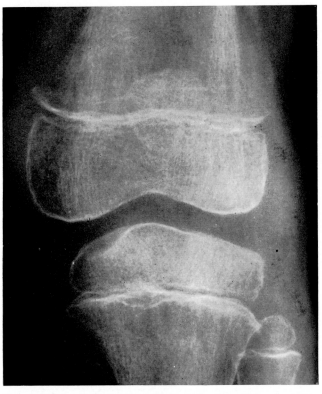

FIG. 167.—Leukaemia. Female aged 5 years. Extensive even trabecular loss in the tibia and femur extending up from the metaphyses for several centimetres. "Corner sign", medial side of femur. Marrow biopsy showed leukaemia with 70 per cent nucleated lymphoblastic cells.

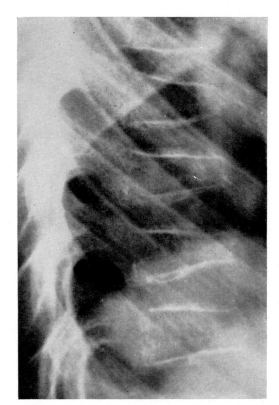

FIG. 168.—Leukaemia. Same patient as in Fig. 167. Even spinal loss of density of vertebral bodies except for end plates, giving a pencilled outline to the bones. Compression collapse of D. 10. Disc spaces wide. Radiographed for backache. Considered possible tuberculosis. E.S.R. 85 mm.; w.b.c. 5,000 per c.mm. Marrow biopsy showed leukaemia.

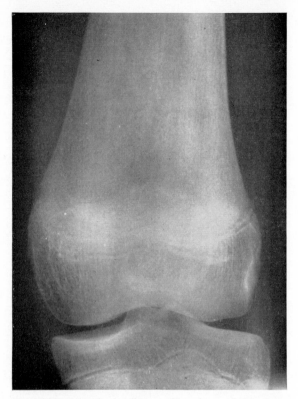

FIG. 169.—Gaucher's disease. Female aged 18 years. Thin cortex and fine trabeculae with ground-glass appearance and flask-like shape of lower end of femur. All major long bones both sides. Weakness, anaemia, and large spleen. Splenectomy. Gaucher cells found. Keratin at fault in reticulum cells.

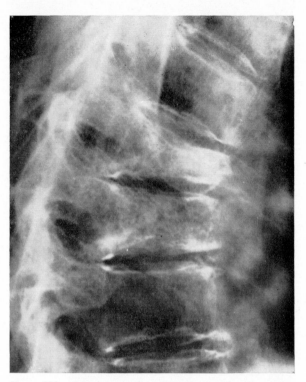

FIG. 170.—Myelomatosis. Female aged 59 years. Wedge-shaped collapse D. 7. Mottled erosion D. 8. Even loss of density D. 6 and 9. Backache some months, treated as spinal osteoporosis. E.S.R. 100 mm. Multiple small erosions of vault of skull, mandible and femora suggested diagnosis which was confirmed by sternal marrow biopsy.

Nutritional vitamin D deficiency

This is seen most often in countries such as England where there is little exposure to sunlight and a low dietary intake of vitamin D. It may also occur in hot climates where thick clothing excludes ultra-violet light. In America, vitamin D deficiency is uncommon as many foodstuffs including milk are fortified. In England, contrary to popular belief, milk is a poor source of this vitamin.

Malabsorption of vitamin D

Vitamin D is fat soluble and therefore diseases of the small bowel, pancreas or biliary tract which produce steatorrhoea may all cause osteomalacia. The list is extensive, but the more common causes include coeliac, Crohn's and Whipple's diseases, intestinal lymphangiectasia, tropical sprue, diverticulae of the small bowel, chronic pancreatitis, fibrocystic disease of the pancreas, and any cause of chronic biliary obstruction. Osteomalacia also occurs following gastrectomy, short-circuiting procedures, or the removal of large portions of the small intestine.

Disturbed vitamin D metabolism

Chronic renal failure—Chronic renal failure is associated with malabsorption of calcium and phosphorus and the development of secondary hyperparathyroidism and osteomalacia (*see* pages 44 and 46). Large doses of vitamin D_3 or very small doses of 1,25-DHCC correct the absorption defect and the serum calcium and phosphorus levels rise. The osteomalacia is also cured, but it is uncertain whether this results from a direct effect of 1,25-DHCC on bone mineralization or is merely due to the associated changes in serum calcium and phosphate levels.

It seems likely that renal failure is associated with a falling secretion rate of 1,25-DHCC due either to a progressive loss of renal tissue or to inhibition of 25-HCC hydroxylation to 1,25-DHCC.

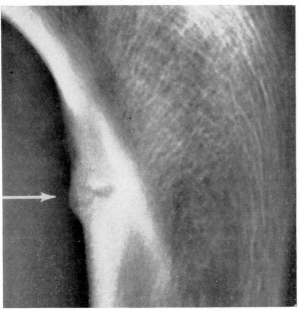

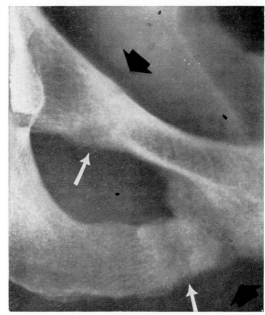

Fig. 171

Fig. 172

FIG. 171.—Osteomalacia with Looser zone. Female aged 37 years. Horizontal hair-line transradiant zone 1 cm. long across cortex in region of lesser trochanter (opposite arrow). Some pain in right thigh. Renal calcifications. Alkali reserve 36 vols. per cent; phosphates 2·3 mg. per cent; alkaline phosphatase and blood urea normal.

FIG. 172.—Osteomalacia—Looser zone pubis and ischium. Female aged 58 years. Linear transradiant zone across pubic bone and ischium (opposite arrows). Pain symphyseal region. Ca. 9·3 mg. per cent; P. 2·6 mg. per cent. Serum alkaline phosphatase 28 K.A. units. Barium meal: deficiency pattern and dilated coils, small intestine.

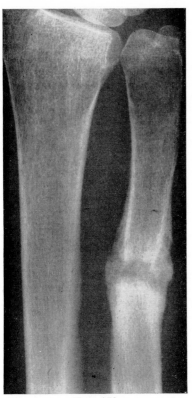

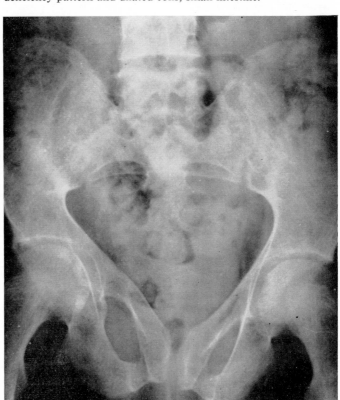

Fig. 173

Fig. 174

FIG. 173.—Osteomalacia. Female aged 65 years. Looser zone 5 mm. wide across ulna. Trabecular pattern thin, cortex thin. Renal tubular phosphate leak. Spine appeared normal.

FIG. 174.—Renal osteodystrophy; osteomalacia; pelvis which is triradiate in shape from softening. Female aged 28 years. Polycystic kidneys. Blood urea 120 mg. per cent; Ca. 8·7 mg. per cent; P. 6·2 mg per cent. Secondary hyper-parathyroidism

Effect of drugs—Phenobarbitone taken over long periods, for instance in the treatment of epilepsy, may produce osteomalacia. The mechanism by which the drug causes osteomalacia is unclear, but may be related to the increased secretion of vitamin D and its metabolites in the bile.

Radiographic appearances of vitamin D deficient osteomalacia

Osteomalacia in children (rickets) is described on page 44. In osteomalacia in adults, there may be no radiographic abnormalities even when there is histological confirmation of the condition.

The earliest evidence of a reduction in bone density is trabecular and cortical bone thinning, which becomes more obvious in advanced cases (*see* Fig. 157). It is more readily seen in the peripheral skeleton, but may be indistinguishable from the osteoporosis produced by other diseases. The diagnostic feature of vitamin D "deficiency" osteomalacia in patients with a widespread loss of bone density is the presence of subperiosteal cortical bone erosions (*see* section on secondary hyperparathyroidism, page 106). Erosions are best seen in the middle phalanges in hand radiographs. They are usually more severe in chronic renal failure than in nutritional deficiency or malabsorption of vitamin D, and are indistinguishable from the erosions of primary hyperparathyroidism.

Chronic renal failure as the cause of osteomalacia is suggested when the bone changes of hyperparathyroidism are very obvious, including in many cases vertebral end plate sclerosis (*see* Fig. 180), sometimes referred to as rugger jersey spine; some submetaphyseal sclerosis of long bones; or the presence of soft tissue or vessel calcification (*see* Figs. 333, 334 and 338). The presence of renal calcification suggests that the renal failure may have been caused by primary hyperparathyroidism.

The osteomalacia of primary hyperparathyroidism may be due to a secondary vitamin D deficiency (*see* page 106).

In severe osteomalacia, softening of bone occurs which may lead to pelvic deformity (Fig. 174) and occasionally to vertebral collapse, bowing of the tibiae, and single or multiple rib fractures. Looser's zones may also be seen.

Looser zones

Looser zones are diagnostic of osteomalacia and not specific to the D deficiency states. They are seen as 1–3 mm. wide transradiant zones extending approximately 1 cm. into the underlying bone at right angles to the cortex, and look like incomplete fractures (Fig. 171). They occur in the ischio-pubic rami (Fig. 172), the axillary borders of the scapulae, the ribs, the femoral necks, the upper third of the femoral shafts and humeri, and the lower third of the tibiae and fibulae. Occasionally they may be seen in the ulna (Fig. 173) and may extend right across the bone. When the metatarsals are involved, the appearances may be those of a stress fracture. Looser zones are frequently bilateral and symmetrical and rarely occur in the absence of an obvious reduction in bone density, although the case shown in Fig. 171 is an exception.

The loss of bone density in osteomalacia due to the vitamin D "deficiency" states is caused by defective mineralization of bone matrix and, while any 1,25-DHCC is present, to continuing and excessive resorption of old bone. It is not yet known whether the mineralization defect arises as a direct consequence of the 1,25-DHCC deficiency or is secondary to the associated changes in serum calcium and phosphate levels. The former suggestion is probably correct, as vitamin D "deficiency" osteomalacia may be seen histologically when there is no obvious serum calcium or phosphorus abnormality. However, a low serum phosphate level will further reduce bone mineralization, since experimentally phosphorus deprivation can produce osteomalacia in the absence of vitamin D deficiency.

Rare causes of osteomalacia

Phosphorus deficiency

Phosphorus deficiency may rarely occur in patients taking purgatives over many years, or it may be due to diminished renal tubular reabsorption of phosphorus as in familial or acquired hypophosphataemia. The low serum phosphate level is probably responsible for the bone mineralization defect. In addition, the function of osteoblasts and other cells may be impaired.

In hypophosphataemia the serum calcium levels are not reduced, secondary hyperparathyroidism does not occur, and subperiosteal cortical bone erosions are not seen.

Hypophosphatasia

Hypophosphatasia is a rare disorder which may be hereditary or acquired and can produce severe osteomalacia (*see* Fig. 164). The cortex is incompletely mineralized and shows a vertical linear pattern with vertical transradiant zones. The trabeculae are thin and few and a Looser zone may be seen. There is one across the fibula in Fig. 164. In this patient the width of the cortex of the second metacarpal was only 2·5 mm. (normal at her age 4 mm.) and the metacarpal index was only 0·3 (normal 0·55). The diagnostic feature of hypophosphatasia is a low serum alkaline phosphatase level. Secondary hyper-parathyroidism does not occur, and therefore no subperiosteal cortical bone erosions are seen.

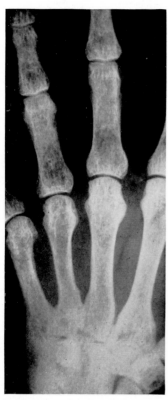

FIG. 175.—Fibrogenesis imperfecta ossium. Male aged 59 years. Hand bones show thin cortex and widely spaced trabeculae. Histological proof. Improved on vitamin D_2.

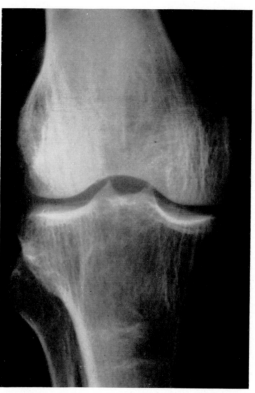

FIG. 176.—Same case as in Fig. 175. Tibia shows widened and widely spaced vertical trabeculae. Cortex normal. Spontaneous fractures which united.

Fibrogenesis imperfecta ossium

Fibrogenesis imperfecta ossium is another rare heritable enzyme defect and was described by Baker and his colleagues (1966). The radiographs show gross thinning of the cortex and widely spaced and thickened trabeculae (Figs. 175 and 176). The distal limb bones tend to be most affected, while the cortex of the major long bones may appear quite normal and the skull is normal.

The underlying abnormality appears to be the production of abnormal bone matrix which fails to mineralize normally. Serum calcium and phosphorus levels are normal and no subperiosteal cortical bone erosions are seen.

Renal tubular acidosis and uretero-colic anastomosis

The precise cause of the osteomalacia in these two conditions is uncertain. In renal tubular acidosis it may be due in part to the lowered serum phosphate level or to a disturbance in vitamin D metabolism. There may be nephrocalcinosis. In some cases correction of the acidosis alone has resulted in healing of the bones, but usually vitamin D is required as well.

In uretero-colic anastomosis, as in chronic renal failure, there is probably a deficiency of 1,25-DHCC. In both conditions, secondary hyperparathyroidism occurs and subperiosteal cortical erosions may be seen.

COARSENED TRABECULAR PATTERN ASSOCIATED WITH DECREASE IN BONE DENSITY

A coarsened trabecular pattern is produced when some of the trabeculae become demineralized and thus invisible in the radiograph, while the remaining ones are widely spaced and stand out more clearly against the relatively transradiant background or are actually thickened in compensation for those lost.

HYPERPARATHYROIDISM

Primary hyperparathyroidism

Hyperparathyroidism exists when there is a sustained and inappropriate high secretion rate of parathyroid hormone in relation to the level of serum calcium. This results in (1) hyperabsorption of calcium by the gut; (2) increased renal tubular reabsorption of calcium and diminished tubular re-absorption of phosphate by the kidney; (3) increased bone resorption and probably bone formation as well. The resulting increase in bone resorption will contribute to the hypercalcaemia only if there is a relative decrease in bone formation—that is, when the matrix synthesis is reduced or its mineralization is delayed or defective. The hypercalcaemia of hyperparathyroidism is thus multifactorial and not due solely to a relative increase in bone resorption.

Radiological appearances

Many patients with hyperparathyroidism have no radiologically detectable bone disease. With higher rates of parathyroid hormone secretion bone abnormalities become visible. These include a coarsened trabecular pattern, usually in association with phalangeal subperiosteal cortical erosions, cyst-like transradiant areas in other bones, and sometimes an obvious widespread reduction in bone density.

Nephrocalcinosis and calculi occur more frequently when there are no abnormalities in the bones in the radiographs. Some patients, particularly young ones, develop sclerosis in the submetaphyseal regions of the bones. Vertebral end plate sclerosis is usually seen only when renal failure is present. At this stage soft tissue, joint cartilage (*see* Fig. 334), pancreatic, vascular and renal calcification may be seen.

Most patients, even those without radiological evidence of bone disease, have histological abnormalities which include an excess of unmineralized bone or osteoid. Although this excess might represent an increase in bone formation, there is some evidence to suggest that these patients are vitamin D deficient. The administration of small doses of vitamin D to patients with primary hyperparathyroidism promotes mineralization of osteoid. In one patient with severe osteitis fibrosa who was similarly treated, healing of the phalangeal erosions occurred (*see* Fig. 204). One mechanism for the development of osteomalacia might be inhibition of 1,25-DHCC production by the high serum calcium and parathyroid hormone levels. Whatever the mechanisms leading to the development of the mineralization defect, its presence has certain practical implications, as pre-operative healing of the bone with vitamin D alone or in addition to phosphate supplements will prevent prolonged post-operative hypocalcaemia in patients with extensive bone disease. These findings are of theoretical importance also, as they imply that bone loss in hyperparathyroidism may be due to defective mineralization and not to the excessive resorption of bone *per se*.

In the absence of a mineralization defect, therefore, subperiosteal cortical bone erosions would probably not occur, and patients with hyperparathyroidism would have a skeleton with a high rate of bone remodelling similar to that seen in early and widespread Paget's disease.

Secondary hyperparathyroidism

Vitamin D "deficiency", whether due to nutritional lack, to malabsorption or to chronic renal failure (*see* page 102), is the commonest cause of secondary hyperparathyroidism. In all these situations there are presumably varying degrees of 1,25-DHCC deficiency. This results in malabsorption of calcium and a lowering of the serum calcium level. Parathyroid hormone secretion is thus increased in an attempt

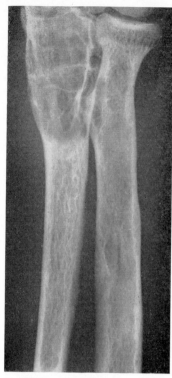

Fig. 177.—Hyperparathyroidism. Male aged 25 years. Coarse trabecular pattern ulna below cystic area. Same case as Fig. 200. Serum Ca. 14 mg. per cent; P. 1·4 mg. per cent.

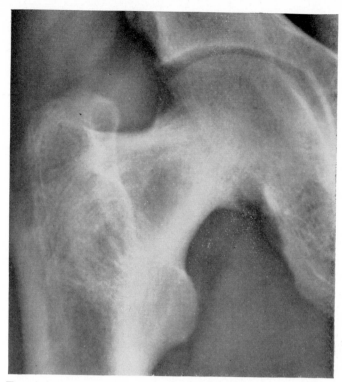

Fig. 178.—Hyperparathyroidism. Male aged 23 years. Coarse trabecular pattern femoral neck rather like Paget's disease. Typical cysts and phalangeal cortical erosions and mottled vault.

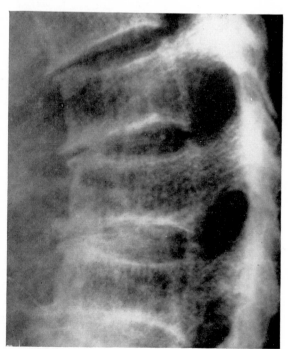

Fig. 179.—Hyperparathyroidism. Female aged 66 years. Coarse pattern in thoracic vertebrae. Slight compression D. 7 and 8. Finger illustrated in Fig. 202b. Pain in thoracic spinal area and weakness, 10 years. Serum Ca. 14·6 mg. per cent; P. 2·2 mg. per cent. Parathyroid tumour removed.

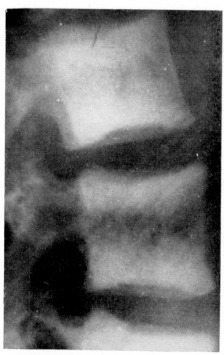

Fig. 180.—Hyperparathyroidism. Female aged 40 years. Rugger jersey appearance with wide horizontal dense bands below end plates and central transradiant band with a faint coarse pattern. Serum calcium 17 mg. per cent. Other bones: cysts, cortical resorption, and mottled vault.

to raise the serum calcium by increasing intestinal calcium absorption and resorption of calcium from bone. Both these actions, however, require the presence of 1,25-DHCC (see page 93), and in the absence of this metabolite, hypocalcaemia may be present even though the level of parathyroid hormone is enormously increased.

The increased secretion of parathyroid hormone also reduces tubular resorption of phosphate and the serum phosphate level falls, except in chronic renal failure when retention of phosphate may occur due to the reduction in glomerular filtration rate. Phosphate retention, by lowering the serum calcium level still further, is probably an important factor in the development of secondary hyperparathyroidism in chronic renal disease. Usually the degree of secondary hyperparathyroidism is greater in chronic renal failure than in nutritional deficiency or malabsorption of vitamin D, and the radiological changes are correspondingly more marked. In all three situations, bone mineralization is defective and osteomalacia invariably occurs.

In the experimental animal, dietary calcium lack produces secondary hyperparathyroidism and the serum calcium level is maintained by increased bone resorption. In the absence of vitamin D deficiency, however, osteomalacia does not develop.

The coarsened trabecular pattern in hyperparathyroidism varies according to the site and is nearly always associated with cyst-like transradiant areas in almost any of the bones, cortical erosions, particularly of the phalanges, or both types of change (see page 120).

The coarsened trabecular pattern is not common in the long bones, but may occasionally be seen associated with cyst-like erosions (Fig. 177). In the region of the femoral neck a very coarse pattern with abnormal orientation of the trabeculae (Fig. 178) may simulate the changes of Paget's disease.

In the vault of the skull a coarsened diploic bone pattern is also the basis for the rather characteristic mottled appearance so often seen in hyperparathyroidism. Detailed study will show a number of 2–3 millimetre ring shadows with a central transradiant zone, or more commonly a number of dense 2–4 millimetre circular shadows, with absorption of the diploic trabeculae around. Often both types of shadow may be seen, and in addition the white line of the cortex of both tables is indistinct or lost.

In the vertebrae the trabecular changes produce a coarse striate pattern and there may be mild compression of the vertebral bodies (Fig. 179). Occasionally there seems to be compensatory bone hypertrophy beneath the end plates (Fig. 180), resulting in a dense band-like horizontal shadow above and below separated by a central band of transradiancy in which the vertical striate pattern may still be seen. These alternating bands of opacity and transradiancy are sometimes referred to as the "rugger jersey" appearance, and are more common when the hyperparathyroidism is secondary to renal disease than when it is from a parathyroid tumour. More rarely, similar dense bands may be seen in a patient with renal disease and phosphate retention, in Paget's disease and in a more exaggerated form in osteopetrosis (see Fig. 102).

HAEMOGLOBINOPATHY (HEREDITARY ABNORMALITIES OF HAEMOGLOBIN)

A coarse trabecular pattern throughout the cancellous bone, due to the loss of some but not all the trabeculae and compensatory thickening of the remaining ones, is seen in sickle-cell anaemia and thalassaemia (including Cooley's anaemia). The changes are extraordinarily even throughout each bone and all or most of the skeleton is affected. The cortex is thinned and there is a characteristic alteration in the shape of the metacarpals which, owing to expansion of the middle part of the shaft, become almost rectangular in form (Fig. 181). In the major long bones, particularly the humeri and femora, the coarsened trabecular pattern is mixed with small 5–8 millimetre circular or oval erosions. The diploic bone of the vault of the skull is widened and shows a coarse, rather nodular pattern. In a minority of cases, vertical linear trabeculae replace the original outer table and give a "sun-ray" or "hair-on-end" appearance (Fig. 182).

The bone changes in both these conditions are the result of marrow hypertrophy induced by the prolonged and excessive haemopoiesis which is needed to keep up the numbers of red cells, whose survival time is half the normal or less.

Either condition may present clinically with a haemolytic anaemia. A patient with thalassaemia usually has a large spleen, and target cells are seen in the peripheral blood.

A patient with sickle cells in the peripheral blood may have severe crises with bone pain, which may be the reason for a bone radiograph. Often the patient is an ill-looking child.

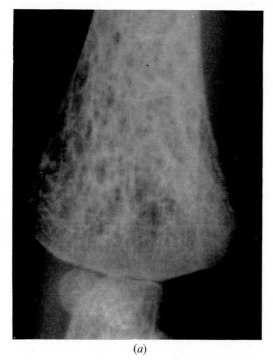
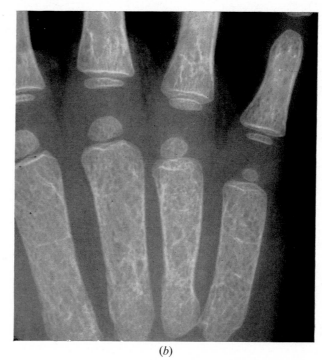

(a) (b)

Fig. 181. (a) and (b).—Thalassaemia—sickle-cell anaemia. Male aged 5 years. Coarse trabecular pattern and thinned cortex with increased width of metacarpals. Symmetrical right and left side in all long bones and pelvis. Skull and vertebrae normal. Cypriot, pale, underweight, enlarged liver and spleen. Hb. 50 per cent, cells very robust.

Infantile Gaucher's disease

In infantile Gaucher's disease there may be multiple trabecular erosions giving a coarse trabecular pattern (Fig. 183). There may in the very late stage be some rather large bone erosions. As in the adult form (*see* page 100), the patient may present with swelling of the abdomen due to a large spleen.

ALIMENTARY TRACT DISORDERS

Sometimes the trabecular absorption resulting from certain alimentary tract disorders referred to on page 102 is uneven and produces a rather coarsened trabecular pattern (Fig. 162). This change is usually seen throughout the limb bones and there are no cyst-like areas or evidence of cortical resorption. In such a case the clinical evidence of the alimentary tract disorder is generally obvious.

HERITABLE ENZYME DEFECT

A coarsened trabecular pattern is one of the features seen in hypophosphatasia. It is referred to on page 105 and shown in Fig. 164.

A similar trabecular pattern is seen in fibrogenesis imperfecta ossium (Fig. 175)—*see* page 105.

A coarse vertical striate trabecular pattern is seen in dysplasia epiphysealis punctata (Fig. 74)—*see* page 44.

PAGET'S DISEASE

A coarsened but irregular trabecular pattern is seen in Paget's disease—*see* page 178.

PATCHY DECREASE IN BONE DENSITY

A patchy decrease in bone density with small erosions distributed over all or most of the skeleton is seen in certain neoplastic diseases, leukaemia and certain anaemias. The hypertransradiant eroded areas, in which the trabeculae have been totally absorbed and replaced by neoplastic, leukaemic or marrow tissue,

109

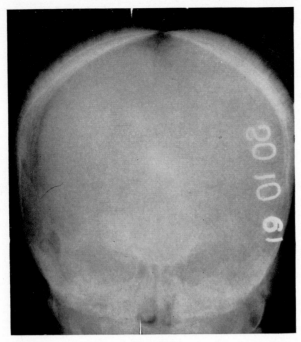

FIG. 182 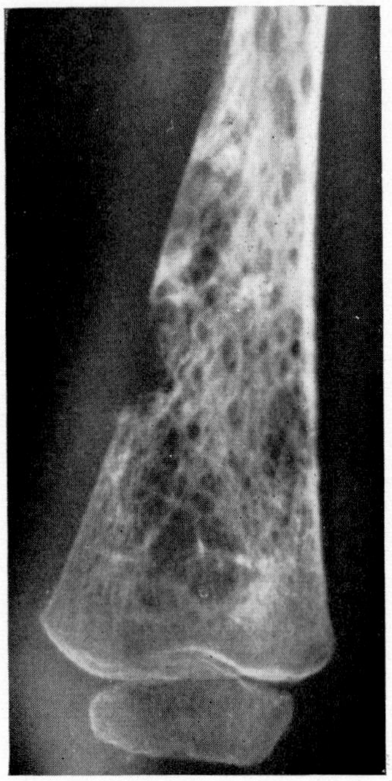   FIG. 183

FIG. 182.—Thalassaemia. Male aged 2 years. Vertical striate pattern beyond line of outer table. Large liver and spleen. 58 per cent of Hb. is foetal. Target cells present.

FIG. 183.—Infantile Gaucher's disease. Female aged 20 months. Multiple small erosions giving coarse trabecular pattern. Present in all bones, and miliary shadows in lungs. Hepatosplenomegaly. P.M.: Gaucher cells causing bone resorption.

may vary from pin-points to large areas several centimetres long and may be closely or widely spaced. If they are almost uniformly small and circular and spaced fairly evenly a few millimetres apart, they will suggest one of the blood disorders. If there is a moderate variation in the size and spacing of the erosions, either myelomatosis or secondary deposits from a carcinoma may be suspected. Gross variation in size and distribution is usually seen only in secondary deposits from a carcinoma.

MULTIPLE SECONDARY DEPOSITS FROM A CARCINOMA

Small secondary deposits may cause small ill-defined areas of erosion with normal trabeculae around, the pattern being that of a widespread patchy loss of density. The erosions may be fairly uniform or may vary greatly, but are most commonly 2–5 millimetres in size and roughly circular or oval in shape. They may be scattered evenly throughout the axial skeleton, ribs and proximal bones of the limbs, with the skull sometimes included and at other times excepted, or they may occasionally be seen only in the skull or pelvis. These small erosions may be the only change or may be associated with some much larger erosions here and there and often with collapse of one or more vertebrae. The erosions are predominantly in the cancellous bone, but there may be erosions of the superficial layer of the cortex or scalloping out of the deep aspect (Fig. 184).

The diagnosis may be made if the presence of a primary neoplasm is known, even if this has been removed many years before, or if a neoplasm is found in some site on careful clinical or radiological examination. The patient is usually a middle-aged woman and the most common site for a primary neoplasm with multiple small secondary deposits in the bones is the breast.

A possible mechanism for the bone erosions is indicated on page 150. It is not uncommon to find widespread secondary deposits in the marrow spaces, particularly in the vertebrae, with no trabecular erosions and therefore no radiological abnormality.

Hypercalcaemia from secondary deposits in the bones

The removal of calcium from the bones by the stimulus or direct action of the neoplastic cells may lead to hypercalcaemia when the calcium liberated exceeds the capacity of the kidneys to excrete it. The blood urea also tends to rise. The serum calcium may rise to levels in the range of 14–20 milligrams per cent. The patient may complain of the symptoms from this, particularly nausea and vomiting, while bone pain may be absent. In such a case the erosions are usually obvious and widespread, but occasionally hypercalcaemia is present when radiologically the extent of the bone erosions is relatively small.

MULTIPLE MYELOMATOSIS

Patchy loss of density may be seen with the multiple erosions induced by myelomatous deposits. These may be indistinguishable radiologically from the erosions of secondary deposits from a carcinoma or other type of malignant neoplasm. Scalloping out of the deep layer of the cortex (Fig. 185) is rather

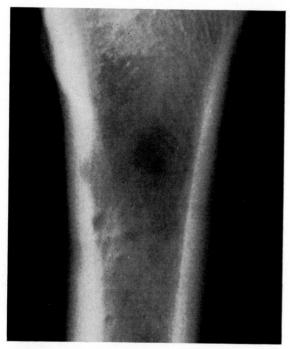

FIG. 184.—Secondary deposits. Female aged 48 years. Small erosions deep in the femur with scalloping out of the deep surface of the cortex as in Fig. 185. Erosions of pelvis. Primary carcinoma of breast.

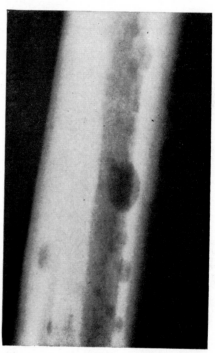

FIG. 185.—Myelomatosis. Male aged 69 years. Well-defined erosions and scalloping out of the deep surface of the cortex of the femur. Also erosions pelvis, skull, ribs. Marrow biopsy: myelomatosis. Serum electrophoresis: excess *gamma*-globulin. E.S.R. 140.

more common than in carcinoma, while if there are in addition some larger erosions, the variation in the range of size of these tends to be less in myelomatosis than in secondary deposits from a carcinoma.

In myelomatosis, patchy loss of density in some bones may be associated with more widespread even loss of density in others, particularly in the vertebrae (Fig. 170), while in the anterior ends of some of the ribs the even trabecular loss may be associated with some cortical expansion giving the rib a "drumstick" shape (Fig. 186), a very uncommon appearance in a secondary deposit from a carcinoma.

The diagnosis of multiple myelomatosis will depend on the biochemical or histological findings. Serum electrophoresis may show a characteristic pattern with an increase in the *gamma*-globulin fraction, or this or a Bence Jones protein may be found in the urine. One or other test is positive in about 60 per cent of cases, while bone marrow biopsy will show characteristic collections of atypical plasma cells replacing the bone marrow, which are pathognomonic of myelomatosis and are found in most cases.

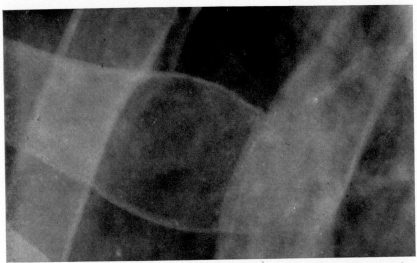

Fig. 186.—Myelomatosis. Male aged 35 years. Spindle-shaped expansion anterior end of rib with absence of trabecular pattern deep in it. The first bone change was erosion and expansion of the posterior part of the right fifth rib. Later erosions of skull, sternum and lumbar spine. *Post mortem:* generalized myelomatous deposits in the bones. *See also* Fig. 239.

Old Age

The generalized even decrease in density which is almost universally seen after the age of 75 years (*see* page 98) often starts at an earlier age, usually in the sixties but sometimes even earlier, as a rather patchy trabecular absorption. Small (3–5 millimetre) areas of erosion with no visible trabeculae are seen surrounded by bone with a thin but otherwise normal trabecular pattern. Such an appearance is common in the upper third of the humerus (Fig. 188).

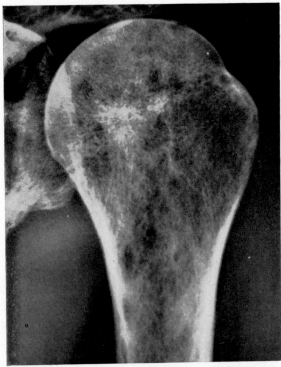

Fig. 187.—Secondary deposit. Female aged 47 years. Small ill-defined erosions (patchy loss of density) in upper third of humerus. Other side normal. Primary carcinoma of breast.

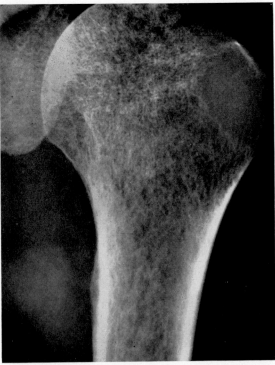

Fig. 188.—Senile osteoporosis. Female aged 61 years. Small erosions in upper third of humerus similar to Fig. 187. Same other humerus. Asymptomatic and no sign of disease.

Distinction from early secondary deposits may be difficult, particularly when a carcinoma is known to be present, as may often be the case in an elderly person. As an additional complication it is not unusual in the more advanced stages of a carcinoma to find a slight general decalcification of the bones which is not due to secondary deposits nor to old age, but is possibly due to excessive osteoclastic activity or to general depression of osteoblastic activity resulting from poor nutrition or from some metabolite produced by the tumour cells.

In senile osteoporosis the changes in the limbs and pelvis are very much the same on the right side as they are on the left, while in secondary deposits the changes are rather less symmetrical in the two limbs. They may be different on the two sides even in senile osteoporosis if for some reason one limb is being used less than the other, but the asymmetry will then be regional rather than a difference in the size and site of the scattered erosions.

In the earlier stages of osteoporosis of the elderly the thinning of the cortex is also apt to be uneven, giving a somewhat scalloped-out appearance to the inner layer. This is not as marked as in the grosser manifestations of myelomatosis or secondary carcinomatous deposits (Figs. 184 and 185), but differentiation from the lesser manifestations of these conditions may be impossible.

HAEMOPOIETIC DISEASES

Small circular erosions 2–3 millimetres in size, usually towards the ends of the long bones, are occasionally seen in leukaemia and even more rarely in association with some anaemias, when they presumably represent islets of trabecular absorption with replacement by hyperplastic marrow tissue.

DECREASED BONE DENSITY IN ONE REGION OR GROUP OF BONES

SPINAL UNDER-MINERALIZATION

The most common cause of spinal under-mineralization is osteoporosis. The spinal condition may be part of a generalized under-mineralization of all or most of the skeleton, as in the senile osteoporosis frequently seen in people over the age of 75 years; or the spine may be the predominant or sole region of osteoporosis, as in some manifestations of Cushing's syndrome (Fig. 158) or in the post-menopausal spinal osteoporosis occurring in some women within an age range of 45–65 years, in which the rest of the skeleton still appears normal for that particular age.

Spinal under-mineralization may also occur in conditions producing osteomalacia, particularly in some severe forms of renal osteodystrophy (*see* page 102).

Finally, it may be seen in leukaemia in children (*see* page 100) or in myelomatosis in elderly persons (*see* page 111).

Whatever the cause of the spinal under-mineralization, the changes are evenly distributed throughout the whole length of the vertebral column and throughout the whole extent of the individual vertebra, but are most easily seen in the lower thoracic and lumbar regions in lateral-view radiographs. In very severe cases the vertebral bodies are exceptionally transradiant and, unless the radiograph is of good quality, may be almost invisible. The cortex and end plates are thin but still contain enough calcium to give a white linear outline to the structureless central parts, in which very few or no trabeculae can be distinguished.

It must be admitted that the x-ray diagnosis of pathological under-mineralization of the vertebrae may be impossible in older persons (*see* page 99). If one takes matched control radiographs of apparently normal persons in the older age groups, the variation in trabecular pattern and thickness of the anterior cortical line of the vertebral bodies is considerable. The trabecular pattern may vary in the same person with the technique used, while the anterior cortical line is only 1 mm. or less in many normal persons. The only reliable evidence, therefore, is compression collapse or a fracture of the vertebral body.

In senile osteoporosis there is no close relationship between the metacarpal cortical index and the degree of vertebral compression, or between the presence of compression and the symptom of backache.

Alterations in the shape of the vertebrae

If the loss of calcium is sufficiently great, the bones will become softened and may then be unable to resist the normal stresses applied to them and there will be consequent alterations in shape. Three forms of altered shape are seen in the vertebral column. In the first the vertebral body gives way to the pressure from the discs on its centre, so that in a lateral view the superior and inferior surfaces are concave and the intervertebral spaces are wider in the middle than at the back or front (Fig. 190). In the second form the whole body collapses and becomes shorter in its height, though the superior and inferior surfaces remain parallel and the disc spaces are normal (Fig. 158). In the third form the decrease in height is most marked anteriorly, so that there is a wedge-shaped collapse with the disc spaces often remaining normal (Fig. 189). Combinations of these forms of collapse in a single vertebra are not uncommon, while all three types of collapse may be seen somewhere in a single vertebral column.

These changes of shape usually occur in only a few of the vertebrae, and it is not uncommon to see two collapsed vertebrae separated by one of normal shape, while in some cases only a single vertebra is flattened.

Pathology

In Cushing's syndrome there are few or no osteoblasts visible in the bone on histological examination (Sissons, 1956), but as the osteoclastic resorption continues at the normal rate, bone under-mineralization occurs.

DECREASE IN BONE DENSITY IN PART OF A LIMB DUE TO DISUSE OR SEPSIS

Disuse of a limb may be temporary, as in immobilization of a fracture or in a septic condition of the soft tissues; it may be prolonged following a nerve injury; or permanent following poliomyelitis or some other neuropathy. The mechanism of the trabecular absorption is uncertain, but Collins (1949) suggested it was due to an imbalance between the osteoblasts and osteoclasts, the activity of the former being depressed due to lack of stimulus produced by normal activity, while the latter remove calcium and eventually matrix from the bone in the usual manner.

Following trauma with fracture and therapeutic immobilization

In regional disuse atrophy following trauma, the loss of density is rather irregular giving the bone a mottled appearance. It involves the cancellous bone rather than the cortex. Not only are the fragments on either side of the fracture line affected, but often other bones situated more distally. The changes are fairly equally distributed throughout the affected bones, except in young adults in whom the areas adjacent to recently fused epiphyses often show a more intense trabecular resorption than the other parts (Fig. 191).

Associated with nearby sepsis

A rather similar regional patchy loss of density is frequently seen when a limb is partly immobilized because of sepsis in the soft tissues. It may also be seen with sepsis even in the absence of therapeutic immobilization, and is then probably due to a limitation of function resulting from the sepsis, to reflex alterations of the vascular supply, or to the chemical or toxic effects of the infection (Fig. 193).

A similar patchy decrease in density or a coarsened trabecular pattern is seen with a septic infection of a nearby joint (*see* Arthritis, Chapter 10, page 183). A coarse trabecular pattern is seen in the bones adjacent to a joint previously damaged by a haemorrhage in haemophilia (Fig. 301), and in the bones adjacent to a joint after recovery from a tuberculous arthritis (Fig. 192) even when the function is good. On the other hand, in the acute active stage of a tuberculous arthritis the loss of density of the nearby bones is much more even and may be so intense that the whole trabecular pattern over a considerable area is completely erased. (For tuberculous arthritis and surrounding bone changes, *see* Figs. 298 and 300.)

Associated with poliomyelitis and neuropathies

Severe regional osteoporosis usually occurs with paralysis of a limb, whether due to poliomyelitis or to some other neurological lesion. The changes tend to be very even and involve both the cortical and the cancellous bone. The cortex is much thinned and the trabeculae of the cancellous bone may become so demineralized that none can be seen at all in the middle two-thirds of the shaft. At the ends of a long bone, a mixture of trabecular absorption, failure of moulding by the normal stresses of activity

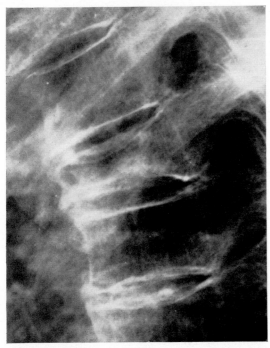

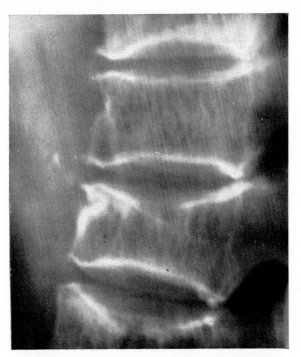

FIG. 189.—Spinal osteoporosis. Female aged 68 years. Some wedge-shaped collapse of D. 7. Poor calcium content of all the vertebrae with few trabeculae. Also collapse of D. 5 and 10. Biconcave indentation into the upper and lower surfaces of the lumbar vertebrae. Hands almost normal. Radiographs taken because of pain from a spontaneous fracture of a rib.

FIG. 190.—Spinal osteoporosis. Female aged 68 years. Tomogram: slightly wedge-shaped collapse of D. 9 with concave indentation into the lower surface and the upper surface of D. 10. Much trabecular absorption. Backache for some years. Some clinical but no radiological improvement after testosterone.

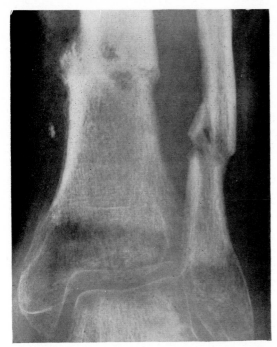

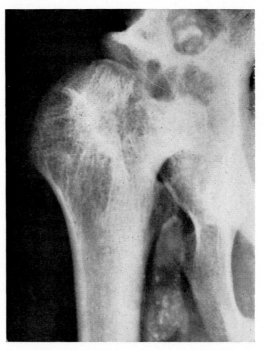

FIG. 191.—Local decalcification. Fracture tibia. Intense decalcification lower fragment with accentuation in region of recently fused epiphyseal line area.

FIG. 192.—Healed tuberculosis hip joint. Coarse trabecular pattern femoral neck. Calcification in abscess below lesser trochanter.

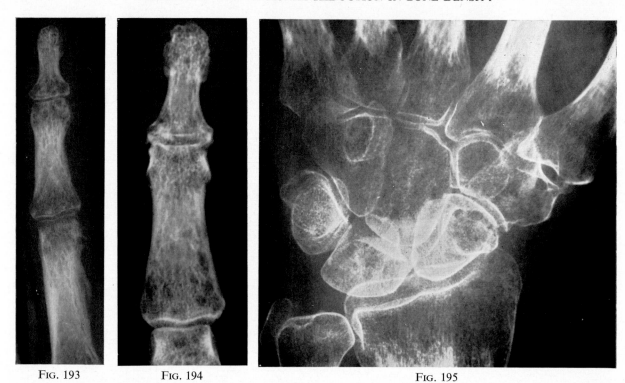

FIG. 193   FIG. 194   FIG. 195

FIG. 193.—Disuse resorption. Male aged 30 years. Patchy loss of density of phalanges. Infection of middle finger with osteomyelitis of proximal phalanx.

FIG. 194.—Südeck's atrophy. Female aged 64 years. Patchy resorption of phalanges.

FIG. 195.—Same case as Fig. 194 showing even resorption of lower end of radius. Some months' severe pain in left arm and wasting. Cause not found.

and thickening of those trabeculae which are still visible will result in a coarse pattern with the lines more widely spaced and less symmetrically arranged than normal (Fig. 9). In a severe case the entire trabecular pattern may eventually disappear.

When the paralysis occurs before mature growth has been reached, the bones of the affected limb cease to grow and remain thinner and shorter than normal.

POST-TRAUMATIC AND IDIOPATHIC ATROPHY (SÜDECK)

Loss of density of the bones of the distal half of an arm or leg may be the result of an idiopathic atrophy such as that described by Südeck (1900). In some cases the changes are patchy, consisting of circular hypertransradiancies some 2–3 millimetres in size scattered throughout the cancellous bone at intervals of 3–4 millimetres (Fig. 194) and affecting perhaps all the bones beyond the middle third of the forearm or tibia. In other cases the loss of density is more severe in certain areas such as the lower end of the radius, where it may be almost even (Fig. 195). In a very severe case it may be even throughout the whole region, with disappearance of most of the trabeculae and thinning of the cortex.

Occasionally the distribution of patchy or even loss of density is more limited, being confined for example to the metacarpal and phalanges of a single digit.

The condition may follow quite a minor traumatic incident without a fracture, or it may occur without an obvious precipitating cause. The limb may be very painful and there may be signs of peripheral vascular insufficiency. Usually there has been no therapeutic immobilization and no restriction of the normal activity of the limb, though some cases may eventually be immobilized because of the intense pain, the loss of density perhaps being intensified because of this. The course is prolonged and, unlike post-traumatic disuse atrophy, the bones do not readily recalcify even when the pain eventually wears off.

Südeck considered the condition to be due to a reflex vascular disorder, but this has not been substantiated and the various theories as to its cause are reviewed by Sweetapple (1949).

116

7—A Relatively Transradiant Area in a Bone

INTRODUCTION

In contrast to generalized decreased bone density, either widespread or confined to a group of bones, is the circumscribed transradiant area without lines of trabeculae in otherwise normal bone. Such an area is commonly isolated, though sometimes associated with other similar areas, and may be produced by a great variety of lesions. These transradiant areas can be grouped radiologically into (1) those which are well demarcated from the adjacent normal bone, some deep in the cancellous bone, some associated with cortical thinning or gross bone expansion and some on the surface of the bone, and (2) those that are poorly demarcated and lie either within or on the surface of the bone.

A single well-demarcated transradiant area within the cancellous bone, sometimes surrounded by a narrow white rim, is an x-ray appearance characteristic of many cysts and innocent tumours—so much so that it is often described in an x-ray report as a bone cyst without further investigation into the underlying pathology. It can in fact represent a very wide variety of pathological conditions including the simple cyst of uncertain aetiology, the cyst-like area in hyperparathyroidism, the cyst-like area due to a developmental defect, the giant-cell or plasma-cell tumour, the granuloma, the infective abscess, the parasitic cyst, the traumatic cyst and the cyst-like space associated with arthritis. Whereas some of these lesions can confidently be described as cysts, the term is obviously inappropriate for others.

The well-demarcated transradiant area with cortical thinning and bone expansion may be a late stage of any of the well-demarcated transradiant areas deep in the cancellous bone, but when the bone expansion is gross the appearances are particularly suggestive of an osteoclastoma or a solitary plasmacytoma. Well-demarcated transradiancies at the surface of the bone usually represent pressure erosions, but may occasionally be due to a developmental defect or, if in a terminal phalanx, an inflammatory or vascular lesion.

A poorly-demarcated transradiant area, either within the bone or on the surface, is typical of a malignant secondary deposit but may also be caused by a primary malignant neoplasm, a haemangioma, a xanthomatous granuloma or an inflammatory (usually tuberculous) lesion.

Beyond this general grouping, the differential diagnosis is usually impossible from the x-ray appearances, although slight clues may sometimes be derived from the shape and site of some of the well-demarcated lesions. There is a tendency, for instance, for the more circular ones to represent true cysts and the elongated oval ones to represent developmental defects. The presence of a rim of dense bone will favour a cyst or a developmental defect, and the absence of such a rim will suggest an osteoclastoma, a xanthoma or a cyst-like lesion with hyperparathyroidism. An erosion transgressing the epiphyseal disc would particularly suggest a chondroblastoma or an osteoclastoma, either of which would be uncommon in the middle third of the shaft, as opposed to a cyst or a granuloma which is not unusual in this site.

A single circular or oval transradiant area in the vault of the skull raises problems of its own and is therefore dealt with separately at the end of this chapter. Although the underlying lesions may be the same as in other bones, their incidence is different. In addition, there are certain lesions which occur in the skull and are not seen elsewhere.

WELL-DEMARCATED TRANSRADIANT AREA WITHIN A BONE

Simple Cysts of Uncertain Aetiology

A single 1–3 centimetre circular or oval well-demarcated transradiant area, lying for the most part in the cancellous bone and having a rim of condensed bone separating it from the surrounding normal trabeculae, is the most characteristic x-ray appearance of a simple cyst of uncertain aetiology (Fig. 196). Variations of this appearance are seen, two common ones being a roughly oval transradiant area with a few thin linear or band-like shadows crossing it here and there and giving it a multiloculated appearance (Fig. 197), and a transradiant zone which is well demarcated from the surrounding bone but not separated from it by a rim of dense bone (Fig. 198). A third variation is a much larger transradiant area which occupies most of the interior of the shaft of a long bone and adjacent to which the cortex is thinned and even slightly expanded; the cortical expansion, however, is slight in relation to the extent of the transradiant area (Fig. 199). Occasionally a cyst-like area of uncertain aetiology causes considerable bone expansion. This special combination of changes is described on page 137 and shown in Figs. 229 and 230.

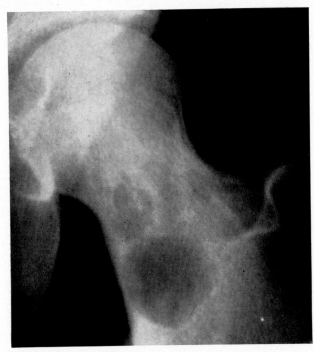

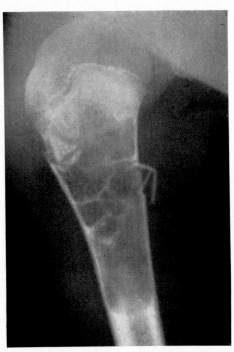

FIG. 196   FIG. 197

FIG. 196.—Cyst of femur. Female aged 18 years. Transradiant area 2 cm. long with very narrow rim of dense bone separating it from the normal trabeculae around. Slight pain in the hip for 2 years. Contents of cyst, marrow-like tissue and mucoid material; wall, sclerotic bone. Normal blood chemistry. Smaller circular transradiancy above it.

FIG. 197.—Cyst of humerus. Female aged 10 years. Transradiant area 6 cm. long in the submetaphyseal region with some line shadows across it but no trabecular pattern within it. Thinning of the cortex over it, and no sclerotic margin around it. Radiographed after a fall, fracture seen. Exploration showed a space with recent haemorrhage into it, and wall of young granulation tissue with some primitive spongy bone. Non-inflammatory.

These cyst-like transradiancies are most commonly seen in the humerus, particularly in a child between 4 and 12 years old, and may be situated either in the upper or in the middle third of the shaft. When present in a child they do not transgress the epiphyseal line. Other sites where such lesions are sometimes seen are the neck or the upper or lower third of the shaft of the femur, and either at one end or in the middle third of the tibia. They are less common in other bones.

The condition is frequently symptom-free and may be discovered from a radiograph taken for some incidental purpose, or because of slight pain following mild trauma with possibly a spontaneous fracture at the site of the cyst, often going through only one part of its shell-like wall (Fig. 197).

There may be no physical signs of the presence of the cyst, and the biochemical and endocrine investigations are within normal limits.

Since the cause of these simple cysts is often uncertain, they may be classified either by the nature of the surrounding membrane or by their contents. A suggested classification is as follows:

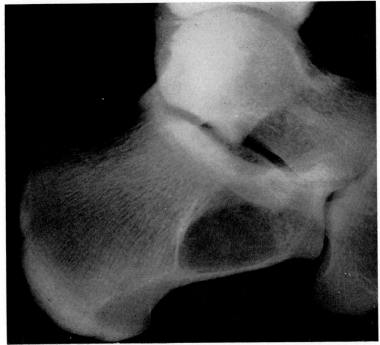

FIG. 198 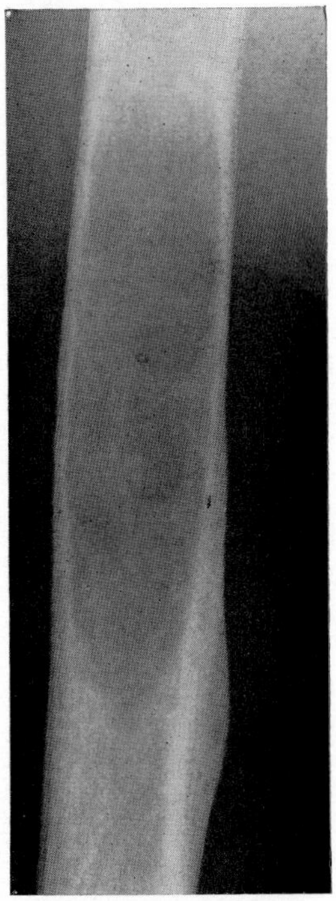   FIG. 199

FIG. 198.—Cyst of calcaneum. Male aged 18 years. Oval transradiant area 3 cm. long without a rim of dense bone. Radiographed because of recent injury. Exploration showed a space with brown fluid in it, presumed to be altered blood, and a wall of fibrous tissue.

FIG. 199.—Cyst of humerus. Male aged 9 years. Transradiant area without trabeculae some 8 cm. long occupying the whole width of the shaft of the humerus. Cortical thinning and slight expansion, and no surrounding rim of dense bone. Exploration showed a space with serous fluid, and a wall of non-specific granulation tissue.

Wall: (1) Lining membrane of fibrous tissue.
        (2) Lining membrane of fibrous tissue with multinucleate cells indistinguishable from osteoclasts.
        (3) No membrane, the wall consisting of partly eroded trabeculae.
        (4) Wall of dense bone with or without a lining membrane.

Contents: (5) Mucinous material.
        (6) Serous fluid.
        (7) Altered blood.
        (8) Marrow and fat.
        (9) Fibrous tissue.

The last type of lesion (9), in which the well-demarcated transradiant area is due to replacement of bone by fibrous tissue, is in fact not a true cyst, but may be a fibrous dysplasia or non-osteogenic fibroma as described under developmental defects on page 124.

The commonest histological finding for a simple cyst is a wall of fibroblastic cells with many giant cells of the osteoclastic type, surrounding mucinous, serous or blood-stained fluid.

OSTEITIS FIBROSA CYSTICA IN HYPERPARATHYROIDISM

The term "osteitis fibrosa cystica" used to be applied to all cyst-like lesions containing fibrous tissue, but has become too vague for this purpose owing to increased knowledge of the varying pathology of such lesions. It is used here solely as a name for the cyst-like lesions seen in hyperparathyroidism, and the other fibrous "cysts" are described under their specific histological titles such as fibrous dysplasia, non-osteogenic fibroma and so on.

For metabolic results of hyperparathyroidism and bone pathology, *see also* pages 92 and 122.

A cyst-like transradiant area is a common finding in hyperparathyroidism and may be seen almost anywhere in any bone, though it is rare in a vertebra or in the vault of the skull. It is not usually separated from the surrounding (normal) trabeculae by a zone of dense bone. It may be circular or oval in shape and may vary in size from a few millimetres to several centimetres. In an advanced case it may occupy the whole length of a major long bone (Fig. 201). There may be strands of opaque bone running across the transradiant area (Fig. 200). These may be caused by uneven thinning of the adjacent cortex, or may represent residual standards of bone running through the absorbed area. There may be one or several such cyst-like transradiant areas either in a single bone or in many bones.

A small transradiant area of 0·5 to 2 millimetres may lie within the cortical bone itself, but larger areas generally occupy the cancellous bone, and if large enough will cause thinning of the adjacent cortex

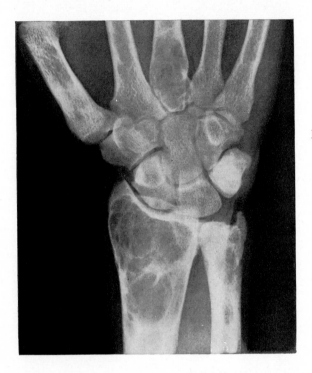

FIG. 200.—Cyst of radius in hyperparathyroidism. Male aged 25 years. Transradiant area without a rim of dense bone. Similar cystic areas in most major long bones; cortical resorption of phalanges as in Fig. 201c; coarse pattern of vertebrae as in Fig. 179, mottled appearance of vault. Serum Ca. 14 mg. per cent; P. 1·4 mg. per cent. Parathyroid tumour in neck removed. Many of the cysts disappeared. Cortical expansion around cystic area in third metacarpal.

(Fig. 200). Often there is no cortical expansion, but this may occur, especially when the transradiant area occupies most of the interior of the bone (Figs. 201 and 202). In a major long bone the expansion of the thinned outer layer may be quite marked (Fig. 205). If the lesion occupies the end of a long bone, the articular cortex usually remains intact (Fig. 200).

Sometimes in addition to the large transradiant area there are multiple small areas of patchy loss of density (Fig. 177) somewhat like those seen in myelomatosis.

Changes in the cortical bone

In addition to the cyst-like transradiant areas, the coarse trabecular pattern in the vertebrae or elsewhere and the mottled appearance of the vault of the skull, very characteristic changes in the cortex of the bones are usually present, particularly in the phalanges. These changes occur most commonly in the middle phalanges of the hand and in the bone around the teeth, though similar appearances may be seen in any of the long bones (Fig. 205). In an affected phalanx, four types of cortical change may be seen: (1) a generalized thinning of the cortex: (2) vertical linear bands of decreased density, giving the cortex a lace-like instead of a homogeneous appearance (Pugh, 1951); (3) small 0·5 to 2 millimetre deep central cortical erosions; or (4) small subperiosteal erosions, that is, erosions of the outer margin of the cortex (Fig. 203). Sometimes one or two of these changes are seen, sometimes all four. The subperiosteal cortical erosions and the lace-like pattern are almost pathognomonic of hyperparathyroidism. In severe cases all the cortical and cancellous bone of the tufts of the terminal phalanges may disappear (Fig. 201b and c). In the mandible the lamina dura and the surrounding bone is often absorbed adjacent to the periodontal membrane, the condition being analogous to the subperiosteal resorption in the phalanges (Pugh, 1954).

Other fairly common sites of cortical erosion are the medial aspect of the tibia some 2 cm. below the knee joint (Fig. 205) and the acromial ends of the clavicles, which may show complete erosion for about 2 cm.

Diagnosis

The clinical symptoms and signs of hyperparathyroidism are often inconspicuous. The characteristic cyst-like transradiancies and trabecular and cortical changes may be found accidentally in a radiograph taken for some incidental purpose such as the investigation of a fracture, backache or dental sepsis or

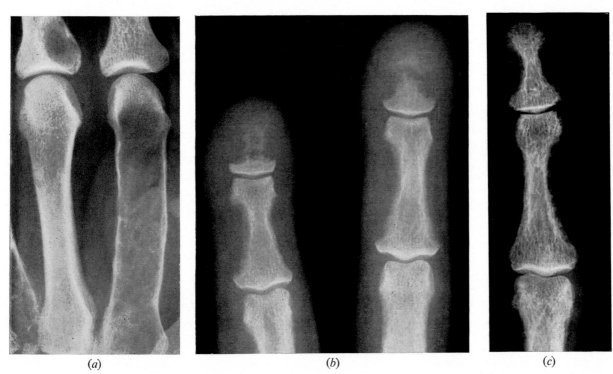

(a)   (b)   (c)

FIG. 201.—(a) Cyst of metacarpal in hyperparathyroidism. Female aged 46 years. Cystic transradiant area occupying most of the shaft of the metacarpal, with cortical thinning and slight expansion. Other bones showed classical changes similar to Figs. 179, 200 and 203. Serum Ca. 17 mg. per cent; P. 1·8 mg. per cent. Renal calcinosis. Limb pains 5 years, recent spontaneous fracture. (b) Hyperparathyroidism. Resorption of part of terminal phalanx and cortical resorption of middle phalanx. (c) Hyperparathyroidism. Female aged 66 years. Similar changes and symptoms to Fig. 203a. Cystic expansion of upper third of fibula, cortical erosion of tibia. Serum Ca. 14·6 mg. per cent; P. 2·2 mg. per cent. After removal of adenoma, Ca. 10 mg. per cent; P. 4·5 mg. per cent. Alkaline phosphatase 36 K.A. units.

the routine exclusion of a chest lesion. In the last instance a cyst-like transradiant area 1–2 centimetres long may be seen in a rib, or quite commonly in the acromial end of the clavicle. Alternatively, a spontaneous fracture through a cystic area may be the presenting symptom, and this usually unites in a normal manner.

In some cases the presenting symptoms or signs are renal, such as the pain of calculi, albuminuria or renal failure. The radiograph may show fine punctate calcifications in the substance of the kidneys (renal calcinosis) or calculi in the calyces or ureter, probably related to the excessive amounts of calcium and phosphorus excreted in the urine.

When either an isolated cyst-like area or renal calcinosis is found during radiography for some incidental purpose, further radiographs of other bones will generally show characteristics change such as cortical resorption in the phalanges, other cyst-like areas, or a coarsened trabecular pattern in the vertebrae or vault. However, in some cases of renal calcinosis there are no radiological bone changes in spite of a blood chemistry typical of hyperparathyroidism. In a suspected case the most appropriate

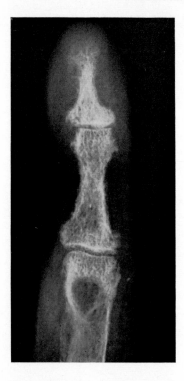

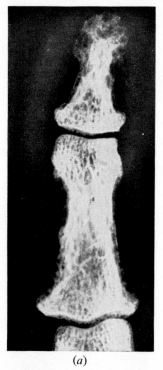

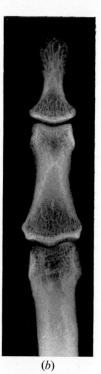

(a)   *(b)*

FIG. 202. — Hyperparathyroidism. Same patient as in Fig. 201c.

FIG. 203.—(*a*) Hyperparathyroidism. Female aged 35 years. Cortical resorption, lace-like pattern in phalanx. Cysts of other bones, backache 9 months. Serum Ca. 15 mg. per cent.; P. 2·1 mg. per cent. Parathyroid adenoma removed from neck. (*b*) Finger of normal adult to show width of cortex.

radiographs to take are an anterior view of both hands, a lateral view of the lower dorsal spine and a lateral view of the skull.

The diagnosis is finally confirmed if, in addition to some of the characteristic bone changes, the serum calcium is raised to 14 milligrams per cent or more and the serum phosphorus lowered to 3 milligrams per cent or less, and if there is clinical or radiological evidence of an enlarged parathyroid gland or of renal disease to which the condition might be secondary. The serum alkaline phosphatase will be raised if bone resorption is active.

Pathology

A cyst-like lesion in hyperparathyroidism will at first show evidence of excessive osteoclastic activity with bone resorption. These areas are later replaced by a vascular fibrous tissue in which there may be some poorly calcified new bone in the form of thin and irregular trabeculae. Many osteoclastic giant cells may be seen. The fibrous tissue may be extensive and form most of the cyst-like transradiant zone seen in the radiograph, or there may be myxomatous degeneration. Owing to the vascularity of the tissue, haemorrhages may occur, producing a truly cystic lesion containing blood-stained or even clear fluid. The mixture of fibrous tissue, giant cells, myxomatous degeneration and haemorrhages, often with some expansion of the bone, produces an appearance which has been described as a "brown tumour". Such a lesion does not in fact represent a tumour, although the x-ray appearances (such as Fig. 200) may simulate those of an osteoclastoma (*see* Fig. 236).

Response to treatment

Following successful treatment either by removal of the parathyroid tumour or by pre-operative vitamin D, the cortical resorption or coarse trabecular pattern may disappear as the normal bone architecture is reconstituted. This process may be more rapid in some bones than in others. The cortical resorption in the fingers, for instance, may disappear before the vertebral or skull changes. Many

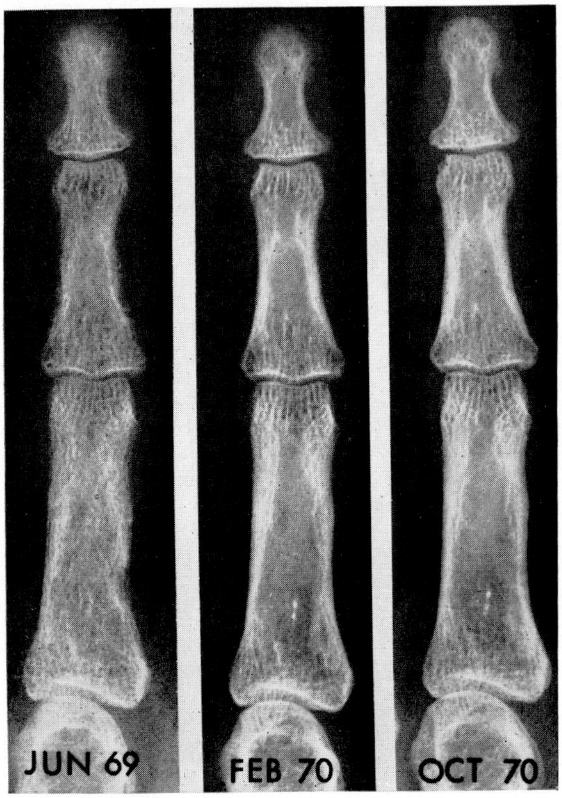

FIG. 204.—Primary hyperparathyroidism. Subperiosteal cortical erosions (June 1969). After therapy with vitamin D (February 1970) and with vitamin D and phosphate (October 1970), showed reformation of cortex and improved mineralization of bone.

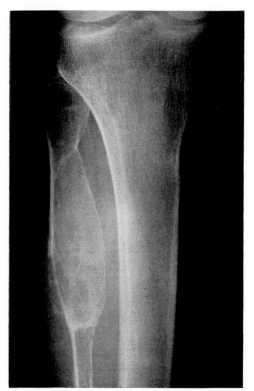

FIG. 205

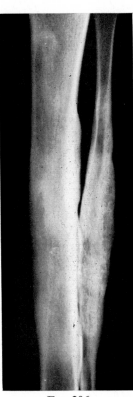

FIG. 206

FIG. 205. — Hyperparathyroidism. Female aged 66 years. Cyst-like lesion of fibula with expanded cortical layer over it. Surface cortical erosion on medial side of tibia. Same case as in Fig. 179. Cortical erosions of phalanges as in Fig. 203.

FIG. 206. — Hyperparathyroidism. Female aged 32 years. Two years after removal of parathyroid tumour. The thickened cortex now has an appearance like dripping candle wax. Same case as in Fig. 114.

cyst-like areas eventually show complete resolution, though some show reconstitution of the bony architecture sooner than others, while some remain unchanged. Much more rarely a transradiant area becomes evenly calcified and opaque (*see* Fig. 114).

Occasionally expanded cortex over a cystic area reforms in rather an exotic manner, the result being a much thickened cortex giving a dripping candle wax appearance (Fig. 206) rather suggestive of melorheostosis (*see* page 87).

The variable histological appearances seen in the cyst-like areas account for the different responses seen in serial radiographs after treatment of the condition.

Hypoparathyroidism

It has been reported by Dent (1957) that the x-ray changes described in hyperparathyroidism may be found in a case in which the blood chemistry indicates hypoparathyroidism.

Developmental Defects

In many cases a circumscribed transradiant cyst-like area is due to a developmental defect whereby a fibrous or cartilaginous mass is formed instead of bone. This type of lesion, though occasionally seen in infancy, usually becomes apparent for the first time in later childhood or young adolescence. It may increase in size for a time, starting at a few millimetres and sometimes reaching several centimetres. It generally ceases to grow after the completion of normal epiphyseal fusion, which occurs between the ages of 20 and 25 years. Thereafter it usually remains stationary and may therefore be seen at any time in later life. Occasionally the lesion may regress, in which case the histology cannot as a rule be proved.

Owing to the early termination of growth, such a developmental aberration can hardly be classified as a bone tumour. It may show many different histological features in different cases, including such conditions as monostotic and polyostotic fibrous dysplasia and the so-called giant cell (osteoclastoma) variants—namely non-osteogenic fibroma, aneurysmal bone cyst, chondromyxoid fibroma and chondroblastoma—as well as the rather more tumour-like masses of a chondroma or a hamartoma.

Fibrous dysplasia

A well-defined 3–10 centimetre oval transradiancy just below the metaphysis in a child, often demarcated by a narrow zone of dense bone from the surrounding trabeculae, may be due to a fibrous dysplasia. In a long bone the lesion usually lies with its long axis parallel to the shaft. Seen at a later stage, the lesion may extend right across a long bone in width and from the metaphysis nearly to the middle third of the shaft in length. When it is extensive, the cortex over it is thinned and may even be slightly expanded; the condition is then frequently mistaken for an osteoclastoma or a fluid-containing cyst (*see* Fig. 197). In another late manifestation, usually seen in an adult, the cortex is unevenly scalloped out and the thicker ridges of cortical bone, viewed end-on, are seen on the radiograph as broad band-like shadows running irregularly across the transradiant zone and giving it a multiloculate appearance (Figs. 207 and 209). This type of lesion is less well defined, and the rim of dense bone may only be present around parts of it, while in other parts it may be quite difficult to judge where the transradiant zone terminates and normal trabeculae begin.

A monostotic dysplasia is seen most commonly in the upper end of the humerus, in the upper or lower end of the tibia, in the neck or upper part of the femur or in an iliac bone—although it may occur in almost any bone. It may even occur within an ossific centre of an epiphysis. The large pseudo-multiloculated type of lesion is seen particularly in the femur (Fig. 207) and the iliac bone (Fig. 208). The biochemistry of the serum is normal except that the alkaline phosphatase may be raised. There may be no endocrine disturbances.

In the polyostotic form, some of the lesions are often in the middle third of the shaft of the long bones. There is thinning and slight expansion of the cortex and the transradiant area, although devoid of trabecular pattern, is rather opalescent and has a ground-glass appearance (Fig. 210); others are similar to Figs. 207 and 208. There may be evidence of sexual precocity as described by Albright and

Reifenstein (1948). The lesions may be bilateral but are not quite symmetrical, and one side may be much more affected than the other.

The condition appears to be a developmental defect in which fibrous tissue is laid down in certain areas instead of bone. Histological examination reveals that the expansion is due to replacement of the normal bone by fibrous tissue of moderate cellularity in which may be seen thin and irregular spicules of bone trabeculae.

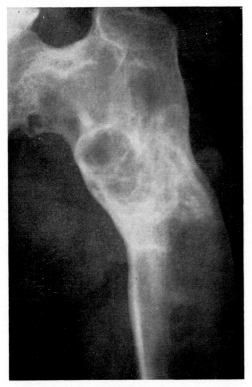

FIG. 207

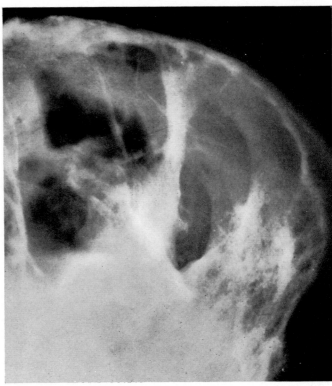

FIG. 208

FIG. 207.—Monostotic fibrous dysplasia. Female aged 33 years. Large transradiant area in upper third of femur with its upper limit at epiphyseal disc, and lower limit poorly demarcated. Cortical thinning and alteration in the shape of the bone. Radiographed because of injury. Blood chemistry normal. Exploration showed solid fibrous tissue with histological appearances of fibrous dysplasia.

FIG. 208.—Monostotic fibrous dysplasia. Male aged 19 years. Poorly-demarcated transradiant areas in the ilium with strands of bone between. Slight intermittent pain in hip region for 2 years. Biopsy—typical fibrous dysplasia.

A cyst-like area of transradiancy due to fibrous dysplasia may develop in an area in which the bone appeared normal in an earlier radiograph. In other cases quite severe changes may be seen by the age of 18 months, though it is unusual to see radiographic abnormalities until about 4–6 years of age.

In a long-term follow up of 37 cases of fibrous dysplasia reported by Harris, Dudley and Barry (1962), 3 patients appear to have died as a result of the disease. In 2 others a sarcoma developed in a region treated by radiotherapy more than 20 years previously. The majority of cases of monostotic fibrous dysplasia and many of those with polyostotic involvement were without symptoms 20–40 years later. In a number of cases there was some progression of the lesion, and among the polyostotic cases further lesions were observed to arise in new sites in 7 patients.

Non-osteogenic fibroma (fibrous metaphyseal defect)

A circular or oval cyst-like transradiancy, usually situated towards the end of the shaft of a major long bone of a limb of an older child or young adolescent, may be due to a non-osteogenic fibroma (fibrous metaphyseal defect) (Jaffe, 1942a; Maudsley and Stansfeld, 1956).

The transradiant zone may be a few millimetres or several centimetres long, and when oval in shape its long axis is parallel to the shaft. It is usually demarcated by a narrow rim of dense bone from the surrounding normal trabeculae (Fig. 211). In some cases it may appear to be multiloculated, but the bony strands projecting into it do not in fact form separate compartments. The adjacent cortex is often thinned and may even show a slight expansion over the transradiant zone, but if the lesion lies deep in the cancellous bone, the cortex will appear normal.

Common sites are the upper end of the humerus, the lower end of the femur, and either end of the tibia. In a young child the lesion may lie immediately below the metaphysis, but, as growth proceeds, the final site may be some distance away.

The central part of the fibroma is filled with material of soft consistency, reddish brown or yellow in colour, with a narrow rim of dense bone beyond which normal bone is found. Histologically the lesion is composed of connective tissue with many plump fibroblasts and with giant cells and foam cells in some areas. The appearances are not uniform throughout, cellular connective tissue being found centrally and more collagenous fibrous tissue peripherally. Because of these variable appearances, this type of lesion is easily confused with a lipoid granuloma in view of the presence of foam cells, with an osteoclastoma because of the many giant cells like osteoclasts found in some parts, and with a fibroma of bone because of the more fibrous areas.

After reaching a certain size, the lesions do not enlarge further, and if treated by curettage they do not recur. Following a spontaneous fracture, or even without the stimulus of trauma, these lesions regress, so that it is probable that they represent a developmental defect and not a true tumour. The term "metaphyseal fibrous defect" may thus be the most appropriate.

Aneurysmal bone cyst

A rather poorly demarcated cyst-like space may be caused by an aneurysmal bone cyst. The radiological appearances closely simulate those of an early osteoclastoma, the eroded area not being separated from the surrounding bone by a zone of dense bone (Fig. 212). In some cases, especially where the lesion is in a long bone, there is marked expansion of the bone around the transradiant area, with a thin white line of surrounding new bone. Malignant change does not occur.

Histologically the lesion is composed of both solid and cystic areas. The latter contain blood-stained fluid, and the walls are formed by fibrous tissue of variable thickness in which there are deposits of haemosiderin and many osteoclastic type giant cells are also seen. Areas of new bone formation are present in the fibrous stroma.

The term "aneurysmal", which is in general use, is somewhat misleading since the bone absorption is not the result of the expansile pulsation of the blood spaces. It is probably a developmental defect, and closely related to a haemangioma in that some of the cystic spaces are lined by endothelium. Its course is more benign that that of an osteoclastoma, with which it has been confused in the past.

Chondromyxoid fibroma

The author has no proven case of this condition, first described by Jaffe and Lichtenstein (1949).

There is an area of bone resorption with cortical thinning and expansion, usually in a bone of the lower limb. Scalloping out of the cortex here and there is described, giving the transradiant zone a trabeculated appearance and thus simulating an osteoclastoma.

The histological features are those of a cellular tumour with a myxomatous stroma and later a tendency to collagenization of the stroma. In some areas the tumour cell nuclei are surrounded by vacuoles so that they resemble cartilage cells and the lesion may be misdiagnosed as a chondrosarcoma. In spite of its cellularity the tumour is benign, and curettage or local removal is curative.

Chondroblastoma

A 1–6 centimetre circular erosion, partly or almost entirely in an epiphysis though often extending a short distance into the metaphysis, will strongly suggest a chondroblastoma. The author has not had a proven case, but the appearances illustrated by Lichtenstein (1952) are identical with those illustrated in Figs. 218 and 330, which were reported by a pathologist to be osteoclastomas. The margins of the transradiant area are well defined and may or may not be surrounded by a narrow rim of dense bone. Sometimes stippled calcifications can be seen within the tumour area. The lesion is seen only in the

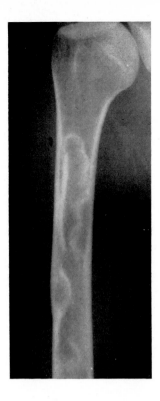

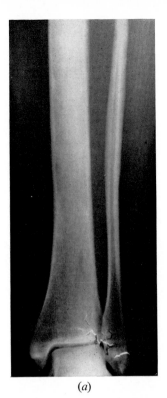

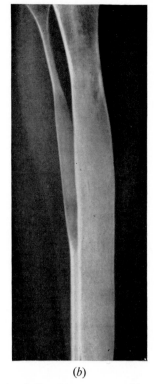

(a)   (b)

FIG. 209.—Fibrous dyspla-
sia. Female aged 27 years.
Cyst-like   transradiant
area in lower two-thirds
of humerus sharply de-
marcated by a rim of
dense bone, and terminat-
ing at region of epiphy-
seal line below. Other
bones affected.

FIG. 210.—Polyostotic fibrous dysplasia. Same case as Fig.
209. (a) Ground-glass appearance with cortical thinning and
slight expansion of middle third of tibia. Other leg similar.
Circular cyst-like area in neck of femur. Blood chemistry
normal. No pigmentation. Menstruation from age of 7
years. (b) Female aged 16 years. Middle third of tibia
expanded with structureless central part. Several bones
affected.

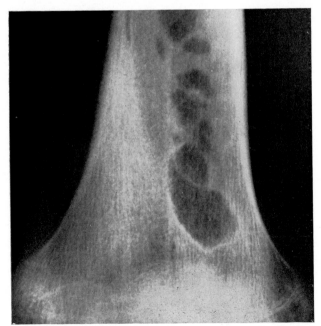

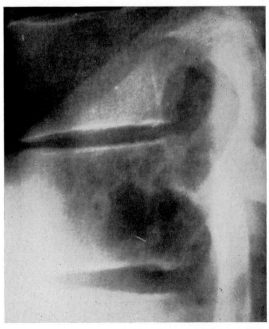

FIG. 211.—Non-osteogenic fibroma (fibrous metaphyseal
defect). Male aged 15 years. Transradiant area in the
lower third of the femur some 8 cm. long and sharply
demarcated from the surrounding normal trabeculae by a
line of dense bone. Slight pain below patella for a year.
Biopsy—non-osteogenic fibroma.

FIG. 212.—Aneurysmal bone cyst. Male aged 26
years. Well-demarcated transradiant area in the
postero-inferior aspect of the body of D. 11.
Spastic paresis of legs and sensory loss to level of
D. 12 for 4 months. Exploration showed a very
vascular tumour with histological appearances of
an aneurysmal bone cyst. Good recovery.

127

epiphyseal region of a major long bone of a limb, particularly the upper end of the humerus or tibia and either end of the femur. It occurs in late adolescence before epiphyseal fusion has taken place, and is benign and usually symptomless.

Histologically the chondroblastoma is a cellular tumour composed of small darkly staining cells. These are regarded as "chondroblasts", as their maturation leads to the development of areas which can be recognized as a cartilaginous matrix and in which patchy calcification can be seen. In addition there are giant cells of the osteoclast type, most numerous around blood vessels. These cells have led to confusion in the past with true giant-cell tumours of bone (osteoclastomas), but the presence of the chondroblasts should indicate the correct diagnosis.

Tuberose sclerosis (mesodermal dysplasia)

Small (1–3 millimetre) cyst-like transradiancies are seen in a phalanx or metacarpal in some cases of tuberose sclerosis. The diagnosis will be suggested if there is mental deficiency, an adenoma sebaceum or a subungual fibroma, a skin nodule, small punctate calcifications in the brain best seen in a lateral view lying just above the sella, and a nodular and honeycomb type of shadow in the lower half of both lung fields. Other x-ray manifestations which are reviewed by Whitaker (1959) and by Hawkins (1959) consist of periosteal deposits on the metatarsals and local thickening of the vault.

Arterio-venous aneurysm

A rather less well demarcated circular or oval transradiancy, often 1–3 centimetres in size, may be the result of a developmental defect of the blood supply within the bone and the production of an arterio-venous aneurysm (Fig. 213). The most common site is the lower end of a femur. There will be clinical evidence of a circulatory disorder in the limb.

Haemangioma

There is some doubt whether a haemangioma represents a replacement of bone by vascular tissue during development or whether it is a vascular tumour. The resulting transradiant area is fairly well demarcated from the surrounding bone, though often less so than other cyst-like lesions (Fig. 214).

This rather uncommon malformation may be single or multiple. It may be seen in the upper or lower ends of the shaft of the femur or tibia, and occasionally in the skull (*see* page 155) and the vertebrae. In the vertebral site a simple coarsening of the trabecular pattern (*see* Fig. 123) is also attributed to a haemangioma, though the evidence for this is inconclusive.

The clinical course seems to be benign and the response to radiotherapy is often slight.

The histological appearances of a haemangioma are characteristic, with large vascular spaces lined by a single layer of endothelium replacing the bone. These cavernous spaces are filled with blood and the whole area is traversed by residual bone trabeculae which tend to run in the direction parallel with the line of maximal stress in the bone.

Chondroma or hamartoma

A cyst-like transradiant area may represent an islet of cartilage, which is of low radio-opacity, in a region which normally contains bone (Fig. 215). This often seems to be a developmental anomaly rather than a cartilaginous tumour, and growth of the cartilaginous mass terminates with the general cessation of bone growth. The lesion may lie deep in the cancellous bone and is sometimes, though not always, surrounded by a narrow rim of condensed bone. When large it may cause thinning and eventual expansion of the cortex, such expansion often being eccentric (*see* page 138).

The lesion is often indistinguishable radiologically from the many other causes of a single well-demarcated transradiant area in a bone, including even a fluid-containing cyst, but in some cases small zones of calcification in the cartilage throw small punctate shadows within the transradiant zone, the so-called "chondroma spots" or "stippling" which are almost specific to this condition (Fig. 216). In certain cases the calcium deposits are more extensive and almost confluent, throwing a much larger, more homogeneous and rather shapeless shadow within the transradiant zone (Fig. 233).

The most common site for a single chondroma or hamartoma is the shaft of a long bone of the hand. Occasionally one is seen in the upper half of a humerus, the region of the femoral neck, the middle third or end of a tibia, or a rib where it usually lies near the neck but may occur in the middle half.

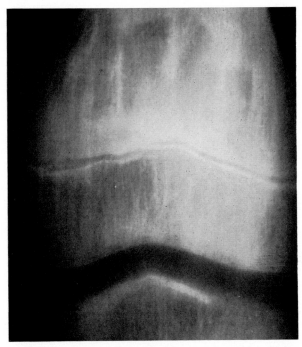

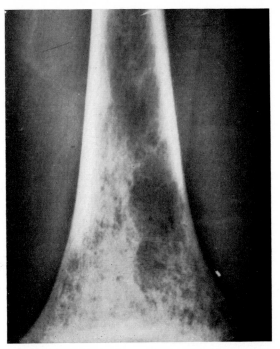

Fig. 213.—Arterio-venous aneurysm. Male aged 11 years. Tomogram showing ill-defined transradiant area in the lower end of the diaphysis of the femur. Arteriogram showed a large vessel to it. Excessive pulsation in right leg. Left ventricular hypertrophy.

Fig. 214.—Haemangioma. Male aged 9 years. Ill-defined transradiant area without trabeculae extending for 10 cm. in lower end of diaphysis of femur, limited by epiphyseal disc. Bilateral and asymptomatic. Biopsy—haemangioma.

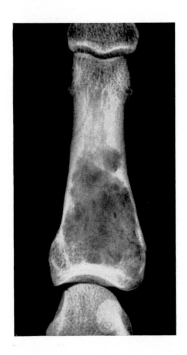

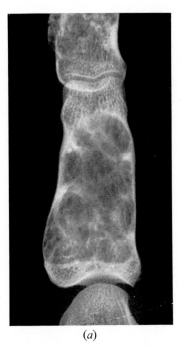

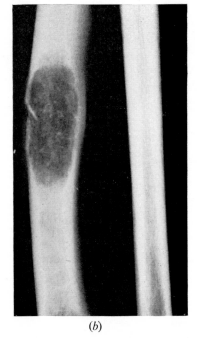

(a)

(b)

Fig. 215.—Chondroma. Male aged 42 years. Transradiant area 2 cm. long in proximal phalanx of index finger, with thinning of cortex over it. Radiographed because of injury. Biopsy—chondroma.

Fig. 216.—(a) Multiple enchondromas in the fingers. Transradiant area in each bone with stippling from calcification in the cartilaginous mass. (b) Enchondroma middle third radius. Transradiant area with stippling. Fracture cortex from trauma.

Multiple chondromas are seen particularly in the phalanges and metacarpals (Fig. 216). Sometimes one or two may be present in one bone in a patient with multiple exostoses in other sites.

Histologically the chondroma is composed of a hyaline cartilaginous stroma containing scanty and regular chondrocytes. Mucoid degeneration may occur in some parts to produce small cystic areas within the cartilaginous parts, while calcification or even ossification may replace areas of the stroma. Sometimes the lesion is composed of a mixture of cartilage, bone, marrow, blood vessels and fibrous tissue, in which case the lesion may aptly be termed a hamartoma.

Neurofibromatosis

A single cyst-like transradiant area or several such areas may be seen deep in a bone in some cases of neurofibromatosis. The pathology is obscure, since it is not always that of a neurilemmoma but often more akin to a fibrous dysplasia.

TUMOURS

Osteoclastoma

If an osteoclastoma is detected at an early stage before the additional cortical erosion or expansion has developed (*see* page 138), it may be seen as a 1–3 centimetre circular or oval transradiancy deep in the bone (Fig. 217). Although the margins may be quite sharp there is no surrounding rim of dense bone, and this serves to differentiate the early osteoclastoma from many other cyst-like lesions and from at least one of the giant-cell tumour variants—namely the non-osteogenic fibroma—in which a rim of sclerotic bone is always seen (Fig. 211). Distinction from the other giant-cell variants may only be possible from the histological appearances (*see* page 125) or from the clinical course, the growth of an osteoclastoma being more rapid and less easily checked by local curettage or radiotherapy. In fact,

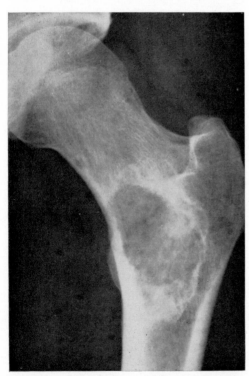

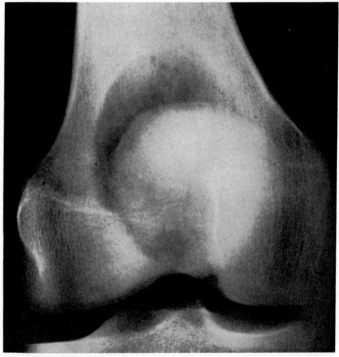

FIG. 217.—Osteoclastoma. Male aged 40 years. Oval transradiant zone some 6 cm. long in the neck of the femur, with slight cortical erosion. Slight pain 10 weeks. Biopsy—grade 2 osteoclastoma with regular spindle cells and osteoclast-like cells. Curetted and replaced with chip grafts. Rapid local spread of erosion; 6 months later large secondary deposits in lungs.

FIG. 218.—Osteoclastoma. Female aged 30 years. Oval 5 cm. transradiant zone in the lower end of the femur extending across epiphyseal disc. In lateral view it lay centrally. Slight pain 3 months, recent swelling. Biopsy—grade 2 osteoclastoma. Curetted, but local recurrence followed, so amputation was performed. Tumour histology the same as the biopsy.

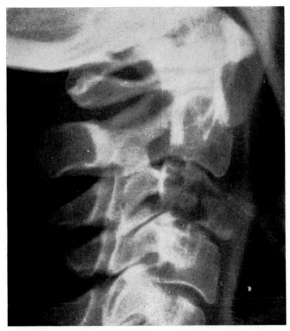

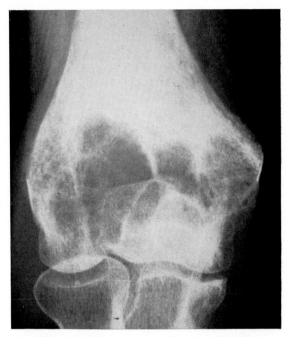

FIG. 219.—Probable osteoclastoma. Female aged 23 years. Erosion of C. 3, with disc narrowing between it and C. 4. Pain in neck for 3 weeks with no unusual features to distinguish it from a disc or other benign lesion. Biopsy—stroma suggests an osteoclastoma, but rather more fibrous tissue than usual. Not a variant. Radiotherapy. No recurrence after many years.

FIG. 220.—Secondary deposit. Female aged 49 years. Fairly well demarcated transradiant areas in lower end of humerus, with no sclerotic margin. Mastectomy for carcinoma 3 years before. Lesion controlled for a time by radiotherapy and removal of ovaries and adrenals. Later more erosion occurred, and gross erosion of the skull, pelvis and other bones was observed.

even when an osteoclastoma is diagnosed at this early stage of local erosion, which rarely happens, it may still not be possible to prevent pulmonary metastases in a very aggressive example nor to improve the local prospects unless the mass can be completely excised.

It may start in an epiphysis (Fig. 330), but is usually observed at a later age and stage when it may be seen to transgress the line marking the site of epiphyseal fusion (Fig. 218). At a still later stage it tends to cause bone expansion as described on page 138.

Although uncommon in a vertebral body, osteoclastomas are occasionally seen in this site and appear as a rather cyst-like transradiant area (Fig. 219), often with little or no evidence of bone expansion.

Solitary plasmacytoma

A single area of transradiancy deep in a bone may be the first evidence of a solitary plasmacytoma. The erosion is roughly oval in shape and 1–3 centimetres long, quite well demarcated and usually without a surrounding rim of dense bone There is a tendency for thinning and expansion of the cortex (Fig 239), though this is often much less marked than in an osteoclastoma of similar size. A rib is a favourite site, so that it may be detected on a routine chest radiograph. The pelvis is another common site. The lesion is seen in a rather older age group than an osteoclastoma, most patients being between 40 and 60 years of age. Although the single erosion may be the sole manifestation for many years, most cases eventually develop generalized multiple myelomatosis (*see* page 111). The appearances of a solitary plasmacytoma cannot be distinguished from a large erosive lesion in a clinically proven case of multiple myelomatosis, in which only on further radiological examination of other bones are smaller erosive lesions seen. In such a case lateral views of the skull and lower dorsal spine and a posterior view of the pelvis and upper femora may be indicated.

Histologically the lesion is characterized by the presence of large and atypical plasma cells, which replace the bone.

Secondary deposit

Occasionally a secondary deposit is seen as a very well defined circular or oval transradiant area deep in the bone. The appearances may be almost cyst-like, but there is no surrounding rim of sclerotic bone (Fig. 220). The diagnosis will be suspected if the patient is known to have a malignant neoplasm in some other site or if there are other secondary deposits in the lung, otherwise one of the many other lesions causing a well-demarcated transradiant area may be suspected. The diagnosis may only be established by a biopsy or by the fairly rapid enlargement of the bone lesion.

HISTIOCYTE AND NON-SPECIFIC GRANULOMAS

Xanthomatous granuloma (histiocytosis x)

A well circumscribed cyst-like lesion in a bone may be due to a xanthomatous granuloma (histio-cytosis x). The transradiant area tends to be oval rather than circular, and in a long bone its long axis is

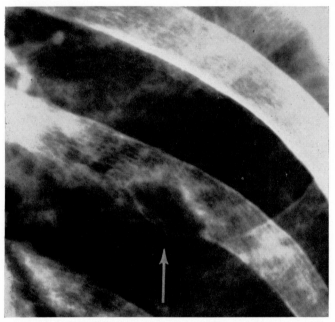

FIG. 221.—Xanthomatous granuloma. Male aged 47 years. Well-demarcated 2 cm. transradiant area in posterior part of left eighth rib. Cortical thinning and expansion (opposite arrow), slight rim of sclerotic bone. Routine chest x-ray, asymptomatic. Biopsy—xanthomatous granuloma.

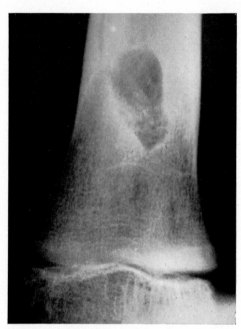

FIG. 222.—Xanthomatous granuloma. Female aged 2 years. Two cm. oval transradiant area in lower end of femur with faint sclerotic margin. Tender swelling in thigh. Multiple erosions of vault up to 6 cm. Biopsy of femur—eosinophil granuloma with foam cells.

parallel to the shaft. It is usually deep in the cancellous bone and is always well demarcated. Although it may sometimes be surrounded by a white line of sclerotic bone (Fig. 221), this is unusual, and it more often resembles a non-cystic erosion in which no such rim of sclerotic bone is seen (Fig. 222).

The transradiancy may reach a size of about 1 centimetre and enlarge no further, or it may grow to several centimetres, particularly in a major long bone or in the vault of the skull. Frequently it enlarges enough to reach the cortex, which is then thinned though rarely expanded over it. Quite often the cortex is sufficiently thinned for a spontaneous fracture to occur, and the resulting secondary subperiosteal callus tends to spread well down over the normal bone as well, an indication that it is not a periosteal new bone formation in direct response to the lesion itself.

Common sites are the submetaphyseal area and the middle third of the femora and tibiae, the ischio-pubic rami, the humerus, the middle third of a rib and the vault of the skull. Less comonly it may be found in almost any bone including the base of the skull, a vertebral body or the sternum, but it is unusual in a hand or foot. In some cases there is one isolated lesion, while in others there may be several separate transradiant areas in a single bone or a single transradiant area in several bones.

The disease may be clinically silent and the lesion discovered accidentally in a radiograph taken for some other purpose, such as a routine chest examination or the exclusion of a fracture after some minor traumatic incident. In some cases there is malaise and fever, particularly in children in the Letterer–Siwe phase.

When the cyst-like transradiant area has been seen and the diagnosis is not obvious, a lateral-view radiograph of the skull and a posterior-view radiograph of the pelvis and femora may be useful to see whether the lesion is isolated or whether others are present. Multiple large erosive-looking lesions with a predilection for the skull, pelvis and upper half of the femora will be very suggestive of a xanthomatosis. A radiograph of the chest is also indicated, since in some cases of xanthomatosis the bone lesion is associated with lung lesions which give a partly nodular and partly honeycomb shadowing in the lower half of the lungs.

Histologically there may be the characteristic foam cells of the Hand–Schüller–Christian phase or the eosinophilic cells when the lesion is an eosinophilic granuloma.

In a long-term follow up of 28 cases with an isolated eosinophilic granulomatous bone lesion, healing was found in all cases, a variety of treatments having been used (McGavran and Spady, 1960).

Non-specific granuloma

Sometimes a cyst-like transradiancy, similar to a xanthomatous granuloma, is seen but histological examination shows a non-specific granuloma which appears not to be a xanthomatous type of lesion. The aetiology is unknown.

HISTIOCYTOSIS (GAUCHER'S DISEASE)

Multiple cyst-like transradiant zones are occasionally seen as a late manifestation in some cases of Gaucher's disease (Fig. 223). They are well-demarcated and circular or oval in shape, and they vary in size from a few millimetres to several centimetres. They are most conspicuous in the major long bones of the limbs. The more usual x-ray changes of Gaucher's disease, the thin trabecular pattern and failure of tubulation (see Chapter 6, page 100, Chapter 1, page 15, and Fig. 169), are invariably present at the same time, particularly in the lower ends of the femora. Occasionally a more isolated oval transradiant area is seen (Fig. 224), while in some cases the cortex shows narrow bands of transradiancy within it running parallel to the bone surface.

SARCOID

A well-demarcated transradiant area in the shaft of a phalanx or the neck or shaft of a metacarpal is sometimes seen in sarcoidosis. The cyst-like area is often 3–5 millimetres in size but may be rather larger, in which case it tends to be elongated in the long axis of the bone and to appear rather trabeculated, probably because of localized indentations into the deep surface of the cortical bone (Fig. 225). After reaching a size of 1–2 centimetres the lesion does not usually progress further.

The transradiant zone may be sharply demarcated by a narrow white rim of sclerotic bone. In some cases there is one isolated lesion and in others similar transradiant areas are seen in several phalanges, metacarpals or metatarsals. More rarely a rather larger cyst-like area is seen in some bone other than those of the hand or foot and is then usually the only osseous manifestation of sarcoidosis.

The bone lesion in sarcoidosis may be symptomless and without physical signs, though occasionally there is pain and swelling of the affected finger. In most cases the bone lesion is associated with other manifestations of sarcoidosis such as irido-cyclitis, small 2–3 millimetre pink or purple skin nodules, or changes in the chest radiograph. The last of these combinations, the bone lesion with chest changes, is not common, a bone lesion being present in only about 2 per cent of cases of intrathoracic sarcoid showing enlarged hilar glands or nodular lung shadows or both.

Since the cause of the condition is generally unknown, the diagnosis rests on a clinical and radiological picture consistent with sarcoidosis, together with a particular histological picture which may be obtained from the biopsy of a skin nodule, an enlarged lymphatic gland or the liver. In the case of a

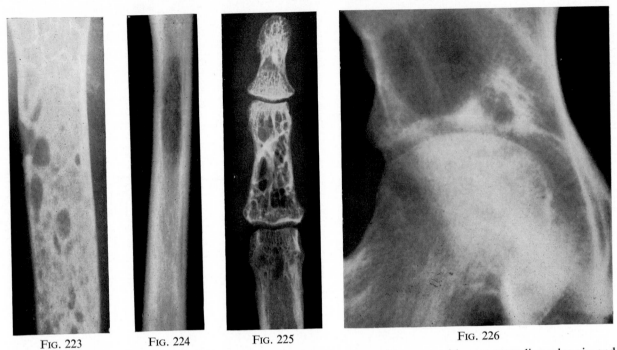

FIG. 223   FIG. 224   FIG. 225   FIG. 226

FIG. 223.—Gaucher's disease. Female aged 35 years. Small deep erosions of humerus with no surrounding sclerosis, and small cortical erosion. Similar appearances other side and in femora, which also show failure of tubulation and trabecular thinning as in Fig. 169. Splenectomy—Gaucher foam cells; also in sternal marrow.

FIG. 224.—Gaucher's disease of femur. Oval transradiant area in upper part. Cortex below split up by vertical transradiant band.

FIG. 225.—Sarcoidosis. Female aged 48 years. Transradiant areas in phalanx with no periosteal new bone. Several other phalanges showed similar changes. Recent breathlessness. Chest x-ray showed nodular shadowing. Lymph node biopsy—sarcoidosis. Mantoux 1:1,000 negative.

FIG. 226.—Tuberculous bone abscess. Female aged 20 years. Transradiant zone, 2 cm., with no sclerotic margin, in ilium above acetabulum. Pain in hip region 3 years. Contents—thick yellow pus: wall caseating tuberculous granulation tissue.

cyst-like lesion in some unusual bone site, the diagnosis may only be made on the bone biopsy. The Kveim test is not as useful for diagnosis as is histological examination of a biopsy specimen.

The Mantoux reaction is often negative but may be positive. In Great Britain the relationship between sarcoidosis and tuberculosis was often very close. Sometimes a known case of sarcoidosis will convert from a Mantoux negative to a positive reaction and eventually show tubercle bacilli in the sputum or in the cyst-like bone lesion. Conversely, a known case of tuberculosis may eventually develop the typical sarcoid type of lesion years later; in fact, calcified hilar glands are not an uncommon finding in a case of sarcoidosis. At the present time this association is less obvious.

The histological features are those of an area of bone which is completely replaced by fibrous tissue in which there are a variable number of circular foci of large pale staining epithelioid cells, with some giant cells of the Langhans type and a few lymphocytes. There is no caseation and no evidence of tubercle bacilli after Ziehl–Neelsen staining.

INFECTIVE CONDITIONS

Tuberculosis

Occasionally a tuberculous bone lesion presents as a well-demarcated 2–3 centimetre circular transradiancy with a white rim of sclerotic bone around it (Fig. 226). There is no periosteal new bone, no local decalcification of the surrounding bone and, in the case of a lesion fairly near the articular cortex, no less of density of the nearby joint space—all features of the more usual type of tuberculous bone lesion. The most common site is a phalanx, where the x-ray appearances are identical with those of a sarcoid type of lesion, but no bone is totally exempt.

The diagnosis may remain unsuspected even when the cyst-like lesion has been demonstrated radiologically. There may be no evidence of any active pulmonary tuberculous lesion and in fact a chest radiograph may appear normal, although more often there are a few small punctate or linear shadows or some dense spots of calcification indicating a probable past tuberculous lesion. The diagnosis of the bone lesion frequently depends on exploration; tubercle bacilli may be found in the contained pus, or caseating tuberculous granulation may be identified by histological examination of a part of the bone cavity wall.

Pyogenic infection

As a rule a pyogenic coccal infection will produce, in addition to the bone abscess, some surrounding sclerosis and perhaps periostitis (*see* page 176). Occasionally these latter changes are so slight that they are not recognized and the x-ray appearances are considered those of a simple cyst. Attention to the quality of the radiographs will often serve to reveal the correct diagnosis.

Fungoid infection

In coccidioidomycosis a cyst-like cavity is sometimes seen in a bone. The diagnosis can only be suggested if the patient resides in an area where this type of infection is endemic. (*See also* Chapter 8, page 165.) A cyst-like lesion in the shaft of the tibia due to cryptococcosis (torulosis) is reported by Durie and MacDonald (1961), and a destructive lesion of the fourth metatarsal by Allcock (1961).

Yaws

In yaws there may be some cyst-like erosions of a long bone.

HYDATID CYSTS

A hydatid cyst may develop in a bone and may frequently produce daughter cysts within the medulla. A single one will cause a 1–2 centimetre well-demarcated transradiant area, and multiple ones much erosion of the cancellous bone and thinning of the cortex. A favourite site is the upper third of the shaft of the femur or tibia (Fig. 227). The bone hydatid cysts, being much rarer than those of the lungs or liver, are usually seen only in parts of the world where hydatid disease is quite common.

POST-TRAUMATIC CYST-LIKE TRANSRADIANCY

Recurrent minor degrees of trauma may result in multiple, small, circular, cyst-like transradiant areas in the cancellous bone. Such transradiancies are rarely more than 3–5 millimetres in size, and may be seen in the carpal bones or the lower end of the humerus in, for example, a pneumatic drill worker.

A small (2–5 millimetre) circular transradiancy with a surrounding narrow rim of sclerotic bone is frequently seen in the scaphoid (Fig. 228) or lunate of otherwise normal persons. Whether such an appearance is the result of trauma or not is unknown, nor is the pathology of the lesion reported. Similar cyst-like transradiancies are not uncommon following a single traumatic incident to the wrist.

HAEMOPHILIA WITH HAEMORRHAGIC BONE CYST

Haemorrhage may occur deep in a bone in a case of haemophilia, presumably the result of a minor traumatic incident. This may lead to an area of bone absorption and a cyst-like space usually full of altered blood. (*See also* Haemophilia with Arthritis, page 188.)

CYST-LIKE TRANSRADIANCY IN ASSOCIATION WITH ARTHRITIS

Circular transradiances, either close below the articular cortex or a short distance away, are common in association with the diminished joint spaces of arthritis and gout (*see* Chapter 10, page 203). In most cases the clinical evidence of a joint lesion together with the diminished joint space makes the diagnosis obvious, but in a few cases the cyst-like areas are a more prominent feature than the joint lesions and their association with arthritis or gout is therefore less easily recognized.

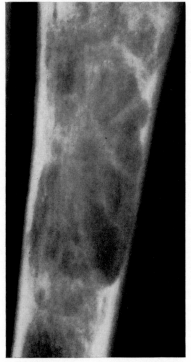

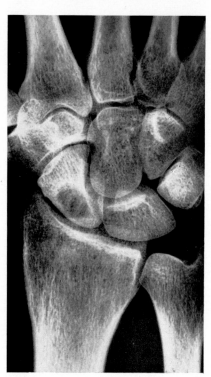

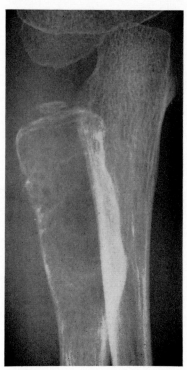

FIG. 227.—Hydatid cyst. Large area of central erosion in tibia with thinning of cortex. Extends throughout middle half. No periosteal new bone. Morbid histological proof.

FIG. 228.—Cyst in the scaphoid. Female aged 54 years. Asymptomatic. No pathology available. No change in 1 month.

FIG. 229.—Cyst of uncertain aetiology. Male aged 7 years. Transradiant area with cortical thinning and expansion of upper end of radius. Metaphysis intact; no periosteal thickening. Contents—blood-stained fluid; wall—no lining, normal bone.

In osteoarthritis of the hip joint, in addition to the diminished joint space and marginal lipping, quite a large (1–2 centimetre) cyst-like, circular or oval transradiancy with a rim of sclerotic bone is not uncommon in the ilium just above the acetabulum (Fig 320) and in the femoral head. A smaller circular transradiancy is very common in osteoarthritis of the first metacarpal–trapezium joint or the metatarso-phalangeal joint of the great toe (*see* Fig. 323), and may be seen in either of the two bones a few millimetres deep to the articular cortex.

In rheumatoid arthritis, 2–8 millimetre cystic erosions are commonly seen in addition to the narrowed joint spaces, marginal erosions and general loss of bone density. They are sometimes surrounded by a rim of sclerotic bone and may lie several millimetres away from the joint itself. They are seen particularly in the bones of the hands.

Occasionally, quite a large well-demarcated transradiant zone is seen close to a joint although the joint space is normal and there is no certain clinical evidence of arthritis (*see* Fig. 313).

Such a cyst-like transradiant area may be the sole evidence of rheumatoid arthritis for a time, the diagnosis being later confirmed by the development of the classical radiographic or clinical evidence of the condition in that or in some other joints, or by a synovial biopsy.

In gout the clearly-demarcated transradiant area of the urate deposit may be seen in a bone either with or without x-ray evidence of arthritis. It tends to lie close to the joint but may be several millimetres away. The transradiancy is usually circular, very clearly defined and some 3–5 millimetres in size. There is often no surrounding rim of sclerotic bone and the lesion looks as if it has been simply punched out of the bone (Figs. 325 and 326). Common sites are the heads of the first metatarsals and the phalanges.

The histology of these cysts varies in the three conditions. In osteoarthritis the sclerotic subchondral bone frequently shows cysts containing a viscid fluid with no soft tissue present, or jelly-like material consisting of oedematous fibrous tissue, or fatty marrow as described by Collins (1949).

In rheumatoid arthritis the "cyst" is usually composed of granulation tissue or fibrous tissue containing lymphocytic aggregations similar to those seen in the pannus found in the joint space. If the transradiant area is large (Fig. 313), it may contain grey or yellow viscid fluid.

In gout the transradiant area in the bone is occupied by tissue which consists of collections of sodium blurate crystals in a fibrous stroma with foreign-body giant cells walling off the crystalline material.

WELL-DEMARCATED TRANSRADIANT AREA WITH CORTICAL THINNING AND GROSS BONE EXPANSION

Many of the cyst-like areas mentioned in the previous section will, if they increase in size, encroach on the cortex, which will first be thinned by absorption and may eventually appear expanded to a greater or lesser degree. The appearance of cortical expansion is often misleading, since the white line of expanded bone overlying the transradiant area of the cyst or tumour usually represents new periosteal bone at the tumour margin rather than the original cortical bone, the latter having become absorbed.

This bone expansion may remain slight or increase until it becomes gross. As a general guide, it usually remains slight in most of the cysts of uncertain origin, in many fibrous dysplasias, in xanthomatous granulomas and in the infections. In some of the cysts, in some developmental defects and in most of the tumours as they enlarge, the cortical thinning and bone expansion may become just as conspicuous a feature as the well-demarcated cyst-like area beneath them.

The most common cause of gross bone expansion round a well-demarcated transradiant area is an osteoclastoma or a solitary plasmacytoma.

SIMPLE CYST OF UNCERTAIN ORIGIN

Simple cysts of uncertain origin, in which bone expansion was not a prominent feature, have been described on page 117. Occasionally a cyst of uncertain origin is seen with considerable expansion of the bone. This may be fusiform (Fig. 229) or more rounded as in Fig. 230. In either case there is a complete covering of dense bone over the transradiant central area, while the trabecular pattern beyond this is quite normal.

HYPERPARATHYROIDISM (OSTEITIS FIBROSA CYSTICA)

A hypertransradiant area with an intact rim of dense bone over it, causing gross expansion of the bone contour, may be seen in some cases of hyperparathyroidism. The most common site is towards the end of a major long bone of a limb, but the lesion may also be seen in a rib. The x-ray appearances are the same as those of an advanced osteoclastoma (see, for example, Fig. 236), but in hyperparathyroidism there will always be additional trabecular or cortical absorption in some other bones (see Chapter 6, page 106, and Chapter 7, page 119).

DEVELOPMENTAL DEFECTS

Monostotic fibrous dysplasia

In many cases of monostotic fibrous dysplasia with cortical involvement there is either no bone expansion or very little, but in others, especially those in the upper third of a femur or the anterior end of a rib, in addition to the transradiant area there is gross expansion.

In the case of a rib the lesion is well demarcated laterally, but antero-medially the mass of fibrous tissue may spread out to occupy a space several times wider than that of the rib end. The mass of tissue may be sufficiently great to cast a shadow in relation to the transradiant lung beneath, and this will obscure any bone transradiancy that might otherwise have been visible (Fig. 231). There may be no clearly defined dense line of bone around the margins of this low-density shadow, but strands of calcium-containing tissue may be superimposed on it.

A lesion in the upper end of a femur tends to be large. Since the fibrous area is not as strong as normal bone, there is often some deformity of the femoral neck and upper third of the shaft as well as cortical thinning and bone expansion (Fig. 207).

In a lesion of the ilium there will often be evidence of bone expansion on palpation which is not seen in the plane of a single posterior-view radiograph (Fig. 208).

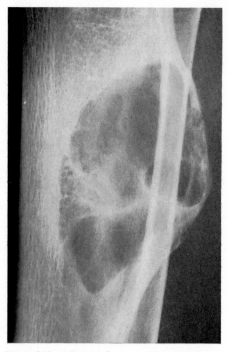

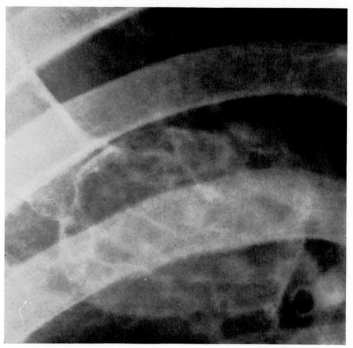

FIG. 230.—Cyst of uncertain aetiology. Female aged 18 years. Five cm. transradiant area in middle third of tibia with cortical thinning and expansion. Contents—brown fluid (altered blood); wall —cellular fibrous tissue and a few osteoclasts.

FIG. 231.—Fibrous dysplasia. Male aged 41 years. Erosion of anterior end of right third rib with low density 5 cm. shadow and a few strands of dense bone running across it. Cellular vascular fibrous tissue, bony spicules, osteoblasts and osteoclasts; fibrous dysplasia.

Giant-cell tumour variants

In the giant-cell variants (*see* page 125), the amount of bone expansion is generally less than in an osteoclastoma which they may otherwise so closely resemble. An aneurysmal bone cyst of a long bone or vertebra is sometimes associated with bone expansion. The cortex is absorbed and there is a thin shell of new bone over the expanded area. This appearance is described by Barnes (1956).

Chondroma

A chondroma may grow sufficiently to cause cortical thinning and eventual gross bone expansion (Fig. 232). It can be seen most commonly in a phalanx, but may occur in any other bone arising from cartilage. If it lies centrally the expansion may be symmetrical on both sides, giving the bone a spindle shape, but if it is eccentric the expansion may be confined entirely to one side. The presence of tell-tale calcifications, appearing either as small spots or as larger amorphous masses within the transradiant area (Figs. 216 and 233), will give the diagnosis, although these are not always present.

NEOPLASM

Osteoclastoma

Although an osteoclastoma is occasionally seen at an early stage as a cyst-like transradiancy deep in the bone (Fig. 218), its growth is rapid and its most usual x-ray appearance, when first seen, is that of an area of localized bone absorption with either a thinned cortex or advanced bone expansion around it. The central area, though sometimes evenly transradiant due to an even trabecular absorption, is more often crossed by a few narrow band-like shadows of residual bony strands which give it a very characteristic foam-like appearance (Fig. 234). At no stage does a barrier of sclerotic bone form between the transradiant tumour and the normal bone adjacent to it.

The cortex adjacent to the transradiant area is first thinned by resorption of its deep surface. As the tumour grows further, the cortex is totally absorbed and replaced by a thin layer of "periosteal" new

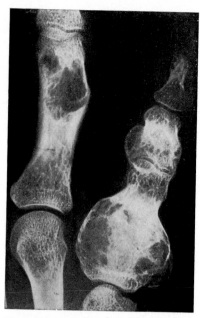

FIG. 232.—Multiple enchondromas in the fingers. Central transradiant area with stippling, cortical thinning and expansion of the shaft. Another finger in the same case (Fig. 216a) showed less expansion, while in yet others there was no stippling in some of the transradiant areas with no trabeculae.

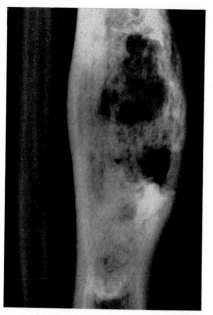

FIG. 233.—Chondroma. Male aged 28 years. Transradiant area 15 cm. long with cortical thinning and expansion in the middle third of the tibia, with areas of increased density within it. Crack fracture at this site 15 years previously. Lump first noticed 7 years ago, now larger. Tumour scraped out and replaced with chip grafts. Biopsy —chondroma.

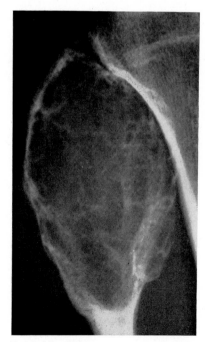

FIG. 234.—Osteoclastoma. Female aged 22 years. Transradiant area 8 cm. long with cortical thinning and expansion of upper end of fibula. Slight pain 3 years, swelling 18 months. Biopsy—osteoclastoma.

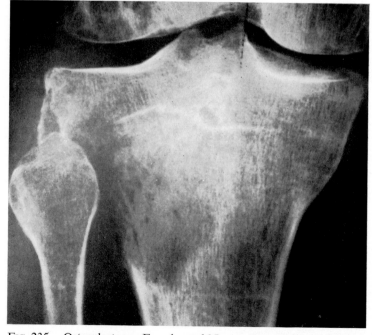

FIG. 235.—Osteoclastoma. Female aged 35 years. Transradiant area 5 cm. long, extending from the articular cortex of the upper end of the tibia across the epiphyseal disc and into the diaphysis. Some erosion of the cortex laterally. Pain 7 weeks. Biopsy—osteoclastoma Grade II.

bone which sharply demarcates the outer margin of the expanded tumour. In some cases a part of the thinned cortex may be totally absorbed before the new bone formation has begun (Fig. 235), but usually the stage of cortical destruction is masked by the formation of new bone just outside and there is a complete white rim of bone over the tumour throughout all stages of its growth (Figs. 234 and 236). Since the lesion tends to lie near the end of the bone, the tumour soon reaches the dense line of the articular cortex, but this is rarely eroded.

If the tumour is placed eccentrically the bone expansion is one on side only, if centrally on both sides, and in either case the tumour eventually extends outwards for a considerable distance beyond the original line of the cortex. An expansion of 1–2 centimetres is usually sufficient for the patient to notice a swelling and seek medical attention, but in a neglected case the tumour continues to grow until the expanded area has reached a size of 10 or more centimetres before it is first seen in a radiograph. Even at this late stage there is usually a thin line of osseous tissue forming the outer margin of the tumour. This line may remain complete, but in some cases gaps appear in it as the tumour enlarges. Such gaps are not necessarily indicative of the aggressive nature of the tumour or of some special type of tumour.

Common sites for an osteoclastoma are the lower or upper end of the femur, the upper end of the tibia and the lower end of the radius; less common sites are the upper end of the humerus, the fibula and the lower end of the tibia, the pelvis, the scapula, and even a vertebral body. Other bones could be affected but very rarely are. It is doubtful whether this tumour occurs in the mandible, though sometimes the histological report gives this diagnosis for what is probably some other lesion.

An osteoclastoma is usually seen in the age group between 20 and 40 years and is not as common as might be supposed from its well-known x-ray appearances, especially if all the giant-cell tumour variants which simulate it are excluded.

Histology

Histologically the osteoclastoma or giant-cell tumour of bone consists of a cellular stroma composed of oval, spindle or round cells together with many giant cells of the osteoclast type. Unlike the many "giant-cell tumour variants" which can simulate it, fibrous tissue, bone formation, foam cells, cartilage or areas of cystic degeneration do not form an integral part of the tumour.

Prognosis

The prognosis following treatment is very variable. Osteoclastomas have been graded by Jaffe, Lichtenstein and Portis (1940) by the regularity and cytological appearances of the stroma, but although the aggressive-looking lesions in Grade III with an almost sarcomatous-looking stroma tend to have a poorer prognosis than those in Grades I and II, this is not always the case.

Many lesions show a strong tendency to local recurrence if treated by radiotherapy or curettage, though little tendency to remote metastases. A few, on the other hand, have identical radiological and histological features and yet produce early metastases, especially in the lungs (Fig. 217). Local treatment by radiotherapy or curettage is unsatisfactory in about 50 per cent of cases if the so-called giant-cell variants (*see* page 125) are excluded. A local recurrence or a definite malignancy may not be apparent until some 10 years after such treatment.

A peculiar feature is the intense trabecular absorption often seen some 6 weeks after radiotherapy (Fig. 237). This may be mistaken for gross malignant aggressiveness, but in most cases considerable recalcification takes place some 6–12 weeks later (Fig. 238). There is some danger of a spontaneous fracture during the stage of intense bone resorption. As a rule the remineralization is incomplete, and from one of the residual eroded areas new foci of bone erosion are apt to develop with the tumour consequently beginning to increase in size again.

Solitary plasmacytoma

A well-demarcated transradiant area with considerable expansion of the surrounding bone is seen in some solitary plasmacytomas. The expansion tends to be less abrupt and rather more spindle-shaped (Fig. 239) than in an osteoclastoma, and the central area less trabeculated or foam-like though sometimes crossed by residual bony sheets. The positive clinical features and the course of the disease are referred to in Chapter 6, page 111.

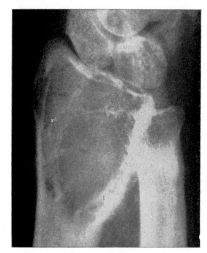
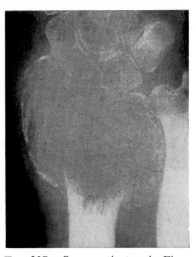
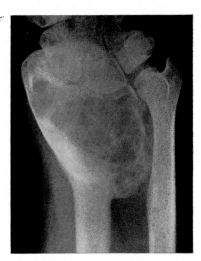

FIG. 236.—Osteoclastoma. Male aged 39 years. Transradiant zone 4 cm. long in submetaphyseal region of radius, with white lines of remaining strands of bone running across it and giving it a foam-like appearance. Cortical thinning and slight expansion. Pain in wrist 1 month. Biopsy—typical Grade II osteoclastoma with spindle-celled stroma and osteoclasts.

FIG. 237.—Same patient as in Fig. 236, 2 months after completion of radiotherapy (2,000 r units over 4 weeks; 250 kVP; 1 mm. Cu/Al filter). This has resulted in a great increase in the erosion, absorption of part of the metaphysis and overlying cortex and some expansion, in part due to compression collapse with shortening of the radius.

FIG. 238.—Same patient as in Figs. 236 and 237, 18 months later. Considerable recalcification with line of metaphysis and outer covering line reconstituted. Further erosion occurred 18 months later, so removal of the lower end of the radius and grafting were carried out.

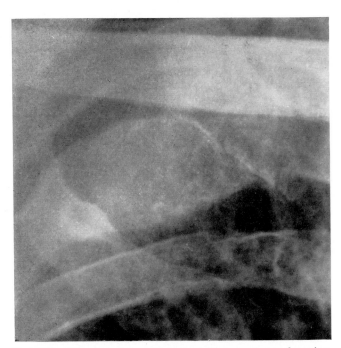

FIG. 239.—Plasmacytoma. Male aged 35 years. Area of erosion 5 cm. long in posterior third of right fifth rib, with cortical thinning and expansion. Same case as Fig. 186. Two years later deposits were present in other bones. *Post mortem*—generalized myelomatous deposits in the bones.

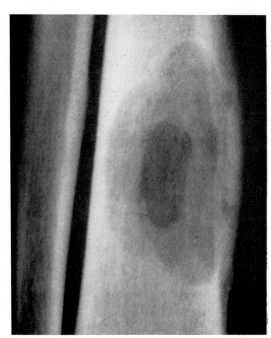

FIG. 240.—Secondary deposit. Male aged 72 years. Well-demarcated oval transradiant area 5 cm. long in the middle third of the tibia without a sclerotic margin and with slight expansion. Hypernephroma 5 years ago. Erosive lesions in other bones and secondary deposits in lungs.

Secondary deposit

Rather uncommonly, some new bone may form over an osseous secondary deposit, resulting in a well-demarcated transradiant area with some bone expansion (Fig. 240). The degree of bone expansion is usually slight.

INFECTION

Tuberculosis of a phalanx

Central erosion with gross expansion of a phalanx, which becomes spindle-shaped, may be the result of a tuberculous dactylitis. The thin outer rim is periosteal new bone, and the lesion is referred to in Chapter 8, page 164, and illustrated in Fig. 273.

WELL-DEMARCATED EROSION OF THE SURFACE OF A BONE

PRESSURE EROSION

Pressure from occupation or nearby bone tumour

A surface erosion of a bone which extends down into the cancellous bone with a clear-cut margin, usually with a narrow rim of sclerotic bone forming its base, is most commonly the result of pressure from either an external or an internal source. A small surface erosion of this kind may be seen as a result of repeated pressure from a wire or string, such as may occur in hat making (Fig. 241). A pressure erosion may be seen adjacent to a benign tumour of a neighbouring bone, and in such a case the exciting cause is obvious. An osteoma of the tibia pressing on and causing erosion of the fibula is an example of this. On the other hand the erosion may be caused by pressure from a radiologically invisible tumour, such as a chondroma, in which the eroded area is clear-cut and sharply demarcated, or a fibrosarcoma or synovioma of the nearby tissues, in which a very superficial cortical indentation is seen (Fig. 242).

Pressure from an aneurysm

An erosion may also be caused by pressure from an aneurysm and is commonly seen in the sternum or vertebrae with an aortic aneurysm. In the sternum the indentation is well-demarcated with a rim or sclerotic bone. In the vertebrae, where the intervertebral disc and cartilage are more resistant to the pounding than the bone, a concave indentation is seen in the anterior or lateral aspect of the vertebral body. This is sharply demarcated by a narrow rim of dense sclerotic bone and may be seen in two of three adjacent vertebrae. If the aneurysm is in the thorax its low-density shadow will suggest the cause of the erosion, but an aneurysm of the abdominal aorta, which may also cause pressure erosions, may be invisible in the plain radiograph.

Pressure from a neurilemmoma, ganglioneuroma or dilated intercostal arteries

A neurilemmoma (neurofibroma) or a ganglioneuroma may cause a similar pressure erosion in a vertebral body or a shallow cortical pressure erosion in a rib. In multiple neurofibromatosis, concave indentations may be seen in several adjacent vertebral bodies (Fig. 243). Again, if the mass is in the thorax it will cast a separate shadow, but if in the abdomen it is unlikely to be visible in the radiograph.

The notching of the under-surface of the middle ribs as a result of the dilated intercostal arteries in coarctation of the aorta is another example of pressure erosion.

Intervertebral disc intrusion (Schmorl node)

A semilunar surface erosion of the upper or lower surface of the body of a vertebra is characteristic of pressure erosion from intrusion of an intervertebral disc into the vertebral body.

The erosion is sharply demarcated from the bone beneath by a linear shadow of sclerotic bone, and is commonly only a few millimetres in size, though it may reach one centimetre or more. When large there is usually associated narrowing of the disc space, since most of the disc substances will lie in the pit in the vertebral body, and the appearances may simulate a tuberculous lesion. The rim of dense bone and the absence of a paravertebral shadow and of clinical evidence of disease will usually serve to differentiate the two conditions.

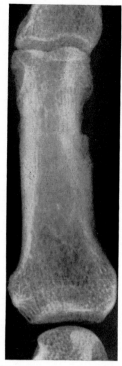

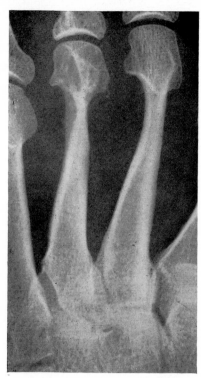

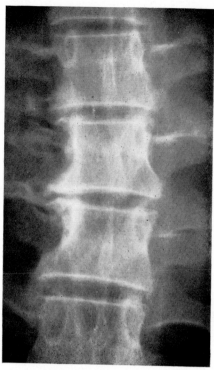

FIG. 241. — Pressure erosion. Male aged 55 years. Surface erosion of medial side of proximal phalanx the right fifth finger. Occupation hat making, during which a thin string presses against this finger.

FIG. 242.—Pressure erosion by fibrosarcoma of the soft tissues. Narrowing of necks and slight separation of distal ends of second and third metatarsals from tumour in the surrounding soft tissues. Biopsy—fibrosarcoma.

FIG. 243.—Pressure erosion in neurofibromatosis. Female aged 41 years. Concave indentation of the right side of the body of the eighth and ninth dorsal vertebrae. The cortical line is intact. The pressure is from adjacent neurofibromas. Cutaneous neurofibromas also present, the condition being familial. Radiographed because of weakness of legs.

The small type of disc intrusion is a common finding in many otherwise normal persons. It is asymptomatic and rarely shows any increase in size once it has been seen in a radiograph.

It is now known, as a result of the routine post-mortem examination of the spine, that Schmorl's nodes or nuclear prolapses are extremely common (Beadle, 1931). The protrusion of the nucleus pulposus into the substance of the vertebral body will often pass unnoticed in a radiograph in the early stages, until later in its development some reactive sclerosis stops its further protuberance and clearly demarcates the area of erosion. (*See also* page 57.)

DEVELOPMENTAL DEFECT AND IMPLANTATION DERMOID

A poorly-demarcated surface indentation of the bone may be caused by a developmental defect, particularly a superficial chondroma (Fig. 244). In the tip of a terminal phalanx the pathology may be that of an implantation dermoid.

HYPERPARATHYROIDISM

Well or poorly demarcated subperiosteal erosions of the cortex of a phalanx are seen in hyperparathyroidism and are described in detail on page 120. Other bones may show similar appearances, particularly the upper end of the tibia (*see* Fig. 205).

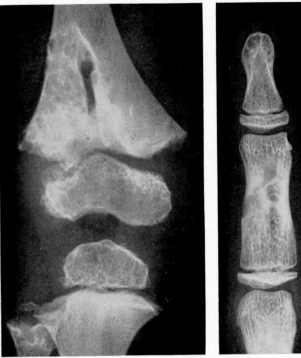

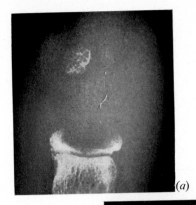

(a)

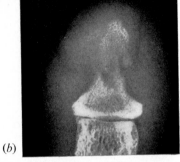

(b)

FIG. 244.—Dyschondroplasia (Ollier's disease). Surface indentation. Male aged 8 years. Superficial chondroma with surface indentation of the side of the phalanx.

FIG. 245.—Osteomyelitis. Male aged 62 years. (a) Acute phase of the infection with erosion of the terminal phalanx and no periosteal new bone. (b) Bone regeneration after control of the infection with the help of antibiotics. Still no periosteal new bone.

URATE DEPOSIT

A well-demarcated surface erosion some 3–8 millimetres in size may be due to a urate deposit (Fig. 325). Such an appearance is seen mainly in the bones of the hands or feet, but occasionally in the elbow (olecranon) or knee region. It is associated with the more characteristic central transradiancies of other urate deposits described on page 203.

RHEUMATOID ARTHRITIS

A surface erosion some distance from the joint, involving both the cortex and the cancellous bone, is sometimes seen beneath a subcutaneous rheumatoid nodule. Generally the clinical findings and the typical appearances of rheumatoid arthritis in other joints will make the diagnosis obvious (Fig. 304).

SURFACE ABSORPTION OF THE TIP OF A TERMINAL PHALANX

Absorption of the distal end of a terminal phalanx is a fairly common form of well-demarcated surface erosion which falls into a category of its own. It may be seen as a result of a pyogenic inflammatory lesion, a leprosy infection, a traumatic amputation, a vascular lesion, a neuropathic disorder, rheumatoid arthritis, hyperparathyroidism, or a developmental defect.

Pyogenic infection

In a pyogenic infection, which is often the result of a local spread of a pulp infection, the erosion of the tip of the terminal phalanx is often without any visible periosteal new bone formation. The diagnosis is usually obvious because of the sudden onset of local pain and swelling.

Leprosy

Absorption of the tip of the terminal phalanx is a common finding in leprosy, and several fingers and toes (Fig. 246) are usually affected. The diagnosis will be obvious from the slow progress of the lesions, the emaciated and ulcerated appearance of the soft parts, and the fact that the disease is endemic in certain parts of the world. The absorption is usually the result of a neglected non-specific infection superimposed on a neurotrophic disorder (Paterson, 1961).

Trauma

After a traumatic amputation of the tip of a phalanx, the remaining bone usually has a flatter surface than is achieved by bone absorption. The history will make the diagnosis obvious.

Vascular disorders and diffuse systemic sclerosis (scleroderma)

Absorption of the tip of one or more terminal phalanges is a common manifestation of certain disorders of the circulation such as primary Raynaud's phenomena of unknown cause (Fig. 247), secondary Raynaud's phenomena due to diffuse systemic sclerosis (Fig. 248), occlusive vascular disease with or without Raynaud's phenomena, and traumatic vascular disease.

In all these disorders the erosion is well demarcated and the remaining bone is usually covered with a narrow rim of dense bone (Fig. 248). There may be associated foci of calcification in the nearby tissues, particularly anteriorly in the pulp. In the early stages both bone absorption and the associated calcifications are best seen in a true lateral view, so that each finger in turn should be placed in a lateral position and radiographed either on a small separate film or on a small separate area of a single long film.

In primary Raynaud's phenomena, perhaps due to overaction of the sympathetic nerves, the vascular disturbance with blueness of the fingers is a well-marked and often long-established feature by the time the bone absorption is seen on a radiograph. In diffuse systemic sclerosis, although the Raynaud type of

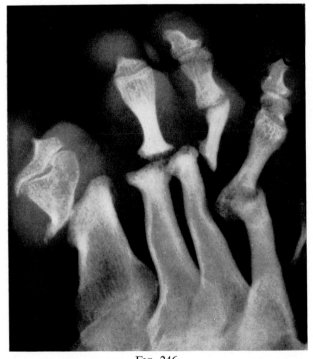
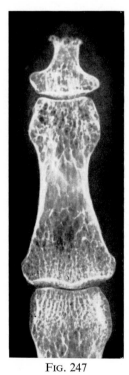
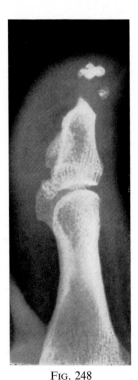

FIG. 246   FIG. 247   FIG. 248

FIG. 246.—Leprosy. Absorption of phalanges and no periosteal new bone.

FIG. 247.—Raynaud phenomena. Female aged 56 years. Absorption of tip of phalanx. Same change in all fingers of both hands. Cracks in fingers and nails and fingers blue and cold 30 years.

FIG. 248.—Diffuse systemic sclerosis. Female aged 33 years. Erosion of tip of phalanx and calcification in the pulp. Fingers blue and cold for 10 years. Cervical sympathectomy performed. Oesophagus wide and inert, colon pouchings. Later, scleroderma of face and arms.

phenomena may sometimes be conspicuous when the bone erosion is first seen, it is more usual for the blueness of the finger tips and the other cutaneous manifestations to appear several years later. Associated calcifications in the surrounding soft parts are relatively rare in primary Raynaud's phenomena and comparatively common in diffuse systemic sclerosis whether associated with blueness of the fingers or not.

When differentiation between these two conditions is difficult, a careful search should be made for other manifestations of diffuse systemic sclerosis, particularly in the skin or alimentary tract. An x-ray examination of the oesophagus with the patient lying down is particularly useful, since normal oesophageal contractions are seen in primary Raynaud's phenomena, whereas if the oesophagus is fibrotic from diffuse systemic sclerosis there are no oesophageal contractions. If the patient is examined standing up, a barium drink will pass down rapidly into the stomach, but if he is examined lying down, the barium will remain in the inert and often somewhat dilated oesophagus until he stands up. In some cases of diffuse systemic sclerosis the oesophagus is normal but atonic inert areas are seen in the colon. These are best demonstrated by a radiograph taken after the evacuation of a barium enema, when the normal areas will be seen to contract down, leaving the inert areas protruding out as 1–2 cm. pouch-like shadows.

Occlusive vascular disease with or without Raynaud's phenomena will usually be obvious clinically. If not, an arteriogram will show the site of the vascular narrowing or occlusion as well as the degree of deficiency of the circulation distal to it, in contrast to the normal vascular pattern seen in primary Raynaud's phenomena.

In a traumatic vascular lesion the cause of the bone absorption will usually be evident from the clinical history of trauma, such as severance of the digital vessels or frost-bite. The bone absorption becomes visible a few weeks after such an incident.

Neuropathic disorders

Absorption of the tip of a terminal phalanx may also be seen in some neuropathies such as diabetic neuritis, tabes, syringomyelia and so on. Sometimes it is difficult to determine how much of the change is neuropathic, how much vascular and how much due to superadded infection through an intact skin.

Rheumatoid arthritis

Absorption of the tip, the proximal end or all of the terminal phalanx may occur in rheumatoid arthritis, this unusual manifestation being described as arthritis mutilans (*see* Fig. 315).

Hyperparathyroidism

In severe cases of hyperparathyroidism with bone involvement there may be cortical and subcortical loss of density of the tips of the phalanges, so much so that they may appear eroded (*see* Figs. 203 and 204). The tips may reappear after successful treatment (*see* Fig. 204).

Developmental defect

Poor development of the distal ends of the terminal phalanges may result in an x-ray appearance similar to that of bone absorption. The end of the bone is absent, and the remaining edge is either sharply pointed or concave with a central indentation. A developmental defect of this kind may be isolated or part of a craniocleidodysostosis. A rather similar appearance is sometimes associated with a grossly swollen finger tip in Maffucci's syndrome (Fig. 340).

Surface Erosion of the Articular Cortex—Osteochondritis Dissecans

A small, 3–8 millimetre erosion of the articular cortex with a normal joint space may be due to a local avascular necrosis (osteochondritis dissecans). The erosion is half-moon shaped, and clearly demarcated from the adjacent normal trabeculae by a narrow 1 millimetre white line of dense bone. In the early stages the lesion may be seen as a semi-circular erosion 2 millimetres wide isolating off a piece of bone facing the articular surface. This central fragment is a sequestrum and may be absorbed or extruded into the joint, where it will be seen as a loose body (Fig. 249). With the disappearance of the sequestrum, the half-moon shaped erosion is clearly visible.

Such a lesion is most common in the condyle of the lower end of the femur, but may also occur in the posterior aspect of the patella or the lower end of the humerus, especially in the capitulum. A rather uncommon site is the upper articular surface of the talus. Once the sequestrum is eliminated by absorption or as a loose body, no further erosion develops. Histological examination of the abnormal area shows the half-moon shaped tissue to be composed of dead bone with disappearance of the osteocytes from the bone trabeculae, but, by contrast, the articular cartilage survives and the cartilage cells appear viable due to their source of nutrition from the joint itself.

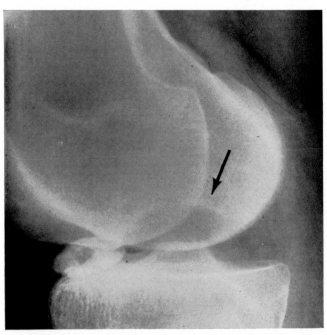

FIG. 249.—Osteochondritis dissecans. Male aged 31 years. Half-moon transradiant area (opposite arrow) from which necrotic fragment separated into joint, visible anteriorly just above tibia, and was later removed. Pain and swelling in knee 4 years; recently locking.

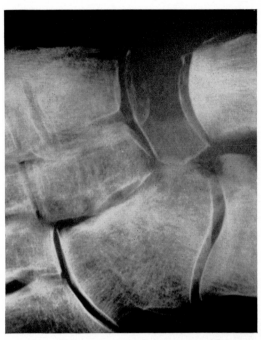

FIG. 250.—Myelomatosis. Female aged 64 years. Surface and deep erosion of the navicular with normal joint space. Also erosion deep in the radius, and later in dorsal vertebrae. Pain in elbow and foot and loss of weight. Sternal marrow biopsy—myelomatosis.

POORLY-DEMARCATED TRANSRADIANT AREA WITHIN THE BONE

The distinction between a well-demarcated and a poorly-demarcated transradiant area within a bone is very obvious in extreme cases, when the latter has no continuous outline or clearly defined limits and the former has a clear-cut outline and often a conspicuous rim of dense bone, but in borderline cases it is often not possible to place a lesion in either of these radiological groups with complete certainty.

The most common cause of a poorly-demarcated transradiant area within a bone is a secondary deposit, and this is very likely to be the diagnosis if the patient is known to have a primary malignant neoplasm elsewhere. A similar appearance may also be produced by a primary neoplasm in the bone, a haemangioma, a xanthomatous granuloma, an unusual manifestation of tuberculosis and, if the lesion is small, a fibrous dysplasia.

MALIGNANT NEOPLASM—PRIMARY BONE OR SECONDARY DEPOSIT

Early changes

A secondary deposit or a primary neoplasm in the bone, if seen at an early stage, often appears as a circular or oval transradiant zone a few millimetres in size, which may be fairly clear-cut but is not sharply demarcated from the surrounding trabeculae. Unless the radiograph is inspected with care, such a lesion may be missed. An erosion in the region of an ischio-pubic ramus or neck of a femur may be attributed to differences in the transradiancy of the overlying soft tissue shadows, such as fat or muscle bundles, or to alimentary tract gas transradiancies. Inspection of the area with a magnifying glass will often show whether the trabecular pattern continues normally in the transradiant area or whether, as in the case of a bone erosion, it stops short. Alimentary tract gas transradiancies tend to be inconstant if the radiograph is repeated, even after a relatively short interval, with an intervening change of posture or a meal. In a chest radiograph a small erosion in a rib may be missed because the attention of the observer is concentrated on the lungs. An erosion in the ilium may be masked by the wing of the sacrum, but will be seen easily if the cortical line and trabecular pattern are scanned with special care. Erosion of the pedicle of a vertebra by a secondary deposit may also pass without being noticed; in this site the integrity of the oval ring shadow of each pedicle should be individually confirmed, so that its absence on one side in one vertebra may be detected (Figs. 251 and 327).

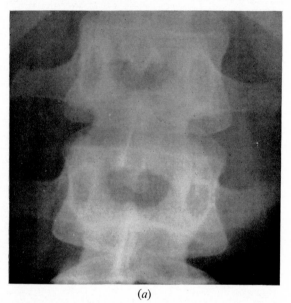
(a)

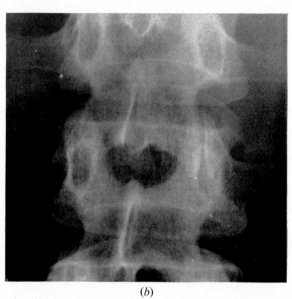
(b)

Fig. 251.—(a) Normal second lumbar vertebra. Bilateral oval line shadows of pedicles of L. 2. (b) Same case 1 year later. Disappearance of oval shadow of pedicle on left side from secondary deposit.

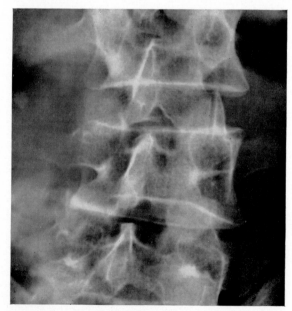

Fig. 252.—Secondary deposit. Erosion on right side of pedicle and cortex of body of L. 4.

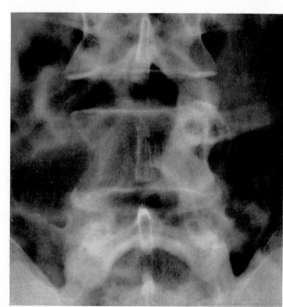

Fig. 253.—Aneurysmal bone cyst. Erosion on right side of pedicle and cortex of body of L. 4. Biopsy proof.

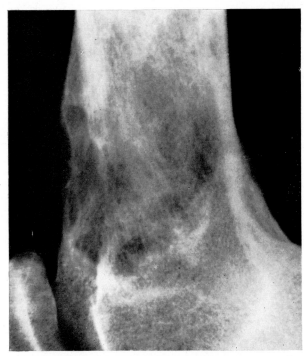

Fig. 254.—Fibrosarcoma. Male aged 65 years. Radio-graphed because of persistent swelling after injury 9 weeks previously. Ill-defined erosion of surface and deeper layers of the lower end of the femur for 8 cm. Biopsy—fibrosarcoma.

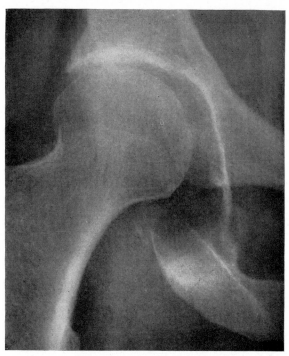

Fig. 255.—Synovioma. Female aged 28 years. Erosion of lower part of the acetabulum. Weakness of hip 6 months; pain 3 months. Exploration showed large tumour near joint invading bone; biopsy—synovioma.

Quite commonly, in bone secondary deposits, malignant cells are present in the marrow spaces and any destruction of the adjacent trabeculae is too slight to be detected in a radiograph. The presence of secondary deposits can frequently be deduced from isotope studies whether the deposits are asympto-matic or are causing bone pain. Confirmation of the diagnosis is often possible since, unless the condition is treated or sometimes even if it is treated, bone erosions will become visible in the radiograph some weeks or months later.

An ill-defined erosion in the base of the skull in the region of the jugular foramen or the base of the sphenoid may be due to a glomus tumour or to direct invasion by a pharyngeal tumour.

Later changes

Since a malignant tumour tends to grow fairly rapidly, the transradiant zone is often one or more centimetres in size by the time it is first seen in a radiograph (Figs. 250 and 254), although it can vary in size from a few millimetres to several centimetres. It is often roughly circular or oval in shape, and if in a long bone its long axis will be parallel to the shaft. It may be confined to the cancellous bone for a time, but tends to cause some absorption of the cortex as it enlarges (Fig. 256). It is usually less well defined than the cyst-like lesions, and the margins are formed by the surrounding unabsorbed trabeculae, the eroded ends of which appear as short fine-line shadows pointing towards the eroded area. There is no sclerosis of the surrounding bone and no periosteal new bone formation. There may be one or there may be several such ill-defined erosions in the same bone (Fig. 256) or in many bones. When multiple as in some secondary deposits, the individual lesions may also vary greatly in size. In multiple myelomatosis, sometimes a very large erosion of several centimetres is associated with many much smaller ones, that is, with a background of patchy areas of trabecular loss; while in multiple secondary deposits from a carcinoma, if one lesion is very large, the range of variation in the size of the other large deposits tends to be greater, and there may or may not be a background of multiple small erosions.

Common sites for these erosions whether single or multiple are the pelvis, femora, humeri, vertebrae and ribs, though such a lesion may be seen in any bone and in any part of a bone. It is very rare in the

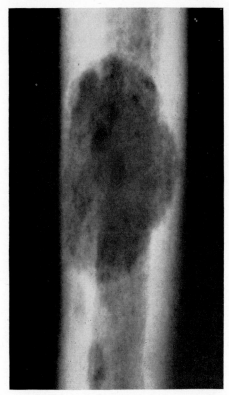

FIG. 256.—Secondary deposits in femur. Male aged 63 years. Deep erosion scalloping out deep layer of cortex, smaller erosion below. Recent leg pain; primary carcinoma of bronchus.

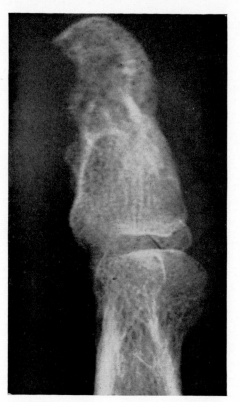

FIG. 257.—Malignant melanoma of skin. Male aged 49 years. Erosion of terminal phalanx by local extension of neoplasm.

bones of a hand or foot, but occasionally an erosion of a phalanx in a foot may be seen when a local neoplasm such as a carcinoma or melanoma of the skin invades the bone by direct extension (Fig. 257).

A malignant lesion near the end of a bone may cause destruction of the articular cortex, but the cartilage is not usually invaded or the joint space narrowed. Occasionally, however, the articular cartilage or, in the case of a vertebral secondary deposit, the intervertebral disc may herniate through the partly destroyed articular cortex or the vertebral end plate into the soft neoplastic mass beneath, causing narrowing of the joint or disc space.

Another consequence of widespread neoplastic invasion is weakening of the bone. This may result in the development of pressure deformities such as the compression collapse of the body of a vertebra (Fig. 40) or the bending of a long bone. A spontaneous fracture is also not uncommon, and the periosteal callus resulting from this may simulate a bone reaction to the tumour (*see* page 166).

Pathology

The underlying pathology is most commonly a secondary deposit from a primary carcinoma in some other site such as the breast, bronchus, alimentary tract or urinary tract. Less commonly it may be a secondary deposit from a carcinoma elsewhere, a myelomatous deposit or, in an adult, a leukaemic deposit. Identical x-ray appearances may be caused by a primary bone tumour, particularly a fibrosarcoma (Fig. 254). A synovioma (Fig. 255) may cause a similar area of bone erosion by direct spread from the synovial membrane into the nearby bone. In a Ewing's type of sarcoma or in an osteosarcoma this type of deep, poorly-demarcated bone erosion is an unusual manifestation, the more usual appearance being a poorly-defined erosion with new bone formation (*see* page 166). It may be caused by a deposit in Hodgkin's disease.

Histologically the eroded area is occupied by the neoplastic cellular masses. Three types of change may be seen at the bone margin as possible mechanisms for the bone absorption. There may be an excess of osteoclasts, suggesting that these have been goaded into activity by the neoplastic cells; there may be only neoplastic cells, suggesting that these are in some way responsible for the bone resorption; or there may be fibroblasts between the neoplastic cells and the bone providing another possible agent responsible for the bone resorption.

FIBROUS DYSPLASIA

In some cases of monostotic fibrous dysplasia, the defect in the bone occupies only a small area a few millimetres long and is often rather poorly demarcated. Although such a lesion is generally seen only in an older child or a young adult, there is no reason to suppose that it may not persist until a later age.

Its relatively slow rate of progression and freedom from symptoms help to distinguish it from a malignant bone neoplasm, but there is always the possibility of its being mistaken for a primary neoplasm or for a secondary deposit of which the primary lesion has not yet been detected. Occasionally pain may be present from some nearby unrelated lesion which itself does not produce any changes in the radiograph, such as a tenosynovitis or synovitis of a nearby joint, and this may lead to confusion with a neoplasm. The more extensive type of fibrous dysplasia described on page 124 will rarely be confused with a neoplasm.

HAEMANGIOMA

A haemangioma may be fairly well demarcated (*see* page 128), but it may also be very poorly demarcated and closely simulate a malignant tumour. Distinction between it and a malignant tumour, including a malignant haemangio-endothelioma, may be possible only by means of a biopsy. In some cases of haemangioma, the whole of one portion of a bone or several adjacent bones may disappear completely (Fig. 258). The relation of such massive osteolysis to haemangiomatosis is discussed by Gorham and Stout (1955).

A case of "massive osteolysis" of a femur due to an angioma of bone is described by Aston (1958).

HAEMANGIOPERICYTOMA

Another rare type of tumour causing a poorly-defined transradiant area is a haemangiopericytoma, which has histological features somewhat like those of a glomus tumour. This may occur in almost any bone, including a vertebra.

IDIOPATHIC BONE RESORPTION

A case of disappearing bones of one arm is reported by Milner and Baker (1958), when there was no evidence that the condition was due to a haemangioma. A similar case in a lower limb is reported by Branco and Horta (1958).

XANTHOMATOUS GRANULOMA

In many cases a xanthomatous granuloma is quite well demarcated (*see* page 132), but since in most cases it is not surrounded by a rim of dense sclerotic bone, the limits of the lesion may be rather indistinct and differentiation from a malignant neoplasm may be impossible from the x-ray appearance. A biopsy may be necessary for the correct diagnosis.

TUBERCULOUS LESION

A tuberculous bone lesion may present as a well-demarcated transradiant area as described on page 134. Rather rarely, the area of trabecular destruction is poorly demarcated: without a surrounding local and regional loss of bone density, and with no periosteal new bone formation. If a lesion of this sort is one or two centimetres in width, distinction from a malignant neoplasm may be impossible from the x-ray appearances and the correct diagnosis can be established only from the clinical course, from the aspiration of pus containing tubercle bacilli, or from the appearance of tuberculous granulation tissue in a biopsy specimen.

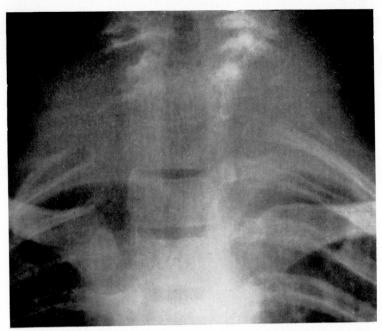

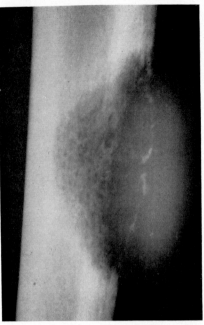

FIG. 258.—Haemangioma. Female aged 2 years. Erosion of lateral aspects of bodies of lower cervical vertebrae and disappearance of posterior parts of upper rib shadows. Biopsy—dilated abnormal blood vessels and marrow spaces; considered haemangioma.

FIG. 259.—Secondary deposit. Male aged 54 years. Poorly-demarcated surface erosion of the anterior aspect of the middle third of the tibia. Primary carcinoma of bladder.

POORLY-DEMARCATED EROSION OF THE SURFACE OF A BONE

An erosion of the surface of a bone may at first be confined to a limited region of the cortex, but this is usually soon destroyed and the erosion extends down into the cancellous bone beneath. Since a deep cancellous bone erosion due to malignant disease may eventually extend to and finally erode the cortex over it, it will often not be possible to see whether the lesion started deep in the bone and extended outwards, or superficially and extended inwards.

A poorly-demarcated erosion starting at the surface of a bone is most commonly the result of a secondary deposit, but it may also be seen in a primary neoplasm of the bone, in a malignant tumour of the synovial membrane or a tendon sheath with local extension into the bone, in a haemangioma, in a xanthomatous granuloma, or as a rare manifestation of a tuberculous bone lesion.

The x-ray appearances often give the impression that a part of the cortical bone and the trabeculae beneath it have simply been erased with a brush or bitten out, for there is no visible reaction whatsoever in the nearby bone, neither sclerosis nor periosteal new bone. The eroded area may be quite small or several centimetres long (Fig. 259).

MALIGNANT NEOPLASM

The first radiological evidence of a malignant bone neoplasm may be erosion of the outer surface of the cortex over a limited area. As the lesion grows to a larger size the whole depth of the cortex will soon be destroyed, and finally the erosion will extend deeply into the cancellous bone beneath (Fig. 254). The actual margins of the eroded cortex will be fairly clear-cut, but the limits of the erosion into the cancellous bone are very poorly defined and the eroded ends of apparently normal trabeculae may be seen forming the margins of the eroded area in one part together with further small areas of erosion lying deep to these.

Such a lesion may occur in any bone, though it is relatively rare in the bones of the hands and feet. Common sites are the femora and pelvis. A primary neoplasm sometimes occurs in the centre of the iliac bone, while secondary deposits are common in any part of the pelvis. Erosion of the ilium behind

152

the sacrum is quite common and easily missed unless carefully sought, since it is usually obscured by the shadow of the overlying sacral wing.

Any part of a bone may be affected, but the lesion is commonly a short distance away from the joint surface or in the middle third. In a vertebral body the surface erosion is usually from one or other side, not from the region of the end plate, and may be accompanied by a low-density para-vertebral shadow due to a surrounding neoplastic mass (Fig. 260).

The underlying pathology is commonly that of a secondary deposit, more rarely that of a primary bone neoplasm such as a fibrosarcoma, and occasionally that of an osteosarcoma, a chondrosarcoma or even a "Ewing's" type of tumour. Direct invasion from a nearby malignant soft tissue tumour—such as a synovioma if near a joint, in the case of a rib, a lung neoplasm—is also a possibility.

The histological features are the same as with a neoplasm deep in the bone (*see* page 167).

XANTHOMATOUS GRANULOMA

A xanthomatous granuloma usually lies well within the bone (*see* page 132), but occasionally it causes cortical as well as cancellous absorption and produces a rather poorly demarcated superficial erosion of the bone which is usually quite large. Radiologically this may be indistinguishable from a malignant neoplasm, the diagnosis being made only when cessation of growth is observed in serial radiographs or when a biopsy is performed.

TUBERCULOSIS

A tuberculous bone lesion, which may be well or poorly demarcated and deep in the bone (*see* pages 134 and 151), may also cause a superficial erosion of the cortex and cancellous bone beneath (Fig. 261), thus closely simulating a malignant neoplasm. This is a rare manifestation. Although the lesion grows very slowly and may even resolve, the correct diagnosis may be achieved only after aspiration of pus containing tubercle bacilli or after a biopsy with evidence of a tuberculous lesion.

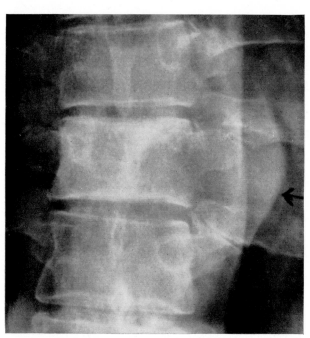

FIG. 260.—Secondary deposit. Male aged 55 years. Poorly-demarcated surface erosion left side of D. 10, with para-vertebral shadow (opposite arrow). Primary spindle cell sarcoma femur.

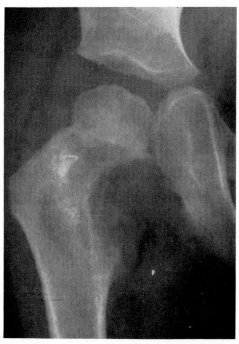

FIG. 261.—Tuberculous lesion. Female aged 3 years. Surface erosion of the femoral neck and lesser trochanter rather poorly demarcated from cancellous bone. Epiphyseal disc intact. Limping for 3 months. W.R. negative. Mantoux positive. Sterile lymphocytic effusion. Final resolution.

A TRANSRADIANT AREA IN THE VAULT OF THE SKULL

A single transradiant area in the vault of the skull may be a few millimetres or several centimetres wide and may have a variety of causes. Radiological diagnosis is sometimes impossible, but information with regard to the site, shape, margins and relationship to the inner and outer table may be sufficient to narrow the list of possible causes very considerably.

Such information is often best obtained from a tangential view, since the standard views may give an image blurred by normal bone on the opposite side, and may fail to demonstrate the relationship of the lesion to the two tables. When interpreting the tangential view, allowance must be made for distortion due to the spherical shape of the bone, for the peripheral part of any lesion more than 2 centimetres wide will not be truly tangential to the x-ray beam and may therefore give a false impression of this relationship. Such distortion will be overcome by a tomogram, as will also any difficulties about the site of any strands of dense bone superimposed on the transradiant area.

There are various characteristics of the vault which influence the x-ray appearances. Since the bones are flat and relatively thin, an acute infective destructive lesion tends to erode the whole thickness of the bone at an early stage. In addition, the vault has a very rich intrinsic blood supply with very vascular tissues external to it. This vascularity assists the formation of viable granulation tissue and favours an osteoclastic rather than an osteoblastic response. For these reasons, and also because the pericranium is not structurally quite equivalent to the periosteum round a long bone, it is rare to see new bone around an infective destructive lesion in the vault.

Similarly, because ossification of the vault takes place in the fibrous stage of the precursor of bone without an intermediate stage, there are no cartilaginous tumours of the vault.

Finally, the proximity of the brain to the vault is responsible for the transradiant zones or digital impressions seen in children and some adults as a result of brain growth and intracranial pulsation, while the proximity of the brain and skin is responsible for certain developmental defects seen only in the skull bones, such as a dermoid or meningocoele.

ANATOMICAL VARIATIONS

Depression for a Pacchionian body

A common cause of a 1 centimetre circular or 1–3 centimetre oval or lobular transradiant zone is a Pacchionian depression. It may be single or there may be several. A common site is the parasagittal region within 3 centimetres of the mid-line, where it may be seen clearly in an anterior-view or posterior-view radiograph. A depression may occur further out and may therefore be seen quite low down in a lateral-view radiograph.

The margin of the transradiant area is sharp and frequently has a surrounding narrow white rim of bone where the ray happens to strike the edge of the depression tangentially, otherwise no such dense margin will be seen. If it can be demonstrated in a tangential view, it will no longer appear as a transradiant area but simply as a shelving depression of the inner table. It is often so deep that there is no space left for the diploic bone, the two tables meeting in the floor of the depression. Occasionally if it is very large the outer table is thinned and may even bulge outwards. Sometimes a venous groove is seen in connexion with the transradiant area.

The arachnoid granulation consists of a large group of arachnoid villi protruding into a widened parietal vein. The vein is flattened between the villi and the vault, which is moulded by the general shape of the granulations.

Emissary veins

A very dark, 2–3 millimetre circular transradiant area with a narrow linear margin of dense bone situated in the parasagittal area near the torcular, and therefore best seen in Towne's projection, may be caused by an emissary vein. Occasionally it may be several millimetres in size.

Diploic venous pool

A 1–2 centimetre, rather irregularly oval transradiant zone in the parietal bone may be due to a normal but large diploic venous pool, and may be recognized by the narrow (venous) band-like transradiancies radiating from it.

Congenital parietal foramen

Two rounded or oval transradiant zones, each about 1 centimetre in size, lying ½–2 centimetres to either side of the mid-line in the upper part of each parietal bone may be caused by congenital parietal foramina. They are best seen in an anterior view, and are much the same size on the two sides.

DEVELOPMENTAL DEFECTS

Meningocoele

A mid-line 1–3 centimetre oval or circular transradiant zone which is sharply demarcated from the surrounding normal bone may be due to a meningocoele. The diagnosis will be suggested if the soft tissue swelling over the defect is either visible in the radiograph or easily felt. The x-ray appearances are indistinguishable from those of a dermoid cyst communicating with the intracranial cavity (*see below*).

Fibrous dysplasia

A circular or oval transradiant area, usually some 2–3 centimetres in size and sharply demarcated by a 2 millimetre surrounding white line of dense bone, is seen in some cases of fibrous dysplasia. A tangential view will generally show some outward bulging of the outer table, which is intact over the lesion. Irregular woolly shadows due to microscopic bony spicules are often seen superimposed on the transradiant zone and these, together with the elevation of the outer table, give the lesion the appearance of a blister of bone. It is unilateral and often in the parietal bone.

Haemangioma

A 1–2 centimetre circular or oval transradiancy, with a clear-cut margin and fine linear shadows radiating across it, will suggest a haemangioma. In a tangential view the fine lines, due to spicules of bone, lie at right angles to the outer table and may have free open ends if the latter is absorbed. Below they extend deeply into the transradiant area.

Intradiploic dermoid and epidermoid

A clearly defined transradiant zone measuring up to several centimetres in size may be due to an intradiploic dermoid. The adjacent tables are expanded and eroded over the lesion, as can be seen in a tangential view. If the tables are destroyed over the central part, the expansile nature of the lesion will still be visible at the margins of the transradiant zones, where elevation of the tables will be seen with eversion of the bone margins.

The usual site is the squamous part of the occipital and temporal bones, but occasionally the lesion may be seen in relation to the posterior wall of a frontal sinus or the upper margin of the orbit.

Extracranial dermoid

A transradiant zone almost anywhere along the mid-line may be caused by a dermoid cyst beneath the galea. There may be thinning of the vault by pressure and the resulting saucer-like depression of the outer table, some 1–2 centimetres across, may be seen in a tangential view. A small defect may be present through which the extracranial dermoid may communicate with an intracranial portion, or the latter may be attached to extracranial tissues by a narrow band passing through a small bone channel. Distinction from a meningocoele is not possible from the radiographs.

ACQUIRED LESIONS

Post-traumatic cyst-like area

A 2–3 centimetre roughly circular transradiant zone may be a late result of trauma. The underlying lesion may be an intradiploic haematoma containing altered blood or a cyst-like area in which the altered blood has become organized into fibrous tissue.

Post-radiation necrosis

An area of a few square centimetres, consisting of small erosions and some sclerosis, may be seen at the site of damage by excessive therapeutic radiation. The erosions appear some weeks, months or even years after the radiation and persist for a long time. Restitution to a normal bone pattern has been observed.

Hyperparathyroidism

Although unusual, a cyst-like transradiant area may be seen in the vault in hyperparathyroidism. It may be the only lesion in the vault or there may be several other cyst-like transradiant areas. In either case it may be associated with the coarse mottled diploic pattern and an indistinct cortical layer as described on page 120. There will invariably be manifestations of hyperparathyroidism in other bones, particularly subperiosteal cortical erosions of the phalanges.

Xanthomatosis (histiocytosis x)

A 1–2 centimetre, roughly circular or oval transradiant area with erosion of the diploë and one or both tables may be caused by a xanthomatous deposit, though more commonly this lesion is larger in size and amorphous in shape. Sometimes multiple lesions of various sizes and shapes are seen together.

The margins are clear-cut and there is no surrounding bone reaction in the great majority of cases. The presence of transradiant areas in other bones (*see* page 132) may suggest the diagnosis, but sometimes this may be made only after a bone biopsy.

Infective conditions

An acute pyogenic osteomyelitis may result in a rather ill-defined area of erosion of the vault without any periosteal new bone formation. The clinical findings will usually give the diagnosis.

Subacute or chronic lesions—whether pyogenic, tuberculous or syphilitic—generally give rise to coalescing areas of destruction, in the margins of which sclerosis may be very slight or even absent. Chronic pyogenic osteomyelitis is nearly always the result of infection introduced by trauma, after surgery, or by spread from an infected sinus or ear. The history will greatly assist in the diagnosis. In syphilis, both congenital and acquired, the vault lesions are only part of a general picture which will be recognized by other clinical features. Tuberculous osteomyelitis of the vault, which is rare in this country, may however give rise to real diagnostic difficulty since the lesions so closely resemble metastases. The response to antituberculous treatment may prove to be a safe method of diagnosis, though biopsy is sometimes undertaken.

Direct trauma

A roughly circular transradiant area in the vault may be the result of a penetrating wound at an earlier date. A bullet track in particular may leave quite a well demarcated hole in the bone. A surgical trephine may also be mistaken for a pathological erosion if the incident has been forgotten and the hair has grown over the scar.

Secondary deposit

A single transradiant area with a relatively poorly demarcated margin is commonly due to a secondary deposit. It may be round, oval or irregular in shape, and quite small like a Pacchionian depression or several centimetres in size. When it is small, only one or perhaps neither of the tables is eroded, but when it is more than a centimetre in size, all the tables are usually destroyed. Sometimes there is only one erosion, sometimes there are several small erosions of similar size, and sometimes there are very many erosions of varying sizes scattered widely throughout both sides of the vault.

The x-ray appearances may be the same whatever the site or the histology of the primary neoplasm, and a secondary deposit from a carcinoma may be indistinguishable from a deposit in myelomatosis whether the lesion is single or there are multiple erosions.

Occasionally, in a secondary deposit from a carcinoma, there may be some faint calcifications in the soft tissues of the scalp over the erosion which will serve to distinguish it from myelomatosis or from the transradiant zone caused by a large Pacchionian depression. These calcifications may be seen only if the radiograph is viewed with a particularly strong light and, if small, a magnifying glass.

In children a secondary deposit from a neuroblastoma may show an erosion and small spicules of new bone at right angles to the vault.

RESPONSE TO AN INTRACRANIAL LESION

Meningioma

A transradiant area in the vault may be caused by erosion from the direct spread of a meningioma, though sclerosis is a much more common reaction of the overlying bone. The erosion may be less clearly demarcated in a slowly-growing tumour than in a rapidly-growing malignant meningioma. Both tables are usually eroded, but in rare cases the erosion is predominantly intradiploic with the transradiant zone visible under an expanded outer table. There may be evidence of hypertrophied vascular channels in the surrounding bone.

There is generally clinical or other radiological evidence of an intracranial lesion, particularly displacement of the calcified pineal to the opposite side or erosion of the sella turcica, especially the dorsum sellae.

DIRECT INVASION FROM SCALP NEOPLASM

Rodent ulcer

A rodent ulcer, if untreated or if it becomes uncontrollable, may eventually spread from the skin into the bone of the vault and cause an irregular localized bone erosion, usually in the frontal region. The cause will be obvious on inspection.

Carcinoma

Similarly to a rodent ulcer, a carcinoma of the skin, if untreated, may grow and eventually erode the bone beneath.

8—Combination of Shadows

PERIOSTEAL OPACITY AND EROSION

The combination of periostitis and erosion is one of the most common non-traumatic bone lesions and occurs in many inflammatory and neoplastic conditions. It is seen in its most exuberant forms in the long bones. When the cause of the lesion is not obvious from the initial clinical investigation the x-ray appearances may repay careful scrutiny, since the balance between erosion and periosteal response often serves as a key to the differential diagnosis. In pyogenic inflammatory conditions of the long bones, the periosteal reaction tends to be equal in severity to the erosion (Figs. 267 and 269), whereas in malignant neoplasms there is greater discrepancy between the two, slight periosteal reaction being seen with marked erosion (Fig. 277) and gross periosteal reaction with slight erosion (Fig. 281).

These generalizations do not hold good in certain atypical manifestations of inflammation or neoplasm. For example, a very similar mixture of gross bone erosion and periosteal new bone is seen in both Fig. 262, a sub-acute osteomyelitis, and Fig. 263, a "Ewing's type" of malignant bone tumour. Similarly, the marked bone erosion with comparatively little periosteal new bone seen in Figs. 264 and 265 is produced in the one case by an unusual type of subacute staphylococcal osteomyelitis and in the other by a "Ewing's type" of malignant bone tumour. In such cases the x-ray appearances are not a reliable indication of the diagnosis (*see also* page 145).

In the flat bones, tarsals, carpals and vertebrae the x-ray appearancse are rather different. In inflammatory conditions there is less periosteal new bone to a given amount of erosion than in a long bone. In this respect the terminal phalanx reacts like a flat bone and the sternum and calcaneum like a long bone. Differentiation is still often possible, since a neoplasm of these bones produces either gross erosion with very little periosteal new bone or a small amount of erosion with abundant subperiosteal calcification.

PYOGENIC INFLAMMATION

Haematogenous infection

The long bones: early changes

In acute haematogenous pyogenic osteomyelitis of a major long bone, particularly from *Staphylococcus aureus*, the earliest change in the radiograph is a faint hazy shadow round the shaft of the bone due to pus and oedema. This, however, very often passes unnoticed, and a negative x-ray report at this early stage should on no account be used as a reason for withholding treatment. The first reliable x-ray evidence is a small area of erosion and periostitis on about the tenth to fourteenth day of the infection (Fig. 266). The erosion may precede the periostitis by a day or two, or the periostitis may precede the erosion, or the two may appear simultaneously.

The erosion may consist of a single poorly-demarcated transradiant zone or several circular or elongated zones, irregular and poorly demarcated, which may be separated by zones of radiographically normal bone. The periosteal new bone in this early stage is seen as a thin linear shadow, parallel to the cortex but separated from it by a transradiant zone which may be anything between 2 and 10 millimetres wide according to the amount the periosteum is elevated by the oedema or pus. This linear shadow may lie directly over an area of erosion or be separated from it by some still normal cortex. Since the periosteum may be raised by inflammatory products for the whole length of the metaphysis, and since the new bone may start anywhere along it, the periosteal new bone may even arise at a slightly different level from the visible erosion.

In the major long bones these early changes are usually seen in the proximal or distal third of the bone, probably because the nutrient artery ramifies in a richer manner towards the bone end. The lesion is also seen, though less commonly, in the clavicles, where it tends to be at one or other end, and in the ribs, where owing to the different circulation it may occur almost anywhere.

If the infection is brought under control at an early stage, either spontaneously or by chemotherapy, the new bone continues to spread medially from the raised periosteum until it joins the cortex, and the erosion remains stationary and gradually becomes ossified again, the normal architecture eventually being restored. When the infection is eradicated by chemotherapy before much erosion has developed, the periosteal deposits are for a time more prominent than the erosions, until they in their turn become absorbed and the original cortex again forms the outer margin of the bone.

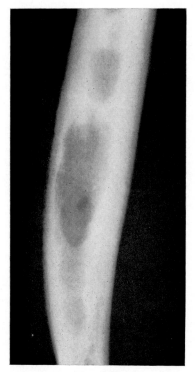

FIG. 262

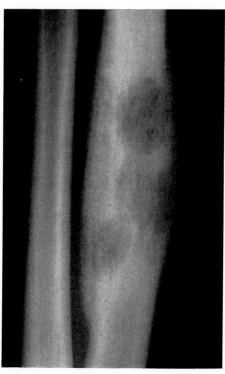

FIG. 263

FIG. 262.—Chronic osteomyelitis. Female aged 19 years. Middle third of humerus showing erosion, sclerosis and periosteal new bone, the latter fused with the cortex. Pain in arm and occasional discharge of pus for 3 years. Cavities with inflammatory granulation tissue. Compare with Fig. 263.

FIG. 263.—Malignant neoplasm. Erosion, sclerosis and periosteal new bone in middle third of radius, rather like Fig. 262. Biopsy—Ewing type of tumour.

The long bones: later changes

If the infection is not adequately controlled by treatment, or if it is less acute so that the patient does not seek treatment until a later stage, the erosions and periosteal new bone increase more or less together until both are quite marked (Figs. 267 and 268) and may rapidly involve the whole of the metaphysis. From about the third week, sequestra may form and become visible in the radiograph (*see* page 175). The periosteal new bone, which is sometimes very abundant and may reach a width of one centimetre or more, becomes fused with the cortex which then appears thickened.

Somewhat rarely the periosteal deposits are formed in layers which have narrow transradiant zones between them, giving the "onion-skin" appearance (Fig. 268). Occasionally these layers, instead of lying parallel to the shaft, are formed in a linear striate manner at right angles to the shaft. These linear shadows are generally joined together at the periphery by vertical linear calcifications giving the so-called "closed feathering pattern" (Fig. 269).

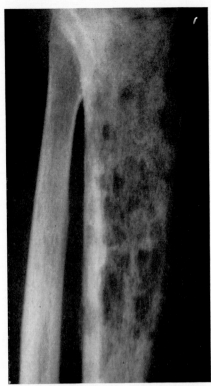

FIG. 264.—Osteomyelitis. Female aged 60 years. Ill-defined erosions of upper third of tibia, with very little periosteal new bone. Some weeks' pain in leg and slight swelling. Explored, staphylococcus grown. Resolution followed. Compare with Fig. 265.

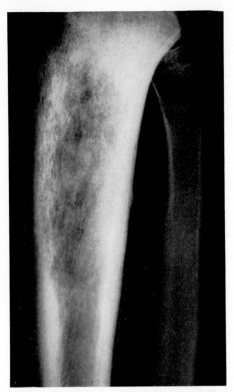

FIG. 265.—Malignant neoplasm. Male aged 19 years. Ill-defined erosions and very little periosteal new bone in upper third of tibia. Compare with Fig. 264. Biopsy—Ewing's type of tumour. Radiotherapy—good response. Secondaries in chest 5 years later.

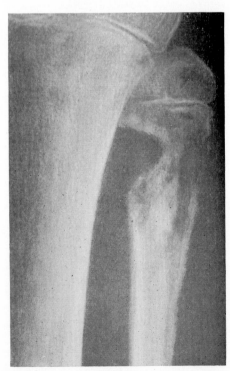

FIG. 266.—Osteomyelitis. Female aged 6 years. Erosion and periostitis in upper end of fibula. Epiphyseal disc intact. Pain and swelling 3 weeks. Resolution after penicillin.

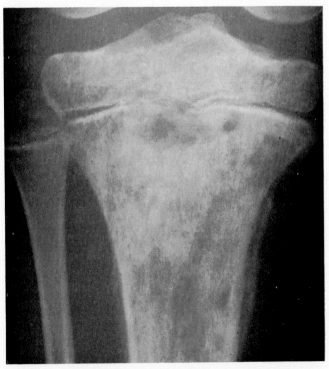

FIG. 267.—Osteomyelitis. Male aged 10 years. Erosion and periostitis in upper third of tibia below epiphyseal disc. Pyrexia and local pain and swelling 2 weeks. Staphylococcus.

In another uncommon form there is marked erosion but only slight periosteal new bone formation (Fig. 264), so that the radiographic appearances are similar to those of an atypical neoplasm. This form of the disease is often subacute and there are no clinical signs to distinguish between an inflammatory lesion and a neoplasm.

The vertebrae and pelvis

An acute osteomyelitis in a vertebral body will cause some narrowing of the disc space by the time that bone changes are visible, but in a mild infection some erosion and periosteal new bone may be seen without obvious narrowing of the disc space, and differentiation from tuberculosis and neoplasm must

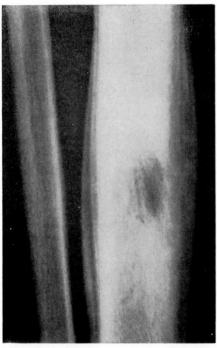

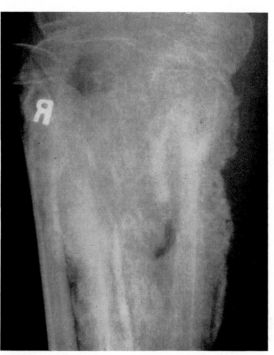

FIG. 268.—Osteomyelitis. Male aged 6 years. Erosion of shaft of tibia and layered (onion skin) periostitis. Staphylococcal.

FIG. 269.—Osteomyelitis. Male aged 9 years. Erosion and periosteal shadow with closed feathering pattern. Long-standing osteomyelitis.

be made. The finding of some periosteal new bone is much in favour of a pyogenic infection. It is usually seen in the posterior view as a narrow linear shadow adjacent to the lateral border of the cortex of the vertebral body on one or other side.

Haematogenous osteomyelitis may also occur in a pelvic bone but is relatively uncommon. There is generally a marked preponderance of periosteal new bone over the erosion, which will result in considerable local thickening of the bone.

Non-haematogenous infection

A non-haematogenous bacterial bone infection may occur as a result of a local spread from an infection nearby or from a penetrating wound or a compound fracture. The organism is variable, though a streptococcal or staphylococcal infection is the most common, and in either case the bone reaction is often much less marked than in the case of a haematogenous infection with the same organism.

The terminal phalanx and skull

In a non-haematogenous infection of a terminal phalanx, usually secondary to a septic pulp or penetrating wound, the periosteal new bone formation is always slight and may even be altogether absent no matter how extensive the erosion may be. A curious feature is that the erosion (decalcification) may be so gross that the outline of the bone may almost disappear, yet as healing proceeds, the trabeculae recalcify and the small amount of periosteal new bone becomes absorbed until the structure of the phalanx is often completely restored.

Similarly, in the skull there is little or no new bone formation no matter how extensive the erosion. However, unlike the terminal phalanx, if the infection is eradicated, regeneration of the eroded bone is slow and generally incomplete.

The mandible

In the mandible the combination of periostitis and erosion from haematogenous infection is much less common than erosion, or erosion and sclerosis, round an infected tooth. The periosteal new bone can best be seen on the inferior aspect of the horizontal ramus in an oblique view, or on the buccal or labial aspect in an infero-superior (occlusal) view. Occasionally, when the infection is in the ascending ramus, it may best be seen on the lateral aspect in an anterior view.

The erosion, for a time at any rate, may be confined to the region of a tooth, but, whether the infection arises in relation to the tooth or from a wound, there may also be widespread poorly-demarcated areas of erosion remote from the tooth. The balance between the erosion and the periostitis is very variable, though as a rule the erosion is the predominant feature. When no obvious dental cause can be seen, especially when the lesion is in the ascending ramus, the possibility that it is due to actinomycosis should be borne in mind. Sequestra may form either in actinomycosis or in a pyogenic infection, and will be seen as isolated undecalcified plaques of bone surrounded by a narrow zone of erosion.

Occasionally in babies or young children the infection may be haematogenous, in which case the unerupted teeth may appear normal, but the periostitis and erosion of the mandible will be the same as those seen in an infection starting from a tooth or an external wound.

The ribs

In infective conditions of the ribs the periostitis tends to be much more marked than the erosion. When it is secondary to a pleural infection, such as a chronic empyema or actinomycosis of the lung and pleura, several neighbouring ribs are usually involved. The lung shadow and the clinical history will generally indicate the cause of the rib changes. More rarely the infection is haematogenous and only a part of a rib is affected, and unless it causes a secondary pleural effusion, there may be no underlying lung shadow. Stab wounds and the procedures adopted during surgical operations on the lungs and heart rarely lead to a rib infection. Occasionally the pressure of a too rigid and injudiciously placed drainage tube during the treatment of an empyema may result in a chronic osteomyelitis of a rib, with erosion and periostitis and even the formation of a sequestrum. Following a partial rib resection for an empyema, the regenerating rib shows an erosion with periosteal new bone formation around it. This appearance may persist indefinitely after the infection has died out and is a common finding in patients often 10–20 years after an empyema treated by rib resection.

Compound fractures with sepsis

In a compound fracture of a long bone with persistent sepsis, calcification in the callus is absent or delayed and the amount of erosion and periosteal new bone formation from the infection is usually very slight. A very small amount of erosion near the end of one of the fragments, either in the cancellous bone or in the cortex, is therefore an ominous radiological finding.

Surgical foreign bodies

In infection round surgical foreign bodies such as traction wires, pins, screws and so on, the erosion is usually slight. The small amount of periosteal new bone around a traction wire may be no more marked than if there were no infective element. Any changes seen which do not appear to be due to the trauma of insertion should therefore be given due emphasis, however slight they may appear.

TUBERCULOUS INFLAMMATION

A combination of bone erosion and periosteal new bone is seen in a tuberculous infection of the shaft of a long bone. In one form the erosion is more obvious than the periosteal new bone (Fig. 270), and the appearances may easily be mistaken for a primary bone neoplasm or a secondary deposit.

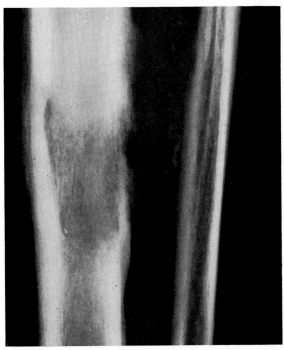

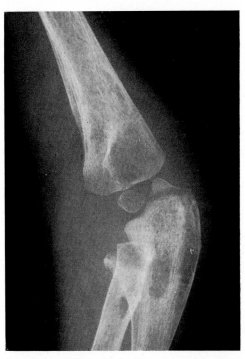

FIG. 270.—Tuberculosis. Female aged 70 years. Erosion and slight periostitis of middle third of tibia. Recent pain and swelling. Biopsy—tuberculosis.

FIG. 271.—Tuberculosis. Female aged 3 years. Much erosion and much periosteal new bone in humerus and ulna. Several bones affected. No sinus in elbow region. Tubercle bacilli found in pus.

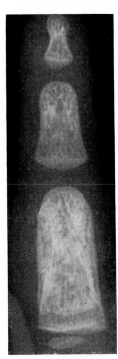

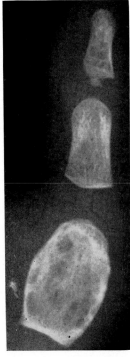

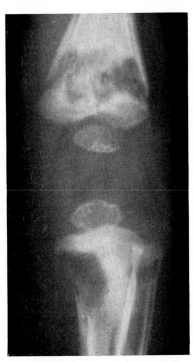

FIG. 272.—Tuberculous dactylitis. Female aged 2 years. Very inconspicuous erosion and some periosteal new bone in proximal phalanx of second finger.

FIG. 273.—Tuberculosis dactylitis. Male aged 2 years. Some erosion and cortical thinning with gross expansion of first metacarpal. W.R. negative. Mantoux positive. Resolution after streptomycin and P.A.S.

FIG. 274.—Congenital syphilis. Female aged 1 year. Submetaphyseal erosion and periostitis of femur and tibia. Similar changes in other leg. W.R. positive. Rapid resolution after penicillin.

In the more usual form the periosteal new bone is relatively the same in extent as the erosion, or may even be the more obvious feature (Fig. 271). In the absence of joint involvement there may be little or no general loss of density of the nearby bone or adjacent bones.

In a tuberculous lesion of the anterior end of a rib, often secondary to an adjacent infected lymphatic gland, the erosion tends to predominate over the periosteal new bone, but in the body of a rib or the phalanx of a child the periosteal new bone may be more obvious than the erosion (Fig. 272). If the periosteal new bone is very abundant the phalanx may become almost spindle-shaped and, if the erosion is slight, may closely simulate a syphilitic dactylitis.

SYPHILIS

Congenital syphilis

Congenital syphilis in young children may have osseous manifestations. A characteristic appearance is seen in the two knee regions, consisting of periosteal new bone deposits adjacent to the shafts of the tibiae and femora and a localized 3–5 millimetre erosion of the cortical and cancellous bone on the medial side of each tibia just below the upper metaphyseal line (Fig. 274). In addition, there may be a 3–5 millimetre transradiant zone parallel to and just beneath the lower metaphysis of each femur and the upper metaphysis of each tibia and, in severe cases, simple periostitis along the shafts of other major long bones and multiple rather poorly demarcated 1–2 centimetre erosions in the skull.

In less typical cases the erosion and periostitis are confined to a single bone and the x-ray diagnosis is less obvious.

Another manifestation is a syphilitic dactylitis, often without changes in the other bones. This condition is characterized by rather more periostitis and less erosion than is generally seen in a tuberculous dactylitis. It is very rare in Western Europe at the present time.

Acquired syphilis

One manifestation of acquired syphilis in adults is a gumma of a single bone. A common site is the anterior aspect of the middle third of the tibia. Radiologically there is a boss of periosteal bone which is fused to the cortex beneath, and some erosion of the deeper layers of the cortex itself (Fig. 275). This latter feature will often distinguish the condition from a simple traumatic periosteal opacity or old subperiosteal haematoma.

In another type of lesion there is a more extensive periosteal reaction and more erosion of the shaft (Fig. 276). The condition then closely simulates a chronic osteomyelitis or an atypical malignant neoplasm.

Yaws

Erosion and periosteal new bone are also seen in yaws. The erosions tend to be small and circumscribed, and the condition is described in detail by Davis (1961).

FUNGUS INFECTION

Actinomycosis

Erosion and periosteal new bone in the mandible, similar to that resulting from a pyogenic osteomyelitis, may be caused by actinomycosis. In some cases the erosion is very marked and the periostitis slight, in others the reverse. A rib, or more often several neighbouring ribs, may be involved secondarily to pleuro-pulmonary actinomycosis, the periosteal new bone tending to be a more prominent feature than the rib erosion. Vertebral involvement can occur.

Madura foot (Written by *J. H. Middlemiss*)

Madura foot is a chronic destructive lesion of the forefoot with much swelling of the soft tissues. The bone resorption may be linear and at right angles to the shaft of the metatarsal, with separate rounded areas of absorption within the medulla and with much soft tissue swelling. This may cause splaying out of the heads of the metatarsals. Periosteal new bone is usually seen only if there is secondary infection.

164

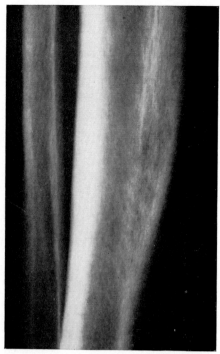 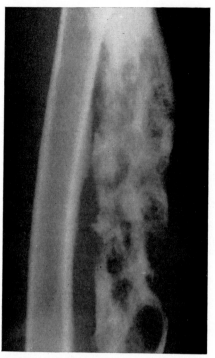

Fig. 275.—Tertiary syphilis. Male aged 80 years. Cortical erosion and periosteal boss of anterior aspect of middle third of tibia. Same in other leg. W.R. positive.

Fig. 276.—Tertiary syphilis. Male aged 53 years. Much erosion and some periosteal new bone in ulna. Very similar to Fig. 262, an osteomyelitis, and Fig. 263, a neoplasm. W.R. positive. Clinical course indicated this diagnosis.

The condition presents as a chronic painless swelling of the foot affecting particularly farmers, peasant herdsmen and others who work barefooted on the land. The patient often allows the swelling to go on for months or years before seeking medical advice. Often superficial nodules form on the surface and open to form sinuses from which comes a purulent discharge containing the characteristic grains of the fungus, which may be either black, yellow or red. Secondary infection of these discharging sinuses is common, and may lead to pain and extension of the inflammatory process. The causative organism is either an aerobic actinomyces (*Nocardia asteroides* or *N. brasiliensis*) or a form of streptomyces giving rise to maduromycosis.

Blastomycosis

Erosion and periosteal new bone can occur in systemic blastomycosis as reported by Martin, Jones and Durham (1914).

Coccidioidomycosis

A lesion in a bone with an x-ray appearance like a staphylococcal osteomyelitis and due to coccidioidomycosis has been reported by Forbus and Bestebreurtje (1946).

CYSTS AND INNOCENT TUMOURS

It is not uncommon to see periostitis in association with the single clearly-demarcated transradiant area of a simple cyst, an eosinophilic granuloma or an osteoclastoma described under "relatively transradiant area" (*see* Chapter 7). The periostitis is generally the result of a mild trauma, and the shadow represents either a subperiosteal haematoma or the callus secondary to a pathological fracture.

Differentiation of an innocent cystic condition with a secondary periosteal opacity from an inflammatory or malignant neoplastic condition with erosion and a periosteal opacity depends on the very good demarcation of the transradiant area and the preponderance of the erosion over the periosteal reaction. If the trauma is surgical, as in the case of a biopsy or a limited curettage, the history and, if available, the histology will give the diagnosis.

MALIGNANT NEOPLASM

The combination of erosion and periosteal new bone formation is not uncommon with a malignant neoplasm, whether of the bone or of the tissues within the bone, or with a secondary deposit. This combination of shadows falls into three groups: a gross erosion with a mere triangular tuft of periosteal

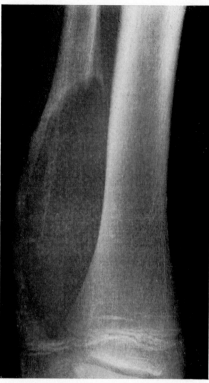

FIG. 277.—Ewing type bone neoplasm. Male aged 15 years. Much erosion of fibula limited by lower epiphyseal disc. Triangular tuft of periosteal new bone on upper anterior margin. Amputation carried out. Histology—tumours composed of darkly-staining small round cells.

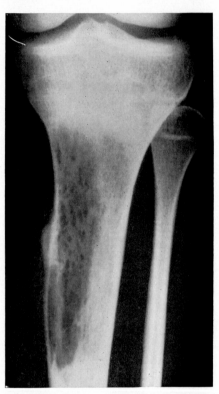

FIG. 278.—Osteosarcoma. Female aged 14 years. Rather poorly demarcated erosion with cortical thinning and very slight expansion of upper third of tibia. First biopsy—osteoclastoma, but rapid spread occurred after curetting and chip grafts and further biopsy confirmed osteosarcoma.

new bone at its margin (Fig. 277); a moderate erosion with a similar tuft of periosteal new bone in addition to much dense bone or feathering around it (Fig. 281); and a conspicuous periosteal shadow parallel to the shaft with very inconspicuous erosion, an appearance seen particularly with a secondary deposit from a neuroblastoma (Fig. 284) or a "Ewing's type" of tumour.

Malignant bone tumours with much erosion

Malignant bone tumours with much erosion and minimal periosteal reaction are the least common of the three types. The usual appearance is that of bone destruction involving the cortical and cancellous bone indiscriminately and often extending over an area of several centimetres. In the main tumour area the destructive process is complete with no strands of bone escaping. At its margins it is poorly demarcated from the surrounding normal bone, where it merges with the jagged ends of uneroded trabeculae and there is no zone of reactive sclerosis to show its limits.

The small triangular tuft of periosteal new bone at the tumour margin is only a few millimetres long and seems to be due to elevation of the periosteum by the tumour between it and the as yet uneroded cortex with which it soon merges (Fig. 277).

It may only be seen at the upper or lower margin of the tumour and in one view, so that in the other view the appearance will be that of an area of erosion only (Fig. 278). The search for such an area of periosteal new bone is therefore of considerable importance in diagnosis. An unusual type is illustrated (Fig. 280) in which the periosteal new bone is not a tuft-like shadow at the margin of the tumour but a thin linear shadow separated from the expanded cortex over the erosion by a small transradiant area. This inconspicuous linear shadow is all that distinguishes it from a simple cyst such as that illustrated in Fig. 229. or an osteoclastoma as shown in Fig. 234.

In some cases the triangular tuft of periosteal new bone is the most conspicuous feature, the erosions being indistinct (Fig. 279). Occasionally the periosteal shadow is partly linear parallel to the shaft and partly showing spicules at right angles (Fig. 280). These may even be joined across the top, giving an appearance of closed feathering (Fig. 281) and very similar to the osteomyelitis illustrated in Fig. 269.

The histological findings in this group are variable, ranging from an osteosarcoma, yet with gross osteolysis, to a chondrosarcoma, a round-cell tumour (Ewing) or a fibrosarcoma, while occasionally a secondary deposit from a carcinoma may show some periosteal reaction near one margin of an area of extensive erosion.

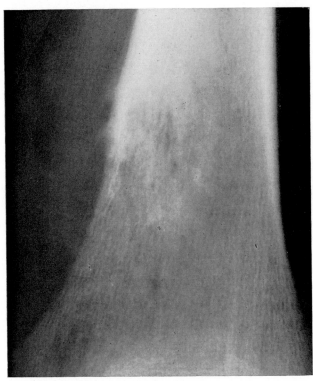

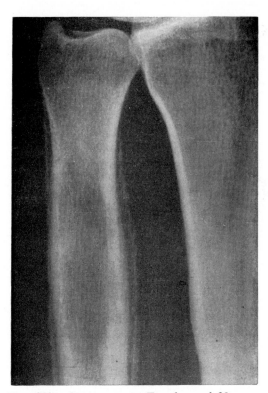

FIG. 279.—Osteosarcoma. Male aged 12 years. Some ill-defined erosion of lower third of femur with triangular tuft of periosteal shadowing on upper medial aspect and very faint calcification in soft parts (not reproducible). Painful swelling 5 weeks. Biopsy—osteosarcoma.

FIG. 280.—Osteosarcoma. Female aged 28 years. Erosion 4 cm. long in the lower end of the ulna with periosteal shadowing in the form of closed feathering, with vertical striae and a peripheral line shadow parallel to the cortex.

Osteosarcoma

An osteosarcoma is a tumour composed of malignant osteoblastic cells. Microscopically the diagnostic feature is the presence of irregular spicules of osteoid tissue formed by and surrounded by neoplastic osteoblasts. The osteoid may partially calcify to form irregular bony spicules; this is responsible for the dense areas or sun-ray spicules seen in those cases with less erosion and much opaque shadowing within or around the bone. Whether the appearances are those of osteolysis or osteosclerosis, the tumour is very malignant, and in a treated series of patients only 10 per cent survived 3 years from the time of diagnosis.

Chondrosarcoma

A chondrosarcoma produces atypical neoplastic cartilage with cells showing irregular and abnormal growth. Mitotic figures are rare, but double nuclear forms are sometimes found. The stroma may show areas of cystic degeneration, calcification or ossification, which will be responsible for any dense shadowing seen in the radiograph. A chondrosarcoma is a less malignant tumour than an osteosarcoma, and in a recent series 50 per cent of the patients were alive 5 years after the initial diagnosis.

Fibrosarcoma

The fibrosarcoma of bone is similar in histological appearances to its more common counterpart arising from the soft tissues. It is composed of cellular fibrous tissue which infiltrates and replaces the bone, and which shows mitotic activity as evidence of its malignancy. The stroma shows a variable amount of collagen formation. Neither cartilage nor new bone formation is seen. It tends to spread readily down the medullary cavity, where the surviving bone trabeculae are surrounded and infiltrated by the tumour tissue. The prognosis, though better than that of an osteosarcoma, is grave—only about 25 per cent of patients surviving for 5 years from the time of diagnosis.

Periosteal osteosarcoma

A further bone tumour entity is the truly periosteal osteosarcoma, sometimes known as a parosteal sarcoma. The tumour forms a mass both outside and in the cortex, and histologically shows a mixture of connective tissues with bone, osteoid, cartilage, fibrous tissue and blood vessels, all of which tend to be well differentiated and readily recognizable. This histological maturity is reflected in the prognosis, which is relatively favourable. Dwinnell, Dahlin and Ghormley (1954) reported a series of 15 patients with only one death directly due to the tumour before the fifth year (the other was due to the amputation procedure). Very late metastases were seen in a few. The lower end of the femur is a usual site.

Ewing's tumour and tumours with similar histology

The histological findings in this group still give rise to considerable controversy, and although many are labelled "Ewing's tumour", some doubt has been cast on the specificity and accuracy of this diagnosis. Tumours in this group have certain features in common, namely destruction of bone; unusual periosteal new bone formation; no obvious evidence of a primary neoplasm elsewhere; and, on histological examination, cells with small darkly-staining nuclei lying within the bone, with no characteristic pattern except a tendency to form solid areas of tumour cells. The differential diagnosis is between a secondary deposit of an undifferentiated carcinoma, a neuroblastoma, a primary reticulum-cell sarcoma of bone, and finally a "Ewing's tumour". Often histological examination cannot differentiate these conditions, though a final diagnosis can sometimes be made at autopsy. In the older age groups the diagnosis usually rests between a primary reticulum-cell sarcoma, with its reasonably good prognosis, and an undifferentiated secondary deposit of a carcinoma with a poor prognosis. Sometimes a positive reticulin staining will suggest a reticulum-cell sarcoma, while sometimes there is an almost epithelial configuration indicating a carcinoma.

In the younger age group, differentiation between a secondary deposit in the bone from a neuroblastoma and a primary tumour of the "Ewing's type" may be impossible. The presence of "rosette formation" will suggest a neuroblastoma, but this feature is often not present. On the other hand, the cells in a neuroblastoma tend to be more irregular in shape and size and to have more intracellular matrix than those of a "Ewing's tumour", which is composed of more regular rounded cells closely packed together with no visible intracellular substance. Often distinction between the two conditions is impossible from the initial histological examination. Of this we can be certain: some cases showing all the histological and clinical features of a "Ewing's tumour" are treated and survive, so that in these cases a secondary deposit from a neuroblastoma can be excluded, and we are left with a primary malignant bone tumour which conforms to the original description by Ewing and which rightly, because we have no better term for it, bears his name.

Malignant bone tumours with much calcification

Malignant bone tumours with relatively little erosion but with ossification or calcification in the tumour, giving a "feathering" or "sun-ray" appearance spreading out from the cortex and a periosteal tuft at the margin (Figs. 281 and 282), are seen more frequently than malignant tumours with much erosion. The "sun-ray" calcification is not a periostitis but is due to the formation of bone by the tumour or of calcification within the tumour. At first it will lie between the cortex and the raised periosteum, which by limiting the outward spread of the tumour causes the rather convex edge to the general

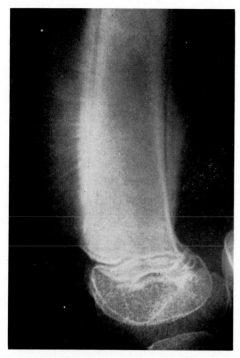

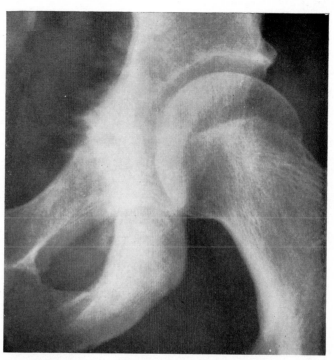

FIG. 281.—Osteosarcoma. Female aged 7 years. Linear periosteal shadow and "sun-ray" calcifications at right angles to cortex of the lower end of femur. Fall 7 weeks previously followed by swelling and then pain. Amputation carried out. Histology—osteosarcoma. Well 14 years later.

FIG. 282.—Secondary deposits. Male aged 53 years. Increased density on medial aspect of acetabulum with linear calcifications vertical to the cortex (sun-ray spicules or feathering). Primary carcinoma of rectum 5 years previously.

alignment of the feathering, until at a later stage the tumour bursts out beyond this barrier. It may then produce a massive low-density shadow far out into the region of the muscles, and the limits of the calcified parts will not be so even.

The feathering may be fine and difficult to see unless the radiograph is of satisfactory quality, or it may be so abundant that it becomes almost confluent, producing a very radio-opaque shadow beyond the limits of the cortex. When it is fine or moderate in extent the ends of the line shadows facing outwards are not joined, but when it is very extensive this feature is not so obvious. The calcification is not always linear in form but may occur in clumps giving the shadows a woolly appearance. A small triangular tuft of periosteal new bone is usually seen at the upper or lower limit of the tumour area.

In these types of malignant bone neoplasm the bone erosion is often inconspicuous, since it tends to be obscured by the overlying tumour ossification or feathering. Nevertheless, unless the feathering is very dense the erosion can always be seen. A shallow external cortical erosion can often be identified (Fig. 279); alternatively, there may be small circular or oval erosions in the cancellous bone. In a relatively early case the faint feathering may be the most obvious evidence of a tumour, but some erosion will always be visible at this stage in radiographs of good quality.

The histological findings in this group are also variable. Most commonly they will be those of an osteosarcoma, but other types of primary bone neoplasm may give similar appearances. Occasionally, feathering with slight erosion of the bone beneath is seen in a secondary deposit (Fig. 282), particularly from a carcinoma of the bladder or rectum or from an osteosarcoma in another bone.

The parosteal osteosarcoma gives a particularly dense shadow adjacent to the cortex with very little evidence of bone erosion, and is therefore sometimes mistaken in the radiograph for an area of myositis ossificans. A similar error may be made on histological examination of a small part of the tumour taken from too small a biopsy, whether it looks in the radiograph like a myositis or shows feathering typical of an osteosarcoma. Fuller histological examination will generally reveal the correct diagnosis.

Malignant bone tumours with much periosteal new bone

Malignant bone tumours with much periosteal new bone occur less frequently than the last group. The predominant appearance is an extensive periosteal shadow due to calcification in the subperiosteal tumour or to excitation of periosteal new bone by the tumour.

The lesion is usually seen only in the middle third of a femur or tibia (Fig. 263), and the periosteal shadow may be laminated, giving an "onion-skin" appearance (Fig. 283). Some slight cortical or cancellous bone erosion may be visible in the routine radiograph or may be seen in a high penetration film or in a tomogram. The periosteal new bone may extend over most of the shaft or be localized over an area of erosion only 1–2 centimetres long (Fig. 284). Such an appearance may be seen in a Ewing's type of tumour or a secondary deposit from a neuroblastoma. Very occasionally an area of deep erosion associated with massive periosteal new bone formation is seen in the upper third of a femur (Fig. 285) in Hodgkin's disease or a secondary deposit from a carcinoma. In the latter case extensive erosive secondary deposits with more usual characteristics will be present in other bones.

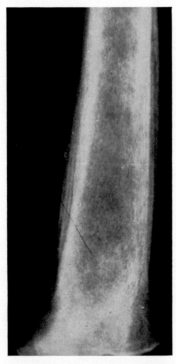

FIG. 283.—Secondary deposit from a neuroblastoma. Male aged 4 years. Erosion of the lower end of the femur with periosteal linear shadow, and linear transradiant zones giving onion-skin appearance. Pain in thigh 1 month. Neuroblastoma near but not in the suprarenal.

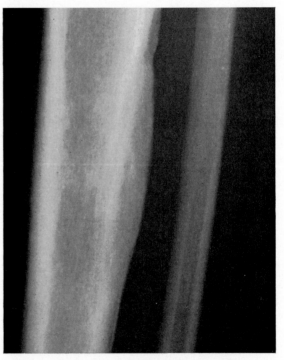

FIG. 284.—Secondary deposit from a neuroblastoma. Male aged 8 years. Slight cortical erosion and dense periosteal shadow on posterior aspect of middle third of tibia. Slight injury 1 year previously with persistent pain since. Some swelling. Biopsy—neuroblastoma. Radiotherapy with resolution for 10 years. Then died from secondary deposits in lungs.

Leukaemia

Multiple erosions in the form of diffuse trabecular absorption of the submetaphyseal regions are seen in leukaemia in children (*see* page 100). They are sometimes associated with narrow linear deposits of periosteal new bone (Fig. 166) induced by subperiosteal infiltration with leukaemic tissue, or perhaps a subperiosteal haemorrhage.

Occasionally, a leukaemic deposit in the bone in an adult results in a localized area of bone erosion some 2–4 centimetres in size. This may show some periosteal new bone nearby, especially if it sustains a spontaneous fracture which induces some callus.

DIFFERENTIAL DIAGNOSIS

The site of the lesion is not often of help in differentiating a malignant neoplasm from an inflammatory or syphilitic lesion. If a phalanx or carpal bone is affected, a malignant neoplasm can almost be excluded as a cause of periostitis and erosion, but in all other sites either type of lesion is possible. Nor does the part of the bone affected give any special clues since neoplastic or inflammatory lesions, though most common in the proximal or distal third of a bone, may also occur in the middle third.

Radiology

The radiological appearances, taken in conjunction with the clinical findings, are often highly suggestive of malignant disease when the erosion is gross and the periostitis slight (as in Fig. 277) or when there is feathering with no clinical evidence of inflammatory disease (as in Fig. 281). They are suggestive of inflammatory disease when there is clinical evidence to support this diagnosis and the periosteal reaction and erosion are well balanced as in Fig. 267. In cases where there is little erosion and much periostitis and the clinical findings are indefinite, the x-ray diagnosis is far less accurate.

Whenever a radiograph of a bone shows the combination of erosion and periostitis and the diagnosis is uncertain, a radiograph of the chest should be taken. There is always the possibility that this may give x-ray evidence of pulmonary secondary deposits, a primary bronchial carcinoma or active tuberculosis, suggesting that the bone condition is malignant or tuberculous. However, it is only fair to state that as a rule it will show no abnormalities and will not assist the diagnosis, at any rate in the early stages.

In many obscure cases radiographs of other bones are useful, since the finding of other areas of erosion will suggest secondary deposits. In these cases a lateral view of the skull and vertebrae and a posterior view of the pelvis and major long bones of the limbs will generally be sufficient.

When no primary lesion can be detected on clinical examination, a radiographic examination of the kidneys, including an intravenous pyelogram, will sometimes reveal an unsuspected renal or suprarenal tumour.

Wassermann and Kahn tests

A Wassermann and Kahn reaction test is often indicated since a positive finding, although rare nowadays, would at least suggest the possibility of a syphilitic lesion.

Bone biopsy

Finally, a bone biopsy may be necessary for diagnosis. The value of this was questioned by Brailsford (1948) because in some cases it produced an initial diagnosis which was proved wrong by the subsequent course of the disease. Nevertheless, in by far the majority of cases accurate results can be obtained. It seems probable that the histological findings are most easy to interpret if the specimen is taken from an area of erosion rather than from an area of reactive sclerosis. Some errors in interpretation can be avoided if the pathologist gives a factual report of what he has seen as well as giving his conclusions, thus showing, for instance, whether a diagnosis of an osteoclastoma is based on the finding of a few giant cells or on the character of the stroma. In many cases a bacteriological examination made at the same time as the biopsy may be helpful, and neglect of this additional examination may often be regretted later on.

The value and accuracy of biopsy findings are increased if they are evaluated in relation to both the clinical findings and the x-ray appearances. When all three are typical and in agreement the degree of accuracy is high, but when there are no obvious clinical clues and there is disagreement between the histological and radiological findings, accurate diagnosis may be impossible and the case should be handled with this initial element of doubt kept in mind. In order to avoid errors, it is important to bear in mind the variable course taken by certain tumours. For example, it is sometimes assumed that an osteoclastoma is always relatively innocent and that a histological diagnosis of this condition is at fault if the local lesion subsequently becomes uncontrollable or if pulmonary secondary deposits appear. In the author's experience such tumours show a great range in the degree of their aggressiveness (*see also* Jaffe, Lichtenstein and Portis, 1940).

PERIOSTEAL SHADOW AND SCLEROSIS

The combination of a periosteal shadow and deep bone sclerosis without obvious erosion is occasionally seen in a long bone. It often presents considerable difficulties of diagnosis, since identical x-ray appearances are seen whether the lesion is syphilitic, bacterial inflammatory or neoplastic. The bone sclerosis (or increased density of the bone) may be situated either adjacent to the deep margin of the cortex or deep in the cancellous bone and separate from the inner table of the cortex. In the first case the cortex has a thickened appearance at the expense of the trabeculae; in the second, the trabeculae appear thickened and the transradiant intertrabecular spaces are encroached upon and become entirely or in part invisible, so that the affected area has a dense homogeneous appearance.

When the deep sclerosis is relatively slight and associated with much periosteal new bone, it may be difficult to say whether the dense homogeneous appearance includes deep sclerosis or whether a normal trabecular pattern is merely hidden by the surrounding shadow of the periosteal new bone.

The periosteal shadow, in its turn, may either be quite clearly demarcated from the outer border of the cortex or be intimately fused to it so that it is impossible to distinguish the two. In either case there will be a bony prominence at the affected area which can be demonstrated by reference to the normal cortical edge above or below. When the lesion occupies the middle third of a long bone it produces a spindle-shaped expansion of the shaft (Fig. 286). This appearance is typical of the periostitis–sclerosis combination. On the whole a sclerotic lesion tends to be more localized than an erosive lesion, thus leading to a local build-up of the periosteal response.

Low-grade Chronic Osteomyelitis

A frequent cause of a localized periosteal new bone formation together with deep sclerosis of the bone beneath is a chronic inflammatory lesion. If the lesion follows on an acute osteomyelitis from which organisms were isolated, the diagnosis will be clear. Sometimes the infection may be subacute or even very chronic—as in the sclerosing osteomyelitis described by Garré—and the diagnosis may not at first be certain.

The periosteal new bone is particularly dense and is often indistinguishable from the adjacent cortex beneath. It tends to be widest near the middle of the lesion so that the bone shows a fusiform expansion (Fig. 286). This, together with the dense appearance of the deep bone, gives an appearance indistinguishable from some forms of malignant neoplasm. The clinical findings are often of no help—these consist of a history of some pain and swelling for weeks or months and a localized, slightly tender, hard swelling which may be felt on palpation. There may be no fever or leucocytosis. It is therefore often necessary to perform a biopsy for the purpose of diagnosis. In an inflammatory lesion the histological features will be quite definite, while bacteriological examination in such cases frequently reveals a staphylococcus.

DIAPHYSEAL DYSPLASIA (ENGELMANN)

Periosteal thickening and deep sclerosis of the middle third of the shaft, resulting in a dense bone with fusiform expansion, has been described by Engelmann (1929), Gulledge and White (1951) and Pugh (1954). The lesion may effect several long bones and is often symmetrical on either side. It occurs in children and is associated with loss of weight and disturbances of the neuro-muscular system.

172

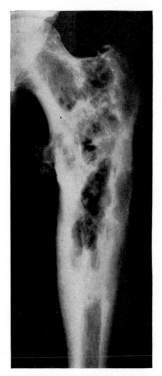

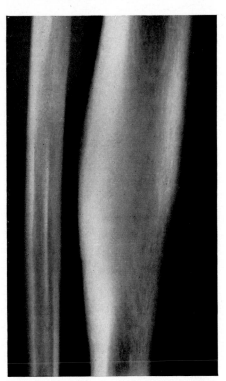

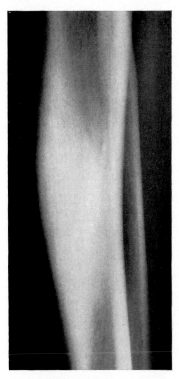

FIG. 285.—Secondary deposit in Hodgkin's disease. Male aged 21 years. Extensive periosteal new bone and deep erosion upper third of femur. Nodes in neck. P.M. proof H.D. of femur, also deposits in the lungs and the lymph nodes.

FIG. 286.—Chronic osteomyelitis. Male aged 19 years. Dense periosteal new bone and sclerosis with spindle-shaped swelling in middle third of tibia. Thought to be a sarcoma, but biopsy showed it to be an inflammatory lesion. No organisms found.

FIG. 287.—Osteoid osteoma. Male aged 13 years. Dense periosteal new bone and sclerosis of middle third of tibia (compare with Fig. 286). Increasing swelling in leg following a kick. W.R. negative. Excision of 5 mm. nidus (invisible in radiograph) carried out. Histology—osteoid osteoma.

A similar appearance may be seen in an adult (Fig. 288), when pain may be the only symptom. A case is reported by Mikity and Jacobson (1958) in which the bone changes were first seen at the age of 29 years and hardly changed over the next 22 years.

Histologically there are sclerosis and hypertrophied trabeculae with no evidence as to the cause of the condition.

OSTEOID OSTEOMA

Occasionally the dense sclerotic bone and abundant periosteal new bone may represent an osteoid osteoma (*see* page 176), the small central erosion so characteristic of this condition being masked by the other two changes. Differentiation from a syphilitic or chronic low-grade coccal lesion such as that illustrated in Fig. 286 is not possible from the radiographs. On the whole the pain is rather more intense with an osteoid osteoma than with other conditions giving a similar x-ray appearance, but this is not true in every case. The erosion containing the central red nidus may not be seen radiographically even in high penetration films and tomograms specially taken for the purpose (Fig. 287), although it is conspicuous and easily found on surgical exploration after paring away some of the dense bone.

SYPHILIS

One cause of this appearance, although a very uncommon one nowadays, is a localized chronic osteitis in tertiary syphilis (*see* page 164). Although some erosion of the cortex may be seen on histological examination, it is invisible in the radiograph owing to the abundance of the sclerosis and periosteal new

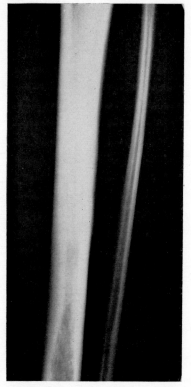

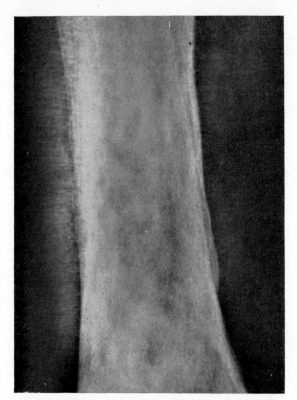

FIG. 288.—Osteosclerosis tibia (? Engelmann's disease). Female aged 35 years. Three months' pain in leg. Blood chemistry normal. W.R. (—). Biopsy—increased vascularity and sclerosis.

FIG. 289.—Urticaria pigmentosa (mast-cell leukaemia). Female aged 67 years. Periosteal new bone with striate calcifications at right angles to shaft. Twelve years' claret-coloured skin eruption. Mast-cell infiltration skin nodules and bone. W.b.c. normal.

bone. Diagnosis is possible only from the clinical history and serological tests, though even here some caution is necessary, since an inflammatory or neoplastic condition is possible in a patient with a positive Wassermann reaction.

MALIGNANT NEOPLASM

Rarely, a malignant neoplasm induces an intense sclerotic reaction with much cortical or periosteal new bone. The radiological appearances, the history and the clinical findings may be the same as for a low-grade bacterial inflammatory sclerosis with periosteal reaction, and the diagnosis may be established only after a bone biopsy.

The histological type may be an osteosarcoma.

Mast-cell (leukaemic) deposits and urticaria pigmentosa

Extensive periosteal deposits and deep sclerosis of the major long bones may be seen in urticaria pigmentosa, both the sclerosis and the periosteal new bone being induced by leukaemic "mast" cell deposits, which are also the cause of small purple skin spots. The periosteal deposits may be of the usual linear type parallel to the shaft, or there may be linear deposits at right angles to the shaft giving a sun-ray appearance (Fig. 289). The distal major limb bones may show a mixture of osteoporosis and periosteal new bone, while the vertebral column and pelvis may show only sclerosis.

The case illustrated is described by Havard and Bodley Scott (1959).

PERIOSTEAL OPACITY WITH EROSION AND SCLEROSIS

In lesions showing erosion and abundant periostitis, slight degrees of sclerosis tend not to be recognized, so that this triple combination of shadows seems more rare than it actually is. In fact, sclerosis is probably quite often present in many cases of osteomyelitis and neoplasia in which periostitis and erosion are thought to be the only changes (Figs. 262 and 263). When the periosteal new bone is less abundant or the sclerosis more marked, the three changes can be separately identified.

The sclerosis, which is the result of osteoblastic activity without corresponding osteoclastic resorption, depends on rather selective stimulation or a particular state of the vascular supply, so that its presence with periostitis and erosion is somewhat haphazard and unaccountable. The bone around the central erosion in which lies the nidus of an osteoid osteoma invariably reacts by sclerosis; on the other hand, though sclerosis is usual in chronic pyogenic or syphilitic infections, it is rather less common in malignant neoplasms.

CHRONIC OSTEOMYELITIS

The same combination of changes is usually present in chronic osteomyelitis, all three being well shown in Fig. 269. The relative amount of each change varies from case to case. Often the periostitis and sclerosis are a more prominent feature than the erosion, which may either be difficult to see or be clearly visible and well-demarcated but relatively small in extent.

Sequestra in osteomyelitis

In the later stages of an osteomyelitis, the radiograph is rarely needed for diagnosis but is often important to demonstrate the presence or absence of sequestra. A sequestrum can be demonstrated when it is denser than the surrounding somewhat demineralized bone and is surrounded by a transradiant zone which in its turn is demarcated by a dense sclerotic zone (Fig. 290). It may be clearly seen in the routine radiographs, but often, owing to the abundant periosteal new bone and sclerosis, it is visible only

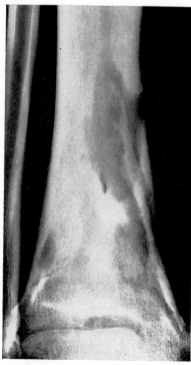

FIG. 290.—Osteomyelitis with sequestrum. Male aged 18 years. Erosion of medial side of tibia with dense linear shadow within it indicating a sequestrum, which was removed. Much sclerosis and some periosteal new bone. Onset of acute osteomyelitis 4 years previously. Finally healed.

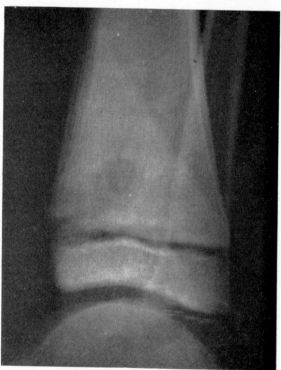

FIG. 291.—Brodie's bone abscess. Male aged 12 years. Circular erosion with sclerosis around and some periosteal new bone anteriorly in lower third of diaphysis of tibia. Some pain and swelling for 2 months. Resolution after penicillin.

when extra radiographs are taken with much more exposure, and with either a coned down x-ray beam of 5–10 centimetres or a clearing grid, to increase the detail and contrast. Sometimes it cannot be seen with certainty except by tomography (*see* page 210).

CHRONIC LOCALIZED BONE ABSCESS

A rather more localized erosion with surrounding sclerosis and only a little periosteal new bone is seen in a chronic bone abscess. The clinical picture is often rather inconspicuous with some pain, swelling and tenderness but with little or no fever or leucocytosis. It is therefore most important for the diagnosis to detect the rather inconspicuous line shadow of the periosteal new bone (Fig. 291). The amount of sclerosis is variable and may be slight, though it is always present and demonstrable as a slight loss of the trabecular pattern in the zone of normal density around the central cavity. Sometimes the sclerosis is much more marked and the erosion inconspicuous, the appearances then being similar to those of an osteoid osteoma.

OSTEOID OSTEOMA

An area of periosteal new bone with dense sclerosis beneath it and a small transradiant zone within the dense area will suggest an osteoid osteoma (Fig. 292).

The transradiant zone is generally eccentric and may lie in the cortex on one side or in the dense bone just beneath the cortex. It may not be clearly seen in a routine radiograph owing to the considerable

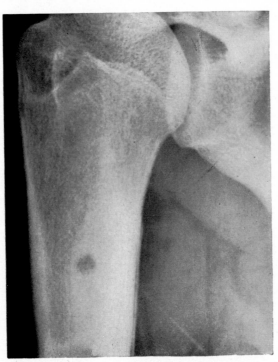

FIG. 292.—Osteoid osteoma. Male aged 23 years. Circular transradiant zone 5 mm. in diameter in humerus with surrounding sclerosis and some periosteal shadowing medially. Increasing pain 8 months. Nidus removed. Histology—osteoid osteoma.

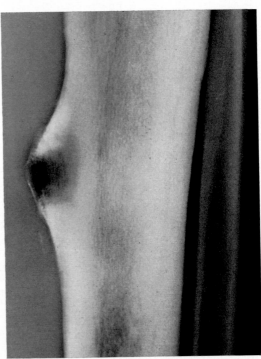

FIG. 293.—Osteoid osteoma. Female aged 31 years. Volcano-shaped raised cortical projection with erosion of its tip and sclerosis of its base. Painful swelling on anterior aspect of tibia, increasing in size, 2 years. Gouged out. Histology—osteoid osteoma.

radio-opacity of the surrounding sclerotic bone, but will usually be visible in an extra radiograph taken with more exposure and the x-ray beam coned down to about 10 centimetres or in a tomogram.

The periosteal new bone, which is homogeneous, often extends 1–3 centimetres in length. It is widest over the transradiant nidus and tapers off in width on either side. There is no transradiant zone between it and the cortex. In some cases the periosteal new bone may become heaped up in the form of a conical projection, with the transradiant zone of the nidus at the top and the sclerotic subcortical bone beneath, resulting in the so-called volcano deformity (Fig. 293).

The sclerotic dense area beneath the cortex usually extends right across the width of the bone.

Common sites are the upper third of the shaft of a humerus or femur, especially the region of the femoral neck, but the lesion may occur in almost any bone including even a vertebra or a phalanx.

In many cases severe and persistent pain in the region of the lesion is the indication for radiography, but in others in which the pain is perhaps slight or absent, the radiograph may have been taken fortuitously or because of slight swelling. The lesion tends to develop slowly over weeks or months, and symptoms may be absent or slight in the early stage, so that by the time a radiograph is taken the bone changes are quite obvious and fairly extensive.

Clinically and bacteriologically there is no evidence that the lesion is inflammatory. At operation the central nidus is pink and soft, and histological examination shows a spherical area of vascular connective tissue in which osteoid tissue is being laid down by active osteoblastic activity. The osteoid tissue forms linear spicules which are partly calcified, while osteoclasts are frequently in evidence. The central nidus is surrounded by dense bone showing no characteristic histological features. Thus the lesion appears to be benign tumour arising from osteoblasts. The removal of the nidus results in the relief of pain and the gradual disappearance of the deep sclerotic and superficial periosteal new bone.

Malignant Neoplasm

A combination of periosteal new bone, deep sclerosis and a surface pressure erosion may be seen in a bone in response to a nearby fibrosarcoma of the soft tissues or a synovioma arising from an adjacent tendon sheath. A metatarsal or femur may be the site of such a lesion. It is sometimes difficult to be sure whether the dense appearance of the bone is due to deep sclerosis or to the overlying dense periosteal new bone.

9—Alterations in the Bone Architecture

The bone architecture as seen in a radiograph of a normal person consists of an outer homogeneous band a few millimetres wide, representing the cortex, and an inner striate pattern made up of fine white lines with dark or relatively transradiant spaces between them, representing the trabeculae.

The cortical architecture is altered by thickening due to the deposition of periosteal new bone or deep sclerosis; thinning due to a cyst-like lesion in the medulla or internal scalloping out by a malignant disease (Fig. 184); and the breaking up of the homogeneous band by transradiant zones into a lace-like pattern as in hyperparathyroidism (Fig. 203).

The trabecular pattern is altered by trabecular mineral loss, or by absorption of some trabeculae with compensatory thickening of others (Fig. 162) as in many forms of under-mineralization.

In fact almost every type of bone disorder causes some alteration in the bone architecture, but most of them are grouped in the previous chapters under such headings as local or general decrease of density, increased density and combination changes. In Paget's disease the alteration of both the cortex and the trabecular pattern is so radical that it merits separate grouping.

PAGET'S DISEASE

Alterations in the bone architecture in Paget's disease may be present throughout the skeleton or in a single bone, and throughout the bone or confined to a half or a third of it. A common finding is to see typical changes in the upper or lower half of a tibia, the affected area ending sharply with a well-defined convex border pointing towards the centre of the shaft with no line of dense bone separating it from the adjacent normal trabeculae.

When the changes are seen in only one bone and the diagnosis of Paget's disease is suspected, further views of other bones will often show the typical alterations of bone architecture to confirm the diagnosis. Any bowing of a bone or local tenderness would be an indication to radiograph that bone, but if there are no clinical clues a lateral view of the skull and a posterior view of the pelvis and lumbo-dorsal region may be worth while.

Cortical changes

In the affected area the cortex is increased in width by the laying down of new bone, particularly on its outer surface. In spite of its increased width the cortical shadow is often grey rather than white, indicating a bone with a relatively low calcium content. It may remain homogeneous or eventually show transradiant areas between the opaque areas of new bone.

The increase in width of the cortex is usually obvious in a long bone, and a tibia or femur may be 6 or more centimetres wide from front to back. In the ischio-pubic ramus the actual increase in width may be less conspicuous, but is none the less noticeable and represents an important diagnostic feature when differentiating the condition from a sclerosing secondary deposit. In a sclerosing secondary deposit there is a similar increase in density of this bone but no increase in width—although deep sclerosis may increase the width of the cortical layer at the expense of the cancellous bone.

Trabecular changes

The trabecular pattern in the affected area is either markedly altered or entirely replaced by structureless bone with a grey homogeneous appearance.

In a long bone, for instance, instead of running in the normal longitudinal and transverse directions, the trabeculae run obliquely making a criss-cross pattern; many of them are thickened, while others are resorbed and produce transradiant zones between the still visible ones (Fig. 294). The trabecular resorption may be so marked that it gives an almost cyst-like appearance, which will be particularly conspicuous if the trabecular pattern around is entirely lost and replaced by homogeneous bone (Fig. 295).

In an affected vertebra the widely-spaced thickened trabeculae may run more or less vertically, giving a coarsely striate pattern, or they may be entirely replaced by structureless bone giving the vertebra an even grey appearance (Figs. 120 and 121).

In the ilia some trabeculae are absorbed, while those remaining are thickened to as much as 3 milli-metres and run as wide line shadows more or less at right angles to the outer cortical line of the iliac

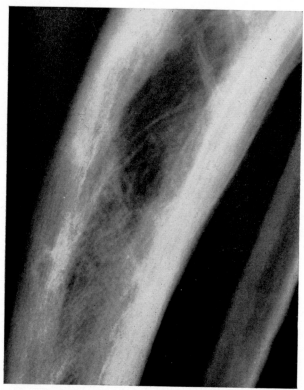

FIG. 294.—Paget's disease. Male aged 66 years. Widened rather striate cortex, absorption of some trabeculae with irregular pattern of new thickened ones. Tibia 4·5 cm. wide, and anterior bowing, noticed by patient for 10 years. Similar changes in femora and pelvis.

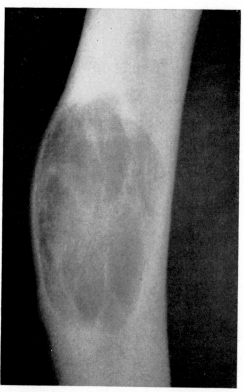

FIG. 295.—Paget's disease. Male aged 67 years. Dense homogeneous bone surrounding 3 cm. cyst-like transradiant area in middle third of humerus. Bone bowed and widened. Similar other side, typical changes similar to Fig. 294 in the tibiae, and thickened mottled vault.

crests. In many cases these are crossed by other coarse line shadows running more or less parallel to the crests. These thickened trabeculae may be spaced several millimetres apart, giving the bone a very coarse striated appearance.

Associated bone deformities

Any bone showing gross alterations in bone architecture tends also to show evidence of softening.

The tibiae and femora commonly show anterior convex bowing, while an affected radius may be bowed laterally and appear rather too long in relation to an unaffected ulna.

The pelvis becomes triradiate (*see* page 25), especially if both sides are affected, but if there are alterations in the trabecular pattern on only one side, there may be indentation of this side only.

Deformities of other bones are seen, such as the increased curvature of an affected clavicle, the flatten-ing and widening of an affected vertebra (Figs. 120 and 121) and platybasia of the skull (*see below*).

Spontaneous fracture

In spite of the increased width of the cortex, the bones are brittle so that minor trauma may result in a transverse fracture, particularly of the upper third of a femur or tibia or the middle third of a humerus. The fracture will unite readily, with abundant calcified callus. Looser zones may be seen.

The skull

The vault of the skull may be increased in thickness to as much as 4 centimetres, the outer table tending to be more thickened and less dense than the inner table, which extends into and may eventually replace the diploic bone. The increase in density of the outer table is often uneven, and the dense areas seen end-on may appear as rather ill-defined circular shadows $\frac{1}{2}$–1 centimetre in diameter, spaced a few centimetres apart and giving the vault a rather woolly appearance. Between the thickened tables, the diploic architecture is lost and the area may be transradiant or may be increased in density with a homogeneous shadowing; this may join the shadows of the thickened tables and produce a vault with a homogeneous grey appearance.

Platybasia

This is common in a badly affected and much thickened skull. There are several ways of demonstrating this change. One is to draw a line backwards from the posterior end of the hard palate to the under-surface of the occipital bone. Normally the tip of the odontoid process of the axis will not project more than 5 millimetres above the line, and is often well below it. In platybasia, whether due to Paget's disease or some other cause of bone softening or to a congenital variation, the odontoid will project 7 millimetres or more above it. If a mid-line tomogram is available, the line may be drawn from the palate to the posterior rim of the foramen magnum. In a normal person the tip of the odontoid will lie well below this line, while in platybasia it will project several millimetres above it.

Osteoporosis circumscripta

In some cases the vault, instead of being thickened, shows a single area of relative transradiancy with loss of diploic structure and thinning of the cortex. This condition may extend from the front to the back of the vault and occupy the upper or the lower half, and is often confined to one side. It is sharply demarcated where it meets the still normal bone, but there is no line of dense bone separating the two. The margin tends to be slightly curved so that the transradiant zone is oval or lobulated in shape.

It may remain unchanged for years, though some cases progress to the more typical appearances of Paget's disease with increased density and thickening of the vault. In most cases there are typical appearances of Paget's disease in some other bone such as a mandible, tibia or pelvis.

Pathology

The basic pathological process of Paget's disease, or osteitis deformans, is the simultaneous occurrence of bone resorption and new bone formation, which remodels the bone and produces a characteristic appearance unlike that seen in any other bone lesion. It is a disease usually found in persons over the age of 40 years, and is not related to hyperparathyroidism or to fibrous dysplasia. The alkaline phosphatase is raised as a result of the active bone resorption, otherwise the blood chemistry is normal.

Calcitonin (*see* page 93) can give a sustained reduction in the rate of bone turnover, especially in Paget's disease, with relief of bone pain if present, and remodelling of bone towards a more normal architecture.

In the early or florid stage of the disease, bone resorption is predominant and the bone is softer and lighter than normal. At a later stage, new bone formation outstrips resorption to produce the large, deformed, thickened bones seen in advanced cases.

Histologically the normal bone architecture is characteristically modified by the presence of large and irregular bone trabeculae, with many osteoclastic giant cells closely applied to the lacunae and apparently absorbing the bone, while in adjacent areas rows of active mononuclear osteoblasts can be seen laying down new bone. This bone matrix is mineralized in an irregular manner as shown by the presence of prominent blue-staining cement lines permeating the substance of the trabeculae and forming a mosaic pattern throughout the abnormal bone. The bone marrow is replaced by a vascular fibrous tissue, and it is the vascularity of this which alters the blood flow through the bone and causes the cardiomegaly which is frequently seen.

Paget's disease and sarcoma of bone

An ill-defined transradiant zone several centimetres in size, seen in a bone severely affected with Paget's disease, will suggest a complicating osteosarcoma. The incidence of this change in Paget's disease is almost 1 per cent, which is far higher than the incidence of a sarcoma in an otherwise normal bone.

If a swelling can be felt over this area, or if the transradiant zone is seen to enlarge in a matter of weeks in serial radiographs, the diagnosis may be obvious, but an ill-defined transradiant zone seen in the initial radiograph may easily be mistaken for an area of bone fibrosis, a common change in Paget's disease.

In most cases the sarcoma results in purely osteolytic changes, but occasionally fine linear shadows may be seen at right angles to the cortex. The cortex is usually eroded beneath these sun-ray spicules, which project out into a soft tissue mass beyond the usual bone contour.

Histologically this neoplasm may be an osteosarcoma, a chondrosarcoma, a fibrosarcoma or even a giant-cell tumour. In the last the prognosis is quite good, but in the others secondary deposits and death are common within a year.

10—Alterations in Joint Space (Arthritis) and Associated Bone Changes

INTRODUCTION

THE DIMINISHED JOINT SPACE

A diminished interval between the articular cortex of the two bones forming a joint, an x-ray appearance commonly referred to as a "diminished joint space", is the hallmark of an arthritis. The diminished joint space represents a loss of articular cartilage which may be brought about by a variety of pathological mechanisms as mentioned below. In suppurative (pyogenic) arthritis the articular cartilage is digested by proteolytic ferments in the pus. In tuberculous arthritis the cartilage is sequestrated by a tuberculous pannus developing on both its articular and subchondral surfaces, and freed from its attachments to the underlying bone, it dies.

In rheumatoid arthritis, not only are the periarticular tissues involved but the cartilage is replaced by a fibrous pannus, resulting in fibrous ankylosis. The pannus may cause resorption of the nearby bone.

In osteoarthritis, the articular cartilage fibrillates and degenerates and becomes worn away until the articular surfaces are formed by eburnated bone.

In gout the cartilage or nearby bone is resorbed as a result of the deposition of sodium biurate crystals in it.

The radiological appearance eventually resulting from destruction of the articular cartilage, whatever the cause, is a loss of space between the articular cortex of the two bones forming the joint, though if the process results in a massive effusion into the joint, the joint space may be increased for a short time.

ASSOCIATED BONE CHANGES

Four types of bone changes may be seen in association with the narrowed joint space. The most common is a small pointed outgrowth of the normal cortical and cancellous bone at the margins of the joint, representing the bony lipping so commonly seen in osteoarthritis.

The second is a localized area of bone resorption or erosion. This may take the form of a pitted erosion of the articular cortex and of some of the bone beneath, a similar erosion of the joint margin affecting both the articular and diaphyseal cortices, or a circular erosion lying deep in the bone, often a few millimetres away from the articular cortex. The deep erosions may be either sharply demarcated by a white linear shadow of dense bone or surrounded by normal trabeculae without any intervening demarcation.

A third bone change is that of a more widespread loss of density extending for some distance away from the joint and perhaps affecting the whole bone or even the whole region, including bones remote from the arthritic area. Such density loss may be either even or patchy.

Finally, there may be some linear periosteal shadowing adjacent to the cortex in the neighbourhood of the affected joint.

DIFFICULTIES OF CLASSIFICATION

The classification of arthritis is controversial except when a specific cause, such as a bacterial infection or a haemorrhage, can be demonstrated. Arthritis of unknown cause has been divided in this book into cases showing the classical clinical and radiological features of "rheumatoid" arthritis and those showing less common and well-known features. For clinical and radiological reasons, ankylosing spondylitis has been considered as a separate lesion, and so also have the various rather rheumatoid types of arthritis which are associated with psoriasis, ulcerative colitis, non-specific urethritis and rheumatic fever.

Diseases of unknown aetiology but of partly known mechanism such as an osteoarthritis, a neuropathic arthritis or an arthritis with a metabolic defect (gout) have been placed in a separate group. A complication of any classification is the fact that, owing to altered function resulting from previous joint damage, osteoarthritis may arise on the site of long-standing arthritis of some other type.

ARTHRITIS OF KNOWN CAUSE

Pyogenic Arthritis (Septic Arthritis)

In most cases of septic arthritis the onset with pain and fever is sudden, the progress of the lesion rapid and the clinical diagnosis fairly obvious. It will be suspected particularly if the patient is known to be suffering from an infection or if there has been a penetrating wound in the neighbourhood of the joint. Occasionally, however, the joint lesion appears to be the primary and only septic infection, and the nature of the acute arthritis may at first be uncertain.

Radiologically, the earlier changes are often a slight opacity of the joint space relative to that on the other side and a faint opacity and swelling of the soft tissue shadows around the joint. The joint space may be increased in width due to a purulent synovial effusion. In some cases this is under such high pressure that the weakened or partly destroyed capsule and ligaments are unable to retain the bones in position, and a pathological dislocation occurs (Fig. 297). In the absence of a dislocation, the joint space will soon be narrowed in spite of the effusion.

With effective chemotherapy the lesion may be arrested at this stage, but often treatment is not instituted early enough or is not sufficiently effective, and a localized area of erosion of the articular cortex or of the bone beneath occurs. This may eventually become quite considerable and, for instance, in the case of a septic arthritis of the hip joint may lead to almost total destruction of the head of the femur or (in a child) the femoral epiphysis.

By the fourteenth day or soon after, a rather patchy loss of density appears deep in the bone, consisting of transradiant areas 3–5 millimetres in diameter and scattered at rather larger intervals. This loss of density extends for several centimetres towards the centre of the shaft of a long bone, and may be seen in nearby bones not actually forming the affected joint in a hand or a foot.

Eventually a small linear shadow of periosteal new bone may appear adjacent to the shaft of one of the long bones forming the joint. This is situated close to the joint but beyond the limits of the attachment of the synovial membrane (Fig. 296). In a subacute infection of a joint this periosteal new bone may be an important feature of the diagnosis, since it is unusual in other forms of arthritis.

As recovery proceeds, the loss of bone density becomes less obvious and finally disappears, and the periosteal new bone fuses to the cortex and becomes absorbed. The joint space, on the other hand, remains diminished or may even disappear completely, with trabecular continuity between the bones indicating bony ankylosis.

A septic arthritis tends to be confined to a single joint, but if it is secondary to a severe septicaemia, several joints may become infected. Sometimes the infection reaches the joint by direct spread from an osteomyelitis of the nearby bone, a common sequence of events in the case of a septic finger. The diagnosis is usually confirmed at an early stage by aspiration and isolation of the organism.

In the case of a septic arthritis from *Bacillus coli* the lesion may be less acute, the radiographic changes less conspicuous, and the whole course of the lesion more chronic.

Pathologically an acute pyogenic arthritis has pus in the joint cavity and there is a purely destructive process of the joint structures. The synovial tissues show an acute inflammatory reaction with increased vascularity and oedema. At an early stage the articular cartilage becomes pitted and then destroyed by the proteolytic ferments in the pus. If uncontrolled, the inflammatory process spreads to involve the subchondral bone, which is replaced by granulation tissue. Subsequent organization of the inflammatory tissue into fibrous tissue and eventually into bone will result in bony ankylosis.

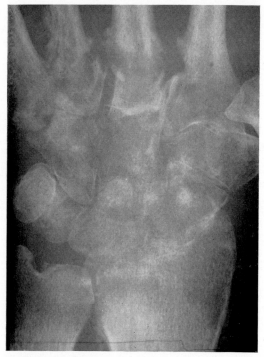

FIG. 296.—Pyogenic arthritis. Loss of wrist joint spaces. Erosions and periosteal new bone in metacarpals and radius. Staphylococcal.

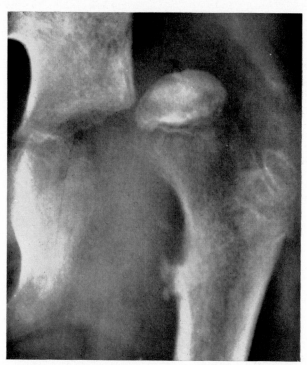

FIG. 297.—Typhoid arthritis. Female aged 6 years. Dislocation of hip, erosion of femoral neck and periosteal new bone. Proved typhoid arthritis. Recovered.

GONOCOCCAL ARTHRITIS

A gonococcal arthritis is a relatively rare condition now owing to recent advances in the control and treatment of the genital infection, but cases still occur, particularly when the genital infection has inconspicuous clinical manifestations and remains unsuspected and untreated.

The x-ray appearances are those of a low-grade septic arthritis. The joint space is often only slightly narrowed. There may be a small area of articular bone absorption or there may be none. A rather characteristic change in the knee is a 5 millimetre punched-out area at the medial margin of the tibia with slight or no periosteal new bone formation near the joint. Patchy regional loss of bone density is often quite marked.

The combination of a painful joint with these radiological features may suggest the diagnosis—particularly if there has been transient pain and swelling of several other joints previously. The organism can rarely be found in the joint fluid, and it is possible that many cases diagnosed as gonoccocal arthritis were in fact Reiter's type of arthritis.

A severe untreated lesion may progress to complete bony ankylosis.

VIRUS ARTHRITIS

A joint space may become diminished and there may be some articular cortical erosion as a result of a severe viral infection such as smallpox (Cockshott and MacGregor, 1959).

TUBERCULOUS ARTHRITIS

A tuberculous arthritis is often confined to one joint, particularly one of the larger joints of a limb, the sacro-iliac joint or an intervertebral disc, but in the widely disseminated type of disease several joints may be affected simultaneously or successively.

The most characteristic changes, in addition to the early diminution of a joint space, are periarticular low-density shadowing due to thickened synovial membrane and effusion, articular cortical erosion, and a very even and often severe loss of density of the nearby bone (Figs. 298 and 300). These changes vary according to the age of the patient and the virulence of the infection: the younger the patient the more conspicuous the trabecular absorption in the bones near the joint, and the more virulent the infection the greater likelihood that changes will be seen in the initial radiograph and the more severe the bone destruction and nearby loss of bone density.

The changes also vary to some extent according to the site of the lesion (*see below*).

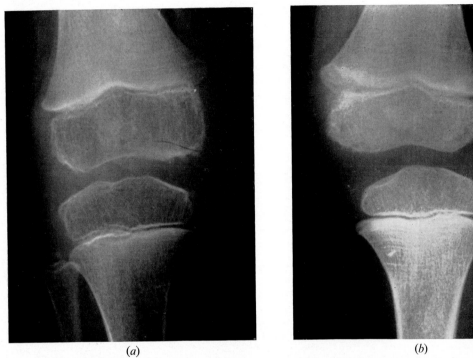

(*a*)   (*b*)

FIG. 298—(*a*) Tuberculous arthritis. Male aged 5 years. Swelling of knee and slight pain 2 months. Slight narrowing of joint space, no erosion, synovial opacity and even loss of bone density shown by comparison with other (normal) side (*b*). In lateral view patella was more ossified than on normal side.

Tuberculosis of the hip joint

The onset of a tuberculous arthritis of a hip joint with pain and limping is often insidious, and in many cases the pain is referred to the knee. In some cases there may be no radiographic changes in the initial radiograph; in others there may be no more than a slight increase in the density and size of the soft tissue shadows round the femoral neck, often less marked than the similar shadow seen in an acute septic arthritis. More often, by the time the initial radiograph is taken there is slight narrowing of the joint space (Fig. 299). This change is soon followed by a general loss of the trabeculae in the femoral head and neck and upper third of the shaft. A small erosion of the femoral head involving the articular cortex may be seen.

If the infection is not brought under control, the destruction of the femoral head will increase and there will be some erosion of the articular cortex of the acetabulum. The widespread even loss of density of the femoral neck and shaft will increase, and the whole trabecular pattern may disappear as if erased with a brush. The cortex is thinned but remains clearly visible and gives a white pencilled outline to the rather transradiant, grey, structureless bone beneath. The joint space becomes greatly narrowed or may disappear almost completely.

At an early stage and in the absence of any radiographic abnormality, the clinical differentiation from other forms of arthritis or, in a child, from an osteochondritis may be very difficult, but it will usually be safe to rest the patient in bed without full immobilization and to observe the hip clinically and with serial radiographs at monthly intervals. Any diminution of the joint space would indicate an arthritis and, if seen in a child or adolescent, might indicate the need for anti-tuberculous therapy even if the diagnosis had not been established. If the diagnosis was then confirmed by satisfactory response or other evidence, the treatment could be continued; if some other diagnosis were made, it could be stopped.

In a rather more advanced stage of the disease, both radiographic and clinical findings will usually point to the diagnosis quite clearly in young people. In the older age groups there may still be uncertainty since the bone destruction and general loss of bone density nearby are less marked, and differentiation from a mono-articular rheumatoid arthritis may be possible only by a biopsy (*see* page 193).

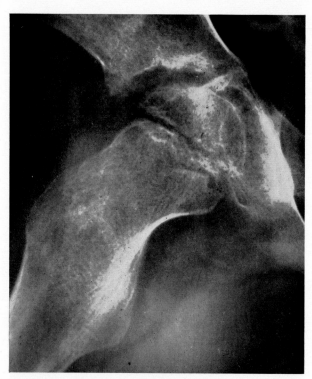

FIG. 299.—Tuberculous arthritis. Female aged 5 years. Narrowing of joint space, small erosion in femoral head and acetabulum. Even general demineralization with loss of trabecular pattern and pencilled outline by thinned cortex. Limp for 6 weeks. Slow improvement on streptomycin and P.A.S.

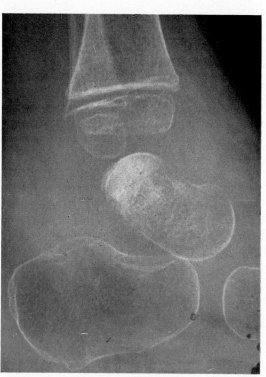

FIG. 300.—Tuberculous arthritis. Male aged 2 years. Erosion of posterior angle of talus and even demineralization of interior of tarsals with loss of most of trabecular pattern. Thinned cortex gives a pencilled outline to the transradiant interiors.

After the diagnosis has been established, further radiographs are indicated only at fairly long intervals, partly because alterations in the x-ray appearances occur very slowly, and partly to avoid inevitable and perhaps excessive gonadal radiation with no useful purpose served.

In cases successfully controlled by chemotherapy, the lesion tends to become stationary in a matter of months and then slowly regresses. During the healing stage a dense 2–3 millimetre line shadow often forms under the edge of the epiphysis of the femoral head and indicates a satisfactory response.

After perhaps a year or more the trabeculae slowly reform in the upper half of the femur, but the pattern rarely returns to normal unless the condition was diagnosed and arrested at a very early stage. More often an abnormal pattern persists, consisting of rather widened and widely spaced trabeculae, with the vertical trabecular lines more conspicuous than the transverse ones (Fig. 192).

Woolly shadows appearing near the upper end of the femur will suggest calcification in an abscess, but this is not a very common finding with modern treatment.

Tuberculosis of the knee joint

In a child a tuberculous lesion of a knee often starts insidiously in the synovial membrane, with slight pain and swelling around the joint and wasting of the leg muscles. With good quality radiographs and with the other knee taken on the same film and using the same exposure as a control, it is often possible to see a slight increase in the radio-opacity of the joint space and a slight increase in the size and opacity of the surrounding soft tissue shadows. This appearance may persist for months, or the lesion may progress more rapidly—in which case diminution of the joint space will soon occur together with an even loss of density of the lower half of the femur and the upper half of the tibia (Fig. 298). In a lateral view the patella will show a similar loss of trabecular structure and radio-opacity. The loss of bone density will be much more marked if the limb has been immobilized. Later, a localized erosion of the articular cortex may be seen, particularly of the upper end of the tibia.

In an adult the synovial opacity and the even loss of bone density tend to be much less marked, and the bone erosion and diminished joint space rather more marked. Distinction from another type of infective arthritis or even a rheumatoid arthritis may be quite difficult even after clinical and serial x-ray observation, and in some cases a biopsy of the synovial membrane may be necessary to establish the diagnosis.

Tuberculosis of a tarsal joint

A tuberculous lesion may start in the tarsal joint or spread to it from a nearby bone. The talo-navicular joint is the one most commonly involved, but the lesion may be seen in any other tarsal joint including the talo-calcaneal joint.

In some cases, particularly in children, the only radiographic change for some months after the onset of pain and swelling of the foot may be a fairly even trabecular absorption of all the tarsal bones (Fig. 300), and perhaps the metatarsals as well. Sooner or later there will be narrowing of whichever joint space is infected, and this will indicate the arthritic cause of the even general loss of bone density throughout the region. Focal bone erosion may occur and be either an obvious or a very inconspicuous feature.

In an adult, a focal bone erosion of one of the tarsals with narrowing of the joint space may be present with very little or no regional even loss of bone density. Such a case may be diagnosed only by means of a biopsy or by aspiration of pus should an abscess form. If the infection is severe with gross narrowing of a joint space, there is a tendency for several other intertarsal joint spaces to be infected and narrowed.

Tuberculosis of a shoulder joint

Tuberculosis of a shoulder joint is rather more common in adults than in children. Pain and limitation of movement are the usual indications for a radiograph, swelling often being absent. There is often slight narrowing of the joint space, but this may not be recognized if comparative views with the other side cannot be obtained. There is little or no demonstrable loss of density in the bones around the joint, but a local erosion of the head of the humerus is often present. This erosion involves the cortex and may spread deeply for almost a centimetre. It is fairly sharply demarcated, but is not limited by a zone of denser bone. There may be more than one such erosion, and considerable deformity of the head may persist after healing.

Calcification in a nearby abscess may occur, particularly in the subdeltoid region, but this is not usual when the infection starts in adult life.

Tuberculosis of a wrist joint

The onset of tuberculosis of a wrist joint is often insidious, with slight pain and swelling and often no changes in the initial radiograph. In a child the only x-ray change may be a slight acceleration of ossification in the carpal bones, which is probably the result of the altered blood supply secondary to the inflammation. One or two centres of ossification may appear in some of the carpals before they are visible in the other normal wrist; alternatively, there may be no additional centres of ossification, but those already present may appear rather larger than the corresponding ossified parts in the normal wrist.

Another relatively early change seen in a patient of any age is a slight diminution of the radio-carpal joint space or some of the intercarpal joint spaces, while a small localized area of bone resorption may be seen near the articular or outer surface of one of the carpal bones, particularly the proximal half of the capitate.

In the absence of therapeutic immobilization there may be no visible even loss of density of the nearby bone, or only very little, but at a later stage or in a more acute lesion it may be present.

In an adult a more destructive type of tuberculous lesion is sometimes seen, with considerable or total loss of both radio-carpal and intercarpal joint spaces and much destruction of one or two of the carpal bones, often starting near the proximal end of the capitate

In older children or young adults the findings, both clinical and radiological, may be very similar to those of a mono-articular early rheumatoid arthritis (Fig. 311). A negative Mantoux reaction and positive Rose–Waaler or latex test will suggest a rheumatoid and not a tuberculous arthritis, although the reverse findings do not exclude a rheumatoid arthritis or an infective arthritis due to a low-grade pyogenic infection.

Pathology

A tuberculous arthritis starts in the subchondral bone or the synovial membrane or in both simultaneously. The synovial membrane is swollen and studded with tubercles. A granulomatous pannus spreads over the surface of the articular cartilage and another layer of granulation tissue involves the bone deep to the cartilage, which thus becomes sequestrated between two layers of granulation tissue, a feature so characteristic of this disease. The adjacent bone becomes progressively osteoporotic as it is replaced by caseous tuberculous granulation tissue, or as a result of disuse. Eventually the joint structures and surrounding tissues become a disorganized mass of caseous material and fibrous tissue, while foci of secondary calcification are common. Some cases may eventually show bony ankylosis, though this is unusual unless there is secondary pyogenic infection.

The histological appearance of the tubercles is quite characteristic, with caseation, and a granulation tissue with epithelioid and giant cells of the Langhans type and some lymphocytes.

The regional lymph nodes frequently show a similar histological change, but since an old tuberculous adenitis may be present near a joint affected by a non-tuberculous arthritis, especially in the inguinal node group, the value of this evidence is often slight.

HAEMOPHILIA WITH ARTHRITIS (HAEMORRHAGE INTO A JOINT)

Haemorrhage into a joint or between the joint cartilage and the articular cortex may lead to a severe and crippling joint lesion, and is seen in some patients with haemophilia.

The joint space may be normal but is often slightly narrowed. Small flat erosions of the articular cortex some 3–5 millimetres long are common. In the early stages there is no alteration of the nearby trabecular pattern, but in a severely damaged joint with diminished function the trabecular pattern becomes widened and coarsened.

In children the haemorrhage may lead to a local growth defect, and a rather characteristic late change is for the normal rounded contour of the lower end of a long bone such as the humerus or femur to be lost and the bone end to be rather square-shaped with deepening of the intercondylar notch (Fig. 301).

On pathological examination, the synovial tissues are stained brown and show fibrous thickening due to the deposition of haemosiderin from the red cells following a haemorrhage into the joint or nearby tissues. In addition there may be multiple erosions in the articular cartilage, while haemorrhages into the subchondral bone may result in small areas of bone resorption with fibrosis.

ARTHRITIS OF UNKNOWN CAUSE

CLASSICAL RHEUMATOID ARTHRITIS

Definition

The term "classical rheumatoid arthritis" is used here to describe one form of arthritis of unknown origin, other forms being considered as variants of this standard type. It may transpire when more is known that there are several different types with different aetiologies, but for the present it is possible to use the clinical and radiological features only as a basis for classification.

The standard type might be described as follows. The patient is a young adult, more often a female, complaining of pains in many joints, particularly the fingers, wrists, elbows, knees and ankles. The same joints are affected in both limbs, though not necessarily with equal severity. There is a spindle-shaped swelling around some of the proximal interphalangeal joints of the fingers, and swelling of the

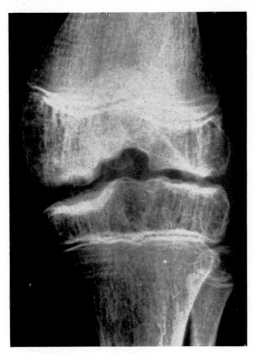 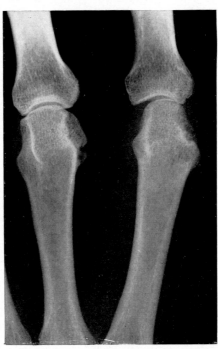 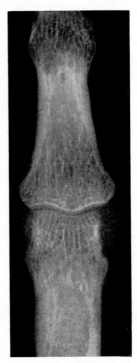

FIG. 301   FIG. 302   FIG. 303

FIG. 301.—Haemophilic arthritis. Male aged 7 years. Slight loss of joint space, articular cortical erosion of femur, rather square-shaped ends of tibia and femur and coarse trabecular pattern. Deep intercondylar notch.

FIG. 302.—Rheumatoid arthritis. Male aged 37 years. Narrow joint spaces at second and third metacarpo-phalangeal joints, with early subcortical erosion of head of second metacarpal and marginal erosion of phalanx.

FIG. 303.—Rheumatoid arthritis. Female aged 30 years. Erosion of either side of head of proximal phalanx and sub-cortical erosions of distal end of middle phalanx (× 2).

second and third metacarpo-phalangeal joints of both hands. The terminal interphalangeal joints are not affected. There is wasting of the muscle and fat of the hands out of proportion to the disuse, and the skin is cold and atrophic in appearance. The erythrocyte sedimentation rate is raised to well over 50 millimetres in 1 hour. The Rose–Waaler test or latex fixation is positive; the percentage positive varies from 93 per cent in cases with biopsy proof and clinical evidence of rheumatoid arthritis to 68 per cent in cases of short duration or doubtful diagnosis. Very few patients with other forms of arthritis give a positive result (Kellgren, Ball and Bier, 1959). There is some constitutional upset, and in a severe case in a young woman there may be amenorrhoea and anaemia. Immunofluorescent techniques have shown *gamma*-globulins fixed to the synovial membrane, suggesting that rheumatoid arthritis represents an immunological disorder.

Radiographs show narrowing of many joint spaces, particularly some interphalangeal, the second and third metacarpo-phalangeal and the wrist joint spaces. Well-marked surface or marginal erosions of the joint can be seen, and there is some trabecular loss throughout most of the bones in or near the joint.

As time goes on, some joints become more swollen and painful, others become affected, and the radiographic changes increase. After months or years the general health of the patient improves, the disease process seems to come to an end, and no further joints are affected. There is permanent fixity of some joints such as the wrists, which show bony ankylosis, while the fingers are fixed in a position of ulnar deviation.

If an early biopsy is available either near the joint margin or from a subcutaneous nodule, it will show characteristic changes.

The diagnosis is usually obvious clinically, so that the chief value of radiology is to show the severity of the damage and the presence or absence of bony ankylosis when fixed flexion deformities are present which it is hoped can be corrected. Occasionally there are few or no symptoms but the classical x-ray changes are seen.

Diminished joint space

The earliest change seen in the radiograph is a slight narrowing of the joint space. This may precede the onset of symptoms or signs, and is usually present when the patient first seeks medical advice. Occasionally, however, it may appear only months or even years after the onset of symptoms, and after a normal initial radiograph. The narrowing is commonly of a proximal interphalangeal joint space, where it is associated with spindle-shaped swelling of the soft tissues around the joint; in the metacarpo-phalangeal joints, particularly of the second and third fingers; and in the radio-carpal, intercarpal or metatarso-phalangeal joints.

In a knee the lateral or medial half may be most affected, so that the narrowing can be detected by comparison with the normal or less affected half. Likewise one knee may be more affected than the other, and early narrowing can be detected by comparing the width of the joint spaces in the two knees.

As the lesion progresses, the joint space becomes still narrower and is finally lost. In some cases fibrous ankylosis ensues, in others complete bony ankylosis with trabecular continuity between the bones (Fig. 307*b*), the latter being a common change in both wrist joints and much less common in a hip, knee, or finger joint.

Erosions

A small bone erosion is characteristic of rheumatoid arthritis and is visible in most cases. It may amount to no more than absorption of a few trabeculae just beneath the cortex near the joint margin, and perhaps be so small that it can be seen only with the aid of a magnifying glass or an enlargement technique (Fig. 303).

More commonly it may be clearly seen as a 2–5 millimetre superficial half-moon erosion, either of the articular cortex (Fig. 306) or of the bone near the margin of the joint (Fig. 302). Alternatively, if it is

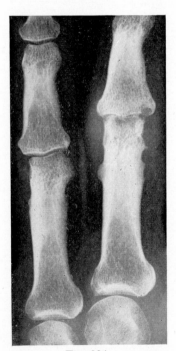 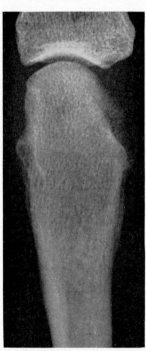 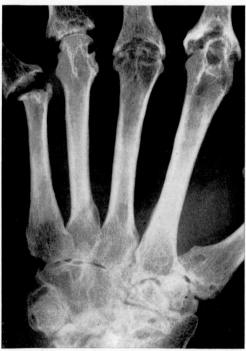

FIG. 304   FIG. 305   FIG. 306

FIG. 304.—Rheumatoid arthritis. Male aged 42 years. Narrow proximal interphalangeal joint space third finger and sub-articular erosions. Also surface erosion of shaft of proximal phalanx both fingers. Six years' arthritis. Serum uric acid 2 mg. per cent. E.S.R. 73.

FIG. 305.—Rheumatoid arthritis. Female aged 36 years. Index finger with narrow metacarpo-phalangeal joint space, sub-cortical trabecular erosion of metacarpal head and periosteal new bone round neck. Recent arthritis hands, later other joints. E.S.R. 27.

FIG. 306.—Rheumatoid arthritis. Female aged 33 years. Narrow joint spaces, small half-moon erosions, especially on fourth metacarpal and adjacent phalanx, and cup-like deformity of phalanx of second finger. Polyarthritis 10 years. Serum uric acid 3·7 mg. per cent.

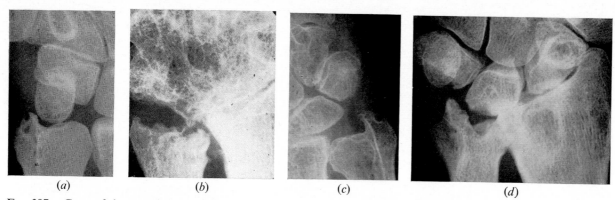

(a)	(b)	(c)	(d)

FIG. 307.—Cases of rheumatoid arthritis all showing erosions of the styloid of the ulna. (a) Small erosion at tip and one deeper. Female aged 34 years. (b) Most of styloid absorbed. Bony ankylosis carpals. Female aged 53 years. (c) Half-moon surface erosion on medial side. Female aged 58 years. (d) Erosions at base on both sides.

seen *en face* or in fact lies deeper in the bone, it will appear as a small circular transradiancy and may lie several millimetres away from the joint surface. It is well defined—either with no rim of dense bone or more rarely with a narrow white line of dense bone separating it from the surrounding trabeculae.

Occasionally it may be very large, reaching a size of a centimetre or more (Fig. 306). It is then identical with the transradiant zone caused by a urate deposit in gout, but can often be distinguished from it by the distribution of the affected joints and the clinical features (*see* page 203).

A moderate erosion on one side of a metacarpal head may result in a beak-like deformity (Fig. 309*b*).

There may be a single erosion or several of them either in the same bone or in the neighbourhood of several affected joints.

Particularly common sites for articular or marginal erosions are the tip or either side of the styloid process of the ulna (Fig. 307), the edges of the second or third metacarpal heads (Fig. 302), or adjacent

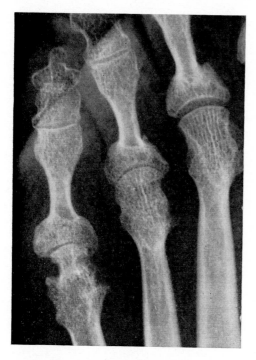

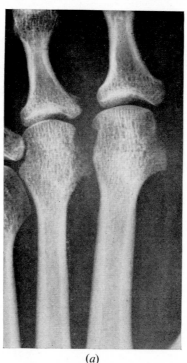

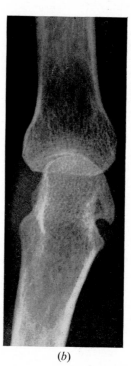

(a)	(b)

FIG. 308.—Rheumatoid arthritis. Female aged 36 years. Metatarsal head erosions, gross in fifth, slight in fourth, and narrow joint spaces. Arthritis 15 years, classical changes hands and wrists.

FIG. 309.—(a) Rheumatoid arthritis. Female aged 43 years. Slight joint space narrowing and erosions on medial side of head of second and third metatarsals. Two years' arthritis, and no radiographic abnormalities in hands, though some swelling. (b) Rheumatoid arthritis. Erosion of head of metacarpal has resulted in a beak-like deformity.

to the articular cortex of the proximal phalanx. In the knee they occur at the lateral or medial margin of the tibia. They are also very common in the heads of the metatarsals (Figs. 308 and 309), and in this site, even when the erosions are large, there may be no pain in this area, though there may be some local tenderness over the metatarsal heads. Small metatarsal head erosions are often seen even when no radiographic changes are visible in painful joints elsewhere, particularly the hands and wrists. The forefoot should therefore be radiographed if remote painful joints appear normal and confirmation of the diagnosis is desired.

In polyarticular rheumatoid arthritis, by the time the patient is attending a hospital out-patient clinic the radiograph will show abnormalities in the hands in 75 per cent of cases. In another 15 per cent there will be metatarsal head erosions even if the hands appear normal, so that the radiograph should show evidence of the disease in 90 per cent of cases if both hands and feet are radiographed. In cases with a normal radiograph, no abnormality may be seen for months or even years, but in most such cases joint cartilage loss and erosions will appear at some time.

Loss of bone density

Loss of bone density in the region of the affected joints is not inevitable even in the active stage of rheumatoid arthritis. Many patients with joint space loss and erosions show none, especially if the limb is being exercised normally. Sometimes there is evidence of trabecular thinning and loss even when the limb is in normal active use.

In some cases there is loss of bone density with thinning of the trabeculae in the juxta-articular region and extending towards the middle of the bone for 1–2 cm. Such a change may be the presenting radiological abnormality, to be followed later by cartilage loss and erosions in or near the joints.

In severely crippled patients there is always a loss of bone density, which may be intense with loss of all the trabeculae and much thinning of the cortex (Fig. 314).

Periosteal new bone

Although not a prominent feature and therefore often unnoticed, a slight thickening of the cortex or a definite line of periosteal new bone may be present around the shaft of a proximal or middle phalanx, around a metacarpal (Fig. 305), or in the supracondylar region of the lower end of the femur.

Abnormal mobility

If the ligaments near a joint are destroyed by the rheumatic process, this may result in abnormal mobility of the joint. Such a finding is sometimes seen in the cervical spine, and if lateral view radiographs are taken in flexion and extension, abnormal backward displacement of the odontoid on the body of the atlas may be seen. In extension the distance between the two bones is only 2 mm. (Fig. 310a), but in flexion it becomes much greater (Fig. 310b).

Pathology

The primary lesion of rheumatoid arthritis is in the collagen of the joint tissues, and the involvement of the periarticular and synovial tissues is responsible for the spindle-shaped swelling so often seen round the proximal joints of the fingers. At the onset the synovial membrane shows villous proliferation with lymphocytic infiltration. A (pink) fibrous pannus spreads over the articular cartilage and slowly replaces this structure on both aspects of the joint, with consequent narrowing of the joint space. Fibrous ankylosis is a common sequel, while in the wrist bony ankylosis is common. The underlying bone is frequently invaded and replaced by similar tissue, and fibrous foci with lymphocytes are responsible for the cyst-like bone erosions so commonly seen in or near the joint.

Histologically, lymphocytic foci and small areas of collagen necrosis surrounded by the histiocytes arranged in a palisade manner are characteristic of rheumatoid arthritis. These may be found at an early stage of the disease in the soft tissues near the joint or in subcutaneous nodules remote from a joint, although a biopsy taken some years after the onset of the condition may show no such specific changes and only some fibrous tissue and lymphocytes.

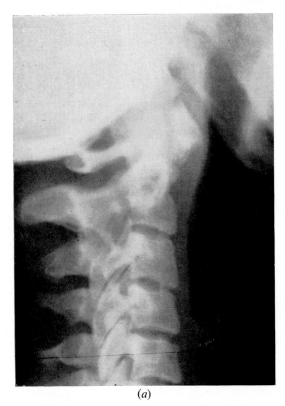
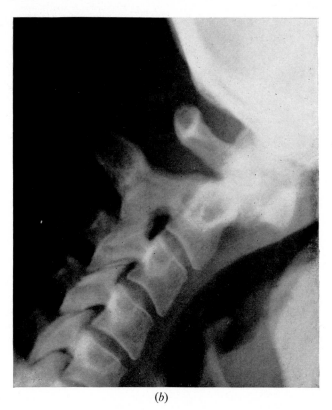

(a)   (b)

Fig. 310.—Rheumatoid arthritis. Lateral view of neck: (a) in extension, odontoid–atlas distance 3 mm.; (b) In flexion, odontoid–atlas distance 6 mm. Severe rheumatoid arthritis in hands and feet.

Unusual Manifestations of Rheumatoid Arthritis

Unusual distribution of affected joints

In some cases the lesion, instead of being a symmetrical polyarthritis, is confined to a single joint for a variable period of months or even years. In a mono-articular lesion the affected joint is commonly the wrist joint (Fig. 311), but it may be a hip, knee, ankle or tarsal joint. The earlier radiological finding is diminution of the joint space, followed by a small, well-demarcated articular or subarticular erosion. General loss of density of the nearby bones may be absent or slight and distinction from an infective, particularly tuberculous, arthritis may be impossible without prolonged observation or a biopsy, though a positive latex and negative Mantoux reaction would indicate the diagnosis.

The lesion tends to progress with further narrowing of the joint space and increasing loss of density of the bones nearby, and an articular cortical erosion may be seen. Occasionally the disease becomes arrested at this phase and the calcium content improves. More often, perhaps after an interval of years, other joints become affected, the x-ray appearances become those of classical rheumatoid arthritis and the diagnosis becomes more obvious. The onset of pain and swelling in the other joints is often quite sudden and may come on in a matter of hours.

At the opposite extreme to the mono-articular type are those—fortunately few—cases in which all or nearly all the joints of the body are affected, including the terminal interphalangeal, sacro-iliac and spinal joints.

Unusual age of onset

Whereas the typical rheumatoid arthritis occurs most commonly in young adults, a variation often known as Still's disease occurs in children, and may give rise to fever and splenomegaly. Again, it may start in one joint (Fig. 312) or it may be polyarticular from the earliest stage.

At the other extreme are those cases which commence in old people. The radiographic appearances may be fairly typical of rheumatoid arthritis, or erosions and loss of bone density may be rather less than in the classical form.

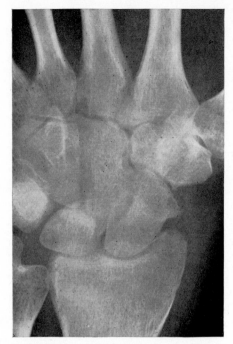

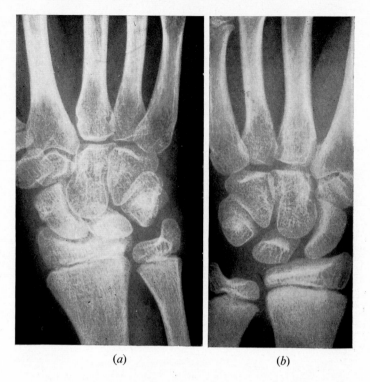

(a)   (b)

FIG. 311.—Mono-articular rheumatoid arthritis. Male aged 22 years. Narrow joint spaces in wrist and rather even loss of density of the carpals and ends of nearby bones. No other joint affected. Pain and some swelling 3 months. G.C. and W.R. negative. Synovial biopsy—sterile. Lymphocytic and plasma-cell congregations of rheumatoid arthritis and not tuberculosis. Two years later, no further joints affected.

FIG. 312.—Still's disease. Male aged 12 years. (a) Narrowing of joint space, patchy trabecular loss in the radial epiphysis and capitate, and slight even loss in other bones left wrist. Polyarthritis narrow second metacarpo-phalangeal joint and recurrent swelling of left wrist for 1 year. Mantoux—negative. (b) Other wrist normal (for comparison).

Milder type of lesion

A variation, in which several joints are affected but the disease is less severe and crippling than classical rheumatoid arthritis, is commonly seen in women soon after the menopause and has been described as post-menopausal arthritis. A similar mild form, seen in patients of any age, is often described as an infective arthritis, meaning not an actual infection of the joint but a change due to some remote hypothetical infection in teeth or sinuses or at some other site. In either lesion there is little or no constitutional upset or wasting of the surrounding soft tissues. The joint spaces are only slightly narrowed, and articular or periarticular erosions are small and inconspicuous. Because there is little diminution of movement there is little or no general loss of bone density.

Unusual radiographic appearances

One variation from the typical radiographic appearances described in classical rheumatoid arthritis is a predominance of erosions, so that in the early stage there may be relatively little narrowing of the joint space, no nearby even loss of bone density or periosteal new bone, but large cyst-like transradiant areas deep in the bone. These may be 1–2 centimetres in size (Fig. 313) and are well demarcated and often oval or circular in shape. They may lie a few millimetres away from the articular cortex, and may thus be confused with other causes of bone cyst (*see* Chapter 7). When they are rather smaller they may be similar to urate deposits.

Sometimes a rheumatic nodule causes a surface erosion of the cortex and bone beneath, some distance from the joint.

If the erosion lies directly beneath the articular cortex and perhaps also erodes it, the adjacent bone may collapse into it producing a ball and socket appearance (Figs. 306 and 314). This is commonly seen when a metacarpal head collapses into the erosion of the proximal end of a phalanx.

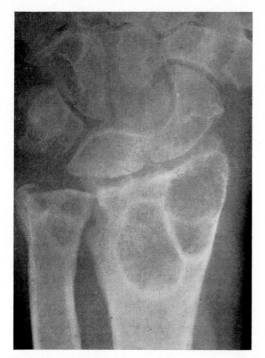

Fig. 313.—Rheumatoid arthritis. Male aged 50 years. Cyst-like erosion of lower end of radius and ulna. No narrowing of the joint space. Aching wrist 2 years. Biopsy—purulent-looking contents (sterile). Fibrous elements, plasma cells and some eosinophils. Later other joints developed typical changes of rheumatoid arthritis.

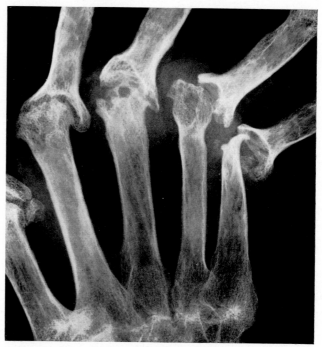

Fig. 314.—Rheumatoid arthritis. Female aged 68 years. Cup and pencil erosion of fifth finger, periosteal new bone on proximal phalanx of fourth finger and even loss of density of all bones. Bony ankylosis of the wrist. Polyarthritis started at age of 38 years. Rose–Waaler test positive.

Another less common variation is excessive absorption of the end of a bone, producing the so-called "sharpened pencil" deformity (Fig. 314). When several bones are affected it has been described as arthritis mutilans (Fig. 315). The eroded pointed end may articulate with a similarly eroded bone (pencil to pencil deformity) or with a cup-like deformity if there is cyst-like erosion of the opposite bone.

Finally there are some cases in which the periosteal new bone around the shafts of the phalanges may be the predominant lesion (Fig. 305). The diminished joint spaces and small erosions will generally make the diagnosis obvious, though for a time distinction from an infective arthritis may be difficult.

ARTHRITIS IN ASSOCIATION WITH OTHER DISEASES

A polyarthritis of unknown aetiology, not very dissimilar to classical rheumatoid arthritis, may appear as a complication in certain chronic diseases. Its slightly different characteristics, together with the fact of the underlying disease, suggest that it is not just a manifestation of rheumatoid arthritis or part of a random association of two diseases but part of a single complex pathological condition.

Arthritis with psoriasis

The arthritis seen in association with psoriasis (Fig. 316) affects particularly the interphalangeal joints of the fingers—unlike classical rheumatoid arthritis which also affects the metacarpo-phalangeal and wrist joints. In psoriasis, narrowing of the affected joint space is present together with articular and marginal erosions somewhat similar to those seen in rheumatoid arthritis, but even loss of density of the nearby bones is not a prominent feature. There is a tendency to marginal splaying out of the base of the terminal phalanges (Fig. 316). At a later stage clear-cut punched-out erosions are seen, and in some cases there is much erosion of the end of the bone forming the proximal side of the joint, giving it a pointed sharpened pencil appearance.

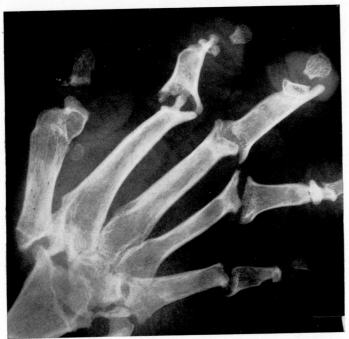
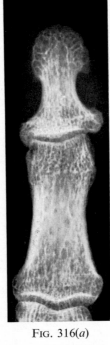
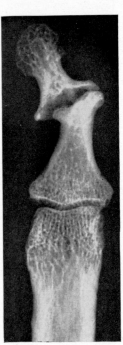

Fig. 315   Fig. 316(a)   (b)

Fig. 315.—Rheumatoid arthritis. Female aged 34 years. Gross bone absorption with pencil-shaped tapering ends (arthritis mutilans). Polyarthritis 6 years and amenorrhoea. Most joints eroded.

Fig. 316.—(a) Psoriasis and arthritis. Male aged 45 years. Terminal interphalangeal joint space narrowed with slight splaying out of the base of the distal phalanx. Psoriasis many years, arthritis for 2 years. (b) Psoriasis and arthritis. Female aged 50 years. Erosion and splaying out of bones of terminal phalangeal joint. Several other joint spaces narrowed in fingers and wrist. Similar appearance great toe. Metatarsal head erosions. Psoriasis 20 years. Nails pitted and brown. Latex—faint positive or negative.

The relationship of the arthritis to the psoriasis is still somewhat uncertain. The spread of the psoriasis to involve the finger nails has been quoted as a link, but this particular change is often not present even in cases showing the joint changes similar to those in Fig. 316, while occasionally the joint changes may precede the skin lesions. In yet other cases with the typical skin lesions, the joint lesions may show the clinical and radiological features of classical rheumatoid arthritis. In one case the patient had psoriasis, ulcerative colitis and the changes of classical rheumatoid arthritis, but since none of these are diseases of known aetiology, it is not possible to say whether the three together represent a single disease or two or three separate ones.

Pathologically in psoriasis there are no specific changes to suggest a rheumatoid arthritis, but there is much fibrosis (Sherman, 1952).

Arthritis with ulcerative colitis

A polyarthritis not very unlike that of rheumatoid arthritis is seen in some cases of ulcerative colitis. The emphasis is on the knees and ankles rather than on the fingers and wrists, though these too may be affected. There may even be changes in the interphalangeal joints of the toes, a rare site in classical rheumatoid arthritis (Bywaters and Ansell, 1958). In some cases there are changes in the sacro-iliac joints similar to those of sacro-iliitis described on page 197, but no involvement of the rest of the spine.

In mild cases there are often no radiographic changes apart from some spindle-shaped swelling of the soft parts round the affected finger joints. In other cases there is some diminution of the joint space with slight even loss of bone density, while in severe cases there may be small articular or nearby erosions like those of a rheumatoid arthritis. Sometimes a small linear shadow of periosteal new bone can be seen adjacent to the shaft of a phalanx.

The Rose–Waaler or latex fixation test is often negative though sometimes positive, the positive reaction suggesting that both diseases are present together. The arthritis tends to be fleeting and to resolve following improvement of the colitis with or without colectomy.

196

Arthritis with non-specific urethritis

Diminished joint spaces with small 1–3 millimetre articular or subarticular erosions similar to those seen in classical rheumatoid arthritis, and affecting the hands and feet in particular, are sometimes found in association with a non-gonococcal urethritis. Whether there is conjunctivitis in addition or not, the association is known as Reiter's syndrome.

Erosion of the styloid of the ulna as in rheumatoid arthritis is common, and there may eventually be bony ankylosis of the wrist bones. Much more common than in rheumatoid arthritis is the presence of periosteal shadows. There may be a thin line shadow adjacent to the shaft of a phalanx or the neck of a metatarsal or metacarpal, or there may be more abundant periosteal deposits, with rather irregular margins and a coarsely trabeculated appearance, lying near the posterior border of the lower end of a tibia or the posterior or plantar aspect of a calcaneum. Near the lower end of the radius and ulna the line shadow may be sufficiently wide to simulate a pulmonary osteo-arthropathy (*see* page 85). In some cases there is narrowing of the joint space and some irregular erosion of the articular cortex of the sacro-iliac joint, which may simulate the changes of a sacro-iliitis (*see below*).

Arthritis with rheumatic fever

The joint swellings of rheumatic fever are not as a rule associated with radiological changes, but occasionally in cases of rheumatic heart disease, changes are seen in the hands which may possibly represent a chronic post-rheumatic arthritis (type Jaccoud) as described by Bywaters (1950). These changes are rather like those of classical rheumatoid arthritis, with a tendency to an erosion of the radial side of a metacarpal head resulting in a hook-like deformity similar to that illustrated in Fig. 309*b*.

Arthritis with systemic lupus erythematosus

The relation of rheumatoid arthritis to lupus erythematosus is uncertain. The rheumatoid serum factor (Rose–Waaler) is positive in about 40 per cent (Kellgren, 1959). The distribution tends to be more like a psoriatic arthritis, with emphasis on the terminal phalangeal joints, but the number of cases seen by the author is too small to warrant any dogmatic statement. Hill (1957) considered the radiographic appearances to be often the same as in classical rheumatoid arthritis, but the erythrocyte sedimentation rate tends to remain high, and severe constitutional disturbances may remain even when the joint lesions appear to be quiescent.

ANKYLOSING SPONDYLITIS (RHEUMATOID SPONDYLITIS—U.S.A.)

Widening of the sacro-iliac joint space, with 5 millimetre pitted erosions of the articular cortex and some slight ill-defined blurring of the adjacent trabeculae for a distance of 1–2 centimetres, is characteristic of the earlier phase of ankylosing spondylitis (Fig. 317). Both joints are usually affected, but the changes are occasionally unilateral. If this is the only radiographic abnormality in a young patient, care must be taken to distinguish it from an exactly similar appearance found in some normal people between the ages of 18 and 24 years. This late adolescent type of joint does not persist in a normal person, so that any such abnormality seen beyond this age will indicate sacro-iliitis.

In most patients with ankylosing spondylitis the onset is after the age of 25 years, so that the typical x-ray appearances of an early sacro-iliitis can usually be easily recognized. In a case where there is any doubt, an oblique view radiograph taken tangentially through the joint is valuable if it confirms the pitted erosions of the articular cortex. For this view the patient is rolled from the supine position about 15 degrees to each side, the right being away from the table top for a radiograph of the right joint and the left away for a radiograph of the left joint. Alternatively, a single radiograph taken with the patient prone and at a tube–film distance of 75 cm. may show both joints almost tangentially owing to the divergence of the rays at this close range. The disease is most common in men.

As the lesion progresses, the joint space narrows and the surrounding sclerosis becomes more marked. Finally the joint space is obliterated and bony ankylosis occurs with resolution of the surrounding sclerosis.

The finding of the characteristic x-ray changes in the sacro-iliac joints together with the clinical evidence of the disease with back pain and stiffness, a raised erythrocyte sedimentation rate and negative

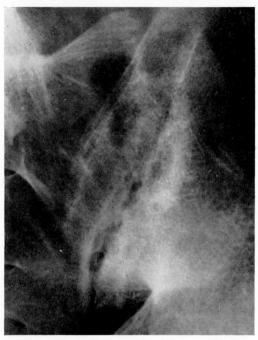

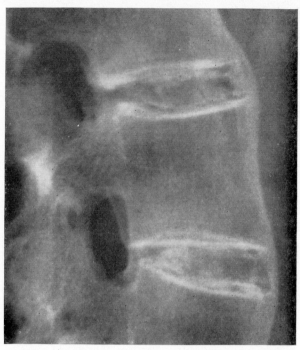

Fig. 317.—Ankylosing spondylitis. Male aged 30 years. Erosions of the articular cortex and sclerosis of the surrounding bone of the sacro-iliac joint. Both sides affected. Increasing stiffness of back for 6 years. E.S.R. 60 mm. Improved clinically after radiotherapy, but radiograph unchanged.

Fig. 318.—Ankylosing spondylitis. Female aged 45 years. Narrow linear shadow joining vertebral bodies anteriorly and being almost a continuation of the cortical line. That is too far posteriorly for only the anterior common ligament. Fifteen years' pain and stiffness of back. Typical changes in sacro-iliac joints like those in Fig. 317.

Rose–Waaler or latex fixation test, is usually sufficient for the diagnosis. Sometimes, however, the clinical findings are slight and accessory x-ray investigations are indicated for changes in other spinal joints or elsewhere. The vertebral bodies tend to lose their trabecular pattern, but retain a well-defined outer cortical line with very clear-cut right angles. A faint hair-line shadow joining the vertebral bodies across a disc space will confirm the diagnosis. In some advanced cases many or all of the vertebral bodies are united by these dense narrow lines of calcified tissue, an appearance described as a bamboo spine (Fig. 318). These lines of calcified tissue are narrower and project less laterally or anteriorly than the complete bridging occasionally seen secondary to a disc degeneration.

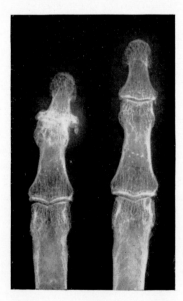

Fig. 319.—Osteoarthritis of terminal joints of fingers. Patient aged 58 years. Some swelling and slight pain.

Other sites where changes may be found include the costo-vertebral and the manubrium–gladiolar (sternal) joints. In fact, attention may first be drawn to the condition by the finding of blurring of these joints in a chest radiograph taken for some other purpose. In advanced cases, irregular erosions and spiky bony protrusions may be seen from the ischial tuberosity and blurring and irregularity of the symphyseal joint are quite common.

In some cases limb joints are also affected and show changes similar to those of rheumatoid arthritis. Narrowing of the hip joint spaces and general loss of trabeculae are most characteristic if there is peripheral joint involvement.

Pathology

In the early stages of the disease the histological appearances are similar to those of a rheumatoid arthritis. In the late stage there is bony ankylosis without evidence of inflammation or other changes to indicate the aetiology. Subcutaneous rheumatoid nodules are rare.

ARTHRITIS OF PARTLY-KNOWN ORIGIN

OSTEOARTHRITIS

Narrowing of the joint space, with no evidence of local decalcification and with a tendency to marginal bony outgrowths or lipping, is a characteristic finding in osteoarthritis. The degeneration, the cause for which is frequently unknown, is primarily in the cartilage—hence the almost invariable narrowing of the joint space. The bony outgrowths or excessive protuberance of the joint margin seem to be secondary to the cartilage degeneration, although such lipping can occur independently of any arthritis as a consequence of normal bone modelling in response to normal or perhaps unusual stresses. Excessive pointing of the tibial spines, for instance, may be the result of strong ligamentous pull and not of arthritis and therefore not the cause of the symptoms.

If the joint space becomes greatly narrowed, the bones may almost touch and become worn down because of the loss of cartilage cover. This together with the compensatory marginal lipping will produce considerable alteration in shape.

Common sites of an osteoarthritis are the larger lower limb joints such as the hips, knees or ankles, but it may also be seen in the vertebral column and in any other joint which happens to be subjected to excessive or unusual stresses, such as the metatarso-phalangeal joint of the great toe in hallux valgus. In some persons the hands, particularly the terminal phalangeal joints, are the only joints affected (Fig. 319) and the larger joints escape.

The hip

Osteoarthritis of the hip is common in the elderly and diminution of the joint space is an early radiographic change. At first marginal lipping may be comparatively slight, but as the lesion progresses it becomes more marked. If the joint space is virtually lost, the bones are almost in apposition with little intervening cartilage and become worn down, the result being a mushroom-like deformity of the femoral head with gross bony lipping at the edges. An almost invariable change is a linear layer of periosteal new bone along the under-surface of the neck of the femur (Fig. 320). This is not found in other joints affected with osteoarthritis, and is apparently related to the capsular thickening usually found round the femoral neck in osteoarthritis of the hip joint.

In many cases there are cyst-like transradiant areas a short distance beneath the articular cortex of the femoral head and acetabulum. In the ilium just above the acetabulum a single circular transradiant area 1–2 centimetres in size may be seen (see Chapter 7, page 135). In the femoral head there may be a single cyst-like transradiant zone, but more often there are two or three 5 millimetre circular transradiant areas. In either site there may be areas of sclerotic bone, and in some cases the relatively hypertransradiant zones between the denser areas may simulate cystic spaces.

The knee

In the knee the cartilage degenerative process may affect mainly the patello-femoral joint, where the narrowing of the joint interval and lipping of the upper and lower posterior angles of the patella may best be seen in a lateral view, or it may affect mainly the tibio-femoral joint. Changes are often seen in both joints, though more obvious in one than in the other. If slight genu valgum deformity is present, the joint space between the tibia and femur may be narrowed only on the inner half and the marginal lipping be confined to the medial edge.

The ankle

In the ankle, lipping is often most marked in the region of the tibia anteriorly, while in the talo-navicular joint it is often most conspicuous on the dorsal aspect.

The toes

Narrowing of the metatarso-phalangeal joint space of the great toe is very common together with some sclerosis of the subarticular bone and lipping of the margins of the bones. One or more 5 millimetre cyst-like transradiant zones may be seen deep in or at the margin of the head of the metatarsal. These are part of the degenerative process and not rheumatoid erosions or urate deposits. There is often moderate or gross hallux valgus which may be a precipitating cause (*see* Figs 58 and 322). On the other hand the toe is sometimes unusually straight and the metatarsal head large and flat, indicating a hallux rigidus (Fig. 323).

The shoulder joint

Narrowing of the humero-glenoid joint space and lipping are not very common except as a post-traumatic osteoarthritis. A much more usual finding in persons with shoulder joint pain is small erosions in the region of the greater tuberosity caused by small areas of bone resorption adjacent to the insertion of the rotator cuff tendon. Marginal lipping of the acromio-clavicular joint is common in the elderly and is asymptomatic.

The wrists and fingers

In many cases there are no abnormalities in the joints of the wrist or hand in spite of gross changes in the lower limb joints. Conversely, there may be narrowing of one or several terminal or middle interphalangeal joint spaces and considerable marginal lipping (Fig. 319) with no or only slight changes in the larger joints of the limbs. The marginal lipping of a terminal interphalangeal joint may produce a visible and palpable swelling of that part of the finger. Narrowing of the joint space between the first metacarpal and the trapezium and gross marginal lipping of both bones are commonly seen in the elderly and usually without symptoms.

The spine

Narrowing of the interspinous small joints with bony lipping is very common in the elderly, particularly in the lumbar region, where it may be most conspicuous in a posterior view taken with the patient supine but rotated 10–15 degrees.

These osteoarthritis changes of the small spinal joints are often overshadowed by the more conspicuous narrowing of the disc spaces with gross marginal lipping of the vertebral bodies, also seen in the elderly and sometimes referred to as spondylosis. In some parts of the vertebral column the marginal bony protuberances in spondylosis are so gross that they meet and fuse, making a convex bridge of bone between two vertebrae either laterally or anteriorly in which an outer cortical layer can be seen with trabeculae beneath.

Precipitating factors

When several joints are affected, age and its accompanying vascular degeneration with partial occlusions is a common aetiological factor. Any calcification seen in nearby main arteries will be evidence of such a process.

When only a single joint is affected, trauma is often an important precipitating factor. The injury may damage the bone or articular cartilage at the time or may precipitate cartilage degeneration at a later date. A fracture some distance from the joint, for example, may unite with some displacement, thus causing unusual stress on the joint. In a similar manner, abnormal stress may be placed on the joint by faulty development during childhood, as with a slipped femoral epiphysis or the large flat femoral head

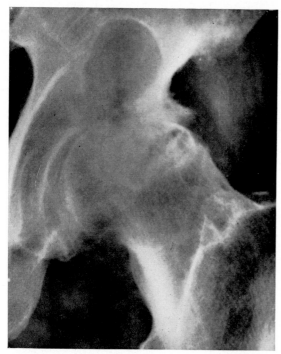

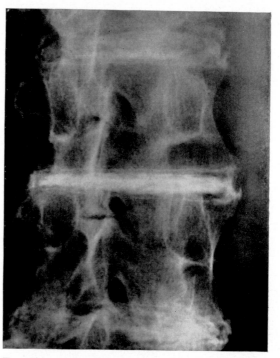

FIG. 320.—Osteoarthritis. Male aged 64 years. Narrowing of hip joint space, cystic area 3 cm. in diameter in bone above joint. Marginal lipping and periosteal new bone on the under-surface of the femoral neck. No loss of bone density. Other hip affected to a lesser extent.

FIG. 321.—Alkaptonuria. Male aged 48 years. Dense band-like shadows of calcification in the region of the intervertebral disc, separated from the end plates by a narrow transradiant zone. Whole spine affected. Only complaint is dark urine, but some kyphosis and stiffness of back.

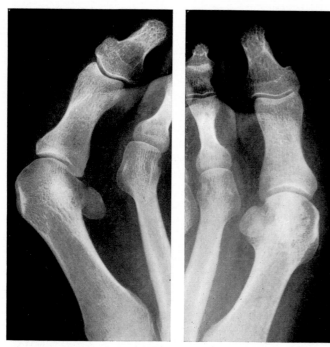

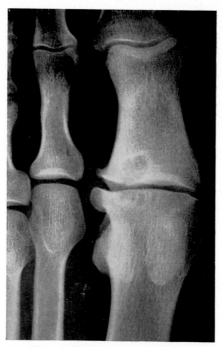

FIG. 322.—Hallux valgus. Female aged 22 years. Valgus deformity shown with slight narrowing of the metatarso-phalangeal joint space. Phalanx displaced laterally on head, which is deformed. Deformity with slight pain. Other side still normal.

FIG. 323.—Hallux rigidus. Female aged 52 years. Straight great toe with narrow metatarso-phalangeal joint space, marginal bony lipping, subarticular cystic areas and wide neck of metatarsal.

and abnormal neck–shaft angle arising from Perthes' disease. In a few cases excessive occupational stress, such as may be incurred by a pneumatic drill worker for example, is an important precipitating factor.

Finally, an osteoarthritis may supervene on a previously damaged joint, particularly an old quiescent rheumatoid arthritis. This would account for the fact that marginal bony lipping is sometimes seen in an otherwise typical case of healed rheumatoid arthritis.

Relationship of x-ray appearances to symptoms

The relation of the x-ray appearances of a diminished joint space and marginal bony lipping to the symptoms in osteoarthritis is often very indefinite, especially in the older age group. In the case of a hip joint the x-ray abnormality may precede the onset of symptoms by many years, but on the whole there is some correlation between the severity of the x-ray changes and the symptoms. In the knee there is rather less correlation and there may be quite severe symptoms and signs with little change in the radiograph, or else a grossly diminished joint space and gross lipping with few or no symptoms.

The acromio-clavical joint frequently shows a narrow joint space and lipping without accompanying symptoms.

The importance of finding these x-ray changes in a joint without symptoms is that they indicate a damaged and fragile joint which is unlikely to be able to stand the strain of any extra effort thrown upon it by therapeutic procedures. Orthopaedic treatment of a hip may thus be considered inadvisable if the knee joint shows such changes. Fractures in or near a joint showing a narrow joint space and lipping must also be treated with special care so that arthritic symptoms are not initiated or accentuated.

Pathology

The primary change is a degeneration of the articular cartilage; this loses its resilience because of a loss of mucopolysaccharide from its substance. (There is a low level of chondroitin sulphate.) Next, superficial fissures are seen in the cartilage running tangentially to the articular surface. As the splits extend deeper they become vertical in the depths of the cartilage. This velvety, fibrillated degenerate cartilage becomes worn away until none remains. By this late stage there is compensatory thickening of the subchondral bone, which becomes smooth and hard to form the eburnated joint surface. New bone forms at its margins to produce the osteophytes which are so conspicuous in the radiograph. The synovial membrane shows a non-specific fibrous thickening, and may contain fragments of degenerate articular cartilage which have become trapped in it.

The cyst-like areas sometimes seen in the bone deep to the articular cortex may be filled by a variety of tissues including mucoid material, jelly-like oedematous fibrous tissue or even fatty marrow (Collins, 1949). When the osteoarthritis is secondary to a previous Perthes' disease, the transradiant zone may contain remnants of cartilage.

INTRA-ARTICULAR LOOSE BODIES

A well-demarcated circular or oval shadow 3–10 millimetres in size, seen between the bone ends in two views, will suggest an intra-articular loose body. There may be only one or there may be several (*see* Fig. 341). If the shadow is even or mottled, it will represent either a calcification in a detached piece of articular cartilage or a piece of ectopic cartilage arising from a hypertrophied synovial membrane. If it has the appearance of bone with an outer cortical line and inner trabeculated cancellous structure, it will suggest either a piece of cartilage converted into bone or a piece of bone extruded as a sequestrum from the region of the articular cortex, such as may occur in osteochondritis dissecans (*see* Fig. 249 and page 146).

Sometimes the joint space is normal, suggesting an independent process; sometimes it is narrowed, either because the loose body initiates an osteoarthritis or because both are the result of some other degenerative process.

A loose body is commonly seen in the knee or elbow joint, but is uncommon elsewhere. It is usually quite obvious in the radiograph, but in some cases may pass undetected unless special views are taken. For instance, if it happens to lie in the intercondylar region of the femur it may only be seen clearly in a view taken with the knee flexed 20 degrees and the central x-ray beam directed at right angles to the top of the anterior margin of the tibia. Such a view should be taken if the history suggests that the joint sometimes becomes locked. Air arthrography is sometimes useful to prove that the shadow does in fact lie within the joint.

NEUROPATHIC ARTHRITIS

Narrowing of a joint space with disintegration of the articular and subarticular bone, with massive marginal lipping and with dense narrow band-like shadows of calcified tissue around the joint (Fig. 324), is very suggestive of a traumatic arthritis resulting from an absence of the normal deep sensory pathways which tend to protect the joint from minor traumatic damage.

Sometimes the neurological lesion is quite obvious clinically, while sometimes it can only be demonstrated with difficulty. In the early stages the radiographic appearances are those of a severe osteoarthritis. Later, the bony disintegration and calcified tissue around the joint will make the x-ray diagnosis more obvious.

Common sites are the hip, knee and ankle joint. Occasionally a lumbar vertebra may be affected, with a narrowed disc space, disintegration of the vertebral body, gross bony lipping and calcification in tissues around. Sometimes the shoulder or elbow is affected.

The lesion is often painless owing to the sensory loss.

METABOLIC DEFECT WITH ARTHRITIS

Gout

Narrowing of a joint space, particularly of a finger or toe, with a sharply defined circular punched-out erosion may be due to gout (Figs. 325a and 326). The erosion, which is often 5–10 millimetres in diameter, may be of the articular cortex or a few millimetres deep to the joint in the head or base of the

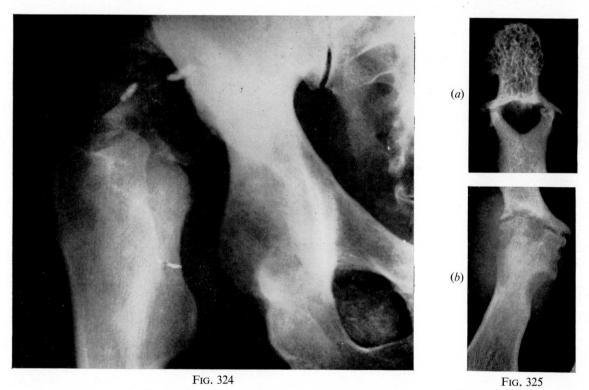

(a)

(b)

FIG. 324   FIG. 325

FIG. 324.—Neuropathic arthritis (Charcot joint). Male aged 56 years. Disappearance of the head of the femur and calcified debris around. Tabes dorsalis. W.R. negative.

FIG. 325.—Gout. (a) Male aged 85 years. Punched-out erosion at distal end of the middle phalanx. Typical gouty tophi and serum uric acid 10 mg. per cent. (b) Male aged 55 years. Superficial erosion of the shaft and articular erosion of the proximal phalanx. Small punched-out erosion of the articular cortex of the terminal phalanx with a narrow joint space. Classical attacks of pain, swelling and redness in the great toe. Serum uric acid 6·5–10 mg. per cent.

shaft. Occasionally it is seen on the external surface of the shaft near the joint and is then saucer-shaped (Fig. 325*b*).

It is not surrounded by a zone of dense bone but by normal trabeculae. General loss of density of the bones nearby is not present, but extensive bony lipping of the joint margins is quite usual. Sometimes the erosions are present without narrowing of the joint space. There is often much swelling of the soft tissues round the joint on one side without any calcification.

In the past there was often confusion between these punched-out erosions, which are occupied by a mixture of fibrous tissue and urate crystals, and the rather similar erosions of rheumatoid arthritis (Fig. 306) or even the cyst-like erosions and lipping of osteoarthritis (Fig. 323). Rheumatoid arthritis

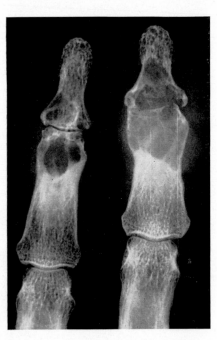

FIG. 326.—Gout. Male aged 51 years. Punched-out-erosions. Some loss terminal joint space. Serum uric acid 12·3 mg. per cent.

and gout rarely coexist, but the cartilage degeneration and lipping of osteoarthritis is a usual complication of urate deposits in or near a joint. Attention should be paid to the distribution, the lesions in gout being often in the terminal and interphalangeal joints and not in the metacarpo-phalangeal and wrist joints as in rheumatoid arthritis. Clinically, the acute episodes of gout with redness and acute swelling around the joint and a satisfactory response to colchicine are different from the ordinary rheumatoid manifestations. The blood uric acid may be raised to a figure of 6–12 milligrams per cent. Occasionally such a high figure is found without radiological manifestations.

Alkaptonuria

Widespread calcification of all or many intervertebral discs is seen in alkaptonuria (Fig. 321). This is a heritable disorder, the defective gene resulting in a deficiency of an enzyme (homogentisic acid oxidase). This defect leads to unaltered homogentisic acid being excreted in the urine, and this is responsible for its dark colour. Faulty metabolites are deposited in the joint cartilages and disc structures, and these may interfere with the collagen. This may lead to the depositing in the affected structure of calcium which may cast a shadow in the radiograph in the intervertebral discs (*see* Fig. 321) or in the knee cartilages, when the appearances would be the same as in Fig. 334.

NARROWING OF THE INTERVERTEBRAL DISC SPACES

Narrowing of the intervertebral disc space may be the result of a degenerative metabolic process similar to that causing an osteoarthritis, but affecting the disc instead of a joint cartilage. Usually several disc spaces are affected. It may also be due to trauma or to an unguarded movement resulting in a disc protrusion, when only a single disc space may be affected. In some cases both types of lesion may be present in different disc spaces, and in either case there may be secondary bony marginal lipping of the vertebral bodies.

Narrowing of a single disc space in a patient under the age of 50 years is more probably due to a protrusion than to a degeneration, and is more likely to be related to symptoms than narrowing of several disc spaces in an older person.

Narrowing of the cervical disc spaces

In the lower cervical region, narrowing of the last 3 disc spaces with quite considerable bony marginal lipping is the rule in persons over the age of 55 years, and is often without symptoms; while if symptoms are present, their relation to the x-ray appearances is hard to assess. Often the local pain disappears but the radiographic changes remain unaltered.

In assessing whether a narrow disc with lipping in the cervical spine is likely to be related to symptoms, the width of the bony part of the spinal canal should be taken into account, since a protruded disc or bony spur at the vertebral margin is more likely to encroach on nerves and give rise to symptoms if the spinal canal is narrow and the distance between the back of the vertebral body and front of the lamina is 1 centimetre or less.

Narrowing of the thoracic disc spaces

In the dorsal spine, narrowing of the disc space is common even in young adults and is invariable in the aged. In the aged it is usually but not always associated with spinal osteoporosis and some increase in the normal kyphosis, while in most persons even by early middle age there is some secondary bony lipping of the anterior angles and a few of the lateral angles as well. In the vast majority of persons with these x-ray appearances there are no symptoms.

Narrowing of the lumbar disc spaces

In the lumbar spine, disc narrowing and often gross marginal bony lipping are the rule in persons over the age of 65 years, and are also without symptoms in most cases. In younger persons from the ages of 30 to 60 years an isolated disc narrowing between L. 4 and L. 5 is often significant, though the x-ray appearances will remain unchanged even when the symptoms disappear. Narrowing of the disc space between the fifth lumbar vertebra and the sacrum is more difficult to interpret, since it may be an anatomical variation, a sort of stage I of a sacralized fifth lumbar vertebra. It is more likely to be due to a disc lesion if there is sclerosis of the bone beneath the end plates of L. 5 or the sacrum, or if there is secondary bony lipping.

11—Some Hints on X-ray Technique

PLAIN RADIOGRAPHS

To Acquire Good Detail

Good detail, which is essential for the demonstration of early trabecular loss or early new bone formation, can be obtained in most cases if the part to be radiographed is adequately immobilized to avoid blurring from movement, if the film is placed as close to the part as possible and if the focal spot of the tube is not too large. On a standard dual-focus tube the 1 millimetre focal spot is more useful than the 2 millimetre one, but if a special tube with an even smaller focal spot is available it will be best for peripheral limb radiography.

Unscreened films with a thick emulsion such as Ilfex, Kodirex and Osray should always be used for this work. Unfortunately films of this type cannot be put through most automatic developing units (1972 models) and must be developed and fixed over a longer time in old-fashioned wet tanks. There is at the moment a great deterioration of quality in many departments because wet developing is not available. It is hoped that a new type of film will become available which can give satisfactory contrast and detail when developed by automatic processors.

A good background blackening and a sharp white trabecular pattern are in the author's opinion desirable for high quality bone work. Excuses for a grey-looking radiograph with poor contrast, such as one showing the soft parts at the same time, are tenable only if on occasion the department can produce radiographs with high contrast. After all, one can always take an additional radiograph to show the soft parts in appropriate cases.

The decline in quality is also partly due to the fact that far too many radiologists go through their training with little or no experience of practical radiography, and with little will to improve quality when they see that it is poor or knowledge of how to do it.

High definition screens instead of standard ones for the thicker parts are usually of little value, since the main factor leading to poor detail is the unsharpness due to scatter rather than screen granularity.

To Acquire Good Contrast

Good contrast, which is an important factor in drawing the observer's attention to a small erosion or poorly-defined area of sclerosis, is obtained by attention to such details as full development, limitation of beam area and avoidance of excessive filtration. Filtration for peripheral limb work should not exceed a total of 2 millimetres Al. This means that if heavier filtration is already on the tube for general radiography, it should be reduced for peripheral limb work, or else another tube with less filtration should be reserved for this type of work.

Care must be taken to follow a standard development technique accurately rather than fall into the habit of bringing the films out of the developer when they "look done". Many films are still seen with poor contrast as a result of insufficient development. The speed of processing is an important factor during operative procedures, and modern high speed developers and fixers used at temperatures around 75°F. ensure full development and fixing in 2–3 minutes.

The use of a high kVp for bone work is a matter of common sense. It is of value to show soft tissues as well as bone, for very high speed radiography in a patient who cannot restrain his movements, or in lower spinal and pelvic radiography to restrict the gonadal dose, but it is neither necessary nor desirable as a routine since the consequent loss of contrast prevents detection of minor bone changes.

The use of a cone or diaphragm to limit the area covered by the x-ray beam and thus limit the area from which scatter rays will cause blurring of the image is useful for the thicker parts, particularly for a bone which is also denser from much sclerosis. A radiograph of a femur or vertebra, for instance, may show much greater contrast if the irradiated area is reduced to a circle some 15 cm. in diameter. Incidentally such a radiograph is less damaging to the patient than one taken with a wider field of irradiation. Occasionally an even smaller field may be appropriate, as in mastoid cell radiography or for a very small area of sclerosis in some other bone.

GOOD POSITIONING

On occasion, good positioning of the patient in relation to the x-ray beam and film is important. For instance, a supraspinatus tendon calcification may pass undetected if it is overlapped by the shadow of the acromion, and the radiograph should therefore be taken with the patient leaning forward to bring the acromion tangential to the x-ray beam (*see* page 216). A lesion in the femoral neck may also pass undetected if the radiograph is taken with the toes everted so that the neck is not parallel to the film.

One radiologist is reputed to have said, "I always judge a department by its thumbs". By this he meant not only dirty thumb-marks on films or cassettes but a lateral view which is slightly oblique, indicating that training and positioning are slipshod, or a grey background suggesting a film with poor contrast.

These comments merely reinforce the ideal that all training radiologists should spend some time taking radiographs and thus be taught to detect and correct faults as they occur.

Dear reader, if you are a trainee, how many hours have you spent in the radiography rooms this month?

MEASUREMENT OF BONE LENGTH

It is sometimes necessary to measure the length of a bone or the whole lower limb by means of radiography. As a rule the length relative to the other limb is more important than an absolute measurement, and the degree of accuracy sought is generally one that will allow an error of up to half a centimetre. Provided that a relatively long tube–film distance of 6–12 feet is used to minimize distortion due to divergence of the rays, and provided that the legs can be placed in nearly symmetrical positions, this presents no great difficulties. If a special long cassette is available such as is often used for total lower limb arteriography, the films can be placed end to end both for radiography and when measuring the image in front of the viewing box. If separate cassettes have to be used, the inevitable gaps between the films can be bridged for the purpose of measurement by placing two opaque line markers 10 centimetres apart, one on each cassette, so that a line shadow is produced across each film. The developed films are placed so that the distance between the line shadows is 10 centimetres, and the appropriate measurements are then made.

If greater precision is required, calculations can be made to allow for divergence of the rays provided that the distance between the bone and the film can be measured. Alternatively the distortion can be overcome by using a narrow transverse beam, radiographing the two ends separately with this central ray, and measuring the distance through which the beam has been moved between the two exposures. The two films are then placed so that the centres of the two narrow areas of exposure lie this same distance apart. The disadvantage of this rather cumbersome method is that it may not reveal the actual site of the shortening if such is present.

TOMOGRAPHY

A standard tomographic attachment on an ordinary x-ray table, such as is frequently used for chest tomography, will suffice for much bone tomography. Greater detail is often desirable, however, and this can be obtained only with more refined tomographic couches with a 50 degrees arc of swing or a figure-of-eight movement.

Ideally the direction of the tube movement should be at right angles to the long axis of a long bone, but this is rarely possible on conventional couches because the connecting rods and tube pillar prevent the patient from being laid across the table. A compromise can sometimes be arranged with the limb lying obliquely across the table.

SELECTION AND SPACING OF LAYERS

Whatever the apparatus used, it is of great importance to select the appropriate layer. This can often be found by measuring the distance from the table top to some palpable or visible anatomical landmark. In the knee region, for example, the lower end of the femur can be felt. On the other hand the shaft of the femur cannot be felt so easily, especially in a stout patient or if there is local swelling of the soft tissues.

The level of the spinal column or sacro-iliac joints can be neither seen nor felt when the patient is supine for a posterior-view tomogram, and the distance of the vertebral bodies from the table top must be roughly calculated from inspection of the size of the patient and how he is lying. In a lateral view of the lumbar or dorsal vertebrae a spinous process can be identified and its distance measured from the table top, but this may be misleading if there is rotation of the vertebrae or scoliosis, since the body of the diseased vertebra might lie a short distance above or below its spinous process.

In addition the lesion may lie to one side of the centre of the vertebral body, so that it is usually necessary to cover a layer range of some 5 centimetres to include the whole vertebral body with certainty, while in the case of a sacro-iliac joint an even wider range may be required.

The spacing of layers is also important. Using an arc of swing of 50 degrees, layers may need spacing every half centimetre to show a small bone lesion.

SIMULTANEOUS MULTISECTION TOMOGRAPHY

Simultaneous multisection tomography is a method whereby five different layers may be tomographed simultaneously with a single exposure and a single swing of the x-ray tube. The method was considered mathematically by Ziedes des Plantes (1933) and applied practically by Watson (1951, 1953). The author examined a series of patients both by this method and by conventional tomography. Although the radiographs by the multisection method had rather less contrast and were greyer than by the other method, the detail was quite as good, and as a rule the lesion was seen equally well. The saving in time and energy is considerable, and for this reason alone the method is valuable. In addition there is a considerable reduction in the amount of radiation received by the patient.

Table 1 shows the total skin dosage of radiation received by patients during a lateral-view tomogram of the thoracic vertebrae taken by both methods under routine working conditions.

TABLE 1

TOTAL SKIN DOSAGE OF RADIATION RECEIVED DURING LATERAL-VIEW TOMOGRAPHY OF THORACIC SPINE (200 mA SECS)

	Type	kVp	Dose per swing: roentgen units	Total dose for five layers in roentgen units
St. Bartholomew's Hospital (Mr. G. S. Innes)	Conventional	75	4	20
	Multisection (five layers)	85	5·1	5·1
Cancer Hospital (Mr. G. Spiegler)	Conventional	80	8	40
	Multisection (five layers)	90	10	10

Simultaneous multisection tomography can be used with most types of x-ray couch provided there is easy access to the clear space beneath the tray of the Potter–Bucky diaphragm.

The apparatus consists of a light-proof box loaded with five or seven intensifying screens to take five or seven films. Transradiant plastic spacers between the intensifying screens are usually 1·1 centimetre thick, but for many bone disorders the spacing can conveniently be reduced to 0·55 centimetre to avoid missing a small lesion. The special series of screens made by Ilford, Siemens, Siriex and others are designed to give an even degree of blackening of all five or seven films.

The tray of the Potter–Bucky diaphragm is withdrawn and the box put in its place so that the uppermost film lies in the same position as the single film would occupy in conventional tomography. The layer reproduced on this top film will then correspond to the layer selector setting, and the other four or six films will reproduce lower layers 1, 2, 3 and 4 centimetres or $\frac{1}{2}$, 1, $1\frac{1}{2}$ and 2 centimetres respectively nearer to the table top level.

The exposure for a five-film multisection box is about double that for a single film tomogram, and for a seven-film box a little over double (*N.B.* The exposure for a single film tomogram is about 10

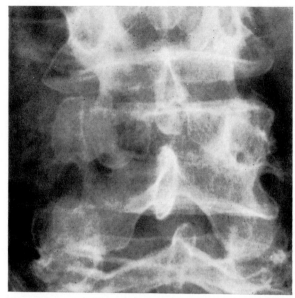

FIG. 327.—Secondary deposit. Male aged 68 years. Plain radiograph showing possible erosion of the right side of L. 4. Pain in the back for 2 months.

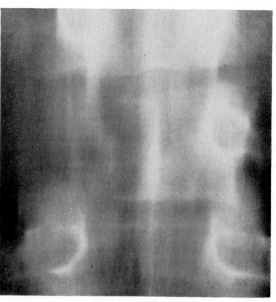

FIG. 328.—Same patient as Fig. 327. Tomogram showing obvious erosion of the pedicle and body on the right side of L. 4.

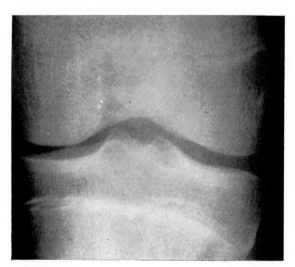

FIG. 329.—Osteoclastoma. Male aged 15 years. Doubtful erosion of the epiphysis of the femur. Pain in the knee 6 months.

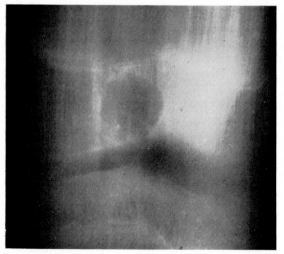

FIG. 330.—Same patient as Fig. 329. Tomogram showing obvious circular transradiant area without a rim of dense bone in the lower femoral epiphysis. Biopsy—osteoclastoma.

per cent more than for a plain radiograph). The increased exposure is best achieved by raising the kVp by 10 or 12 kilovolts rather than by doubling the mA or time. For most parts this will present no difficulties, but for a lateral-view tomogram of the lower spine in a large person or a lateral view of the upper thoracic vertebrae through both shoulders, a single film technique may be necessary unless the apparatus is capable of working at 110 or 120 kVp.

VALUE OF TOMOGRAPHY

Tomography is of value in many disorders of the larger bones when the lesion, though suspected clinically, cannot be seen clearly or cannot be seen at all in the plain radiographs.

It is particularly useful for lesions in the vertebral column. In the cervical spine a posterior-view tomogram will sometimes show a lesion in the lateral mass of the vertebra which cannot be seen with certainty in a plain posterior-view radiograph owing to the obliquity of the bone in relation to the x-ray beam, or to the shadows of overlying articular facets.

In the lumbar or dorsal spine a posterior-view tomogram is often of value to show whether a pedicle is intact or eroded when it appears indistinct in the plain radiograph. A lateral-view tomogram is often of value to show or exclude erosion or sclerosis of the vertebral body when the vertebra is obscured to some extent in the plain radiograph by the overlying shadows of the ribs, or the shadows or trans-radiancies of the thoracic or abdominal contents. It is surprising how large a lesion can sometimes be detected by a tomogram (Fig. 328) which cannot be seen clearly even on a review of the plain radiograph (Fig. 327).

When an angular kyphosis or severe scoliosis is present, tomograms are often of value to show the nature and extent of any bone erosions which may not be demonstrable in the plain radiographs, either because of the oblique lie of the individual vertebra in relation to the x-ray beam or because they are obscured by the shadows of the overlying ribs which are much crowded together.

A paraspinal abscess or neoplastic mass may be excluded or demonstrated with certainty in a case where there is some doubt from inspection of the plain radiographs.

A bone lesion in the sacro-iliac region may also be seen best by tomography, which is therefore indicated if there is pain and localized tenderness over one joint, or if a lesion is suspected from the plain radiographs but the area is obscured by intestinal shadows or transradiancies.

Tomography of a rib is indicated when a lesion is suspected but cannot be seen clearly or with certainty in the plain radiographs, where it may be obscured by overlying pulmonary shadows.

Although used less frequently for limb bones, tomography is nevertheless valuable in some cases. Sequestra in chronic osteomyelitis may be shown plainly when they are invisible or very unclearly demonstrated in the plain radiographs. This is an important use for tomography.

The central transradiant nidus of an osteoid osteoma may sometimes be clearly seen even if there is much surrounding sclerosis obscuring it in the plain radiograph.

The extent and margins of an erosion in a major bone of a limb or the clavicle may be plainly visible in a tomogram. For instance, the erosion of an osteoclastoma in the lower epiphysis of the femur is clearly shown in the tomogram in Fig. 330, but is very indistinct in the plain radiograph in Fig. 329.

INJECTION OF SINUSES

It is often necessary to inject a sinus with a contrast medium in order to determine its extent and its connexion, if any, with the underlying bone. Iodized oil[1] or propyliodone in oil[2] is suitable. The opening of the sinus should be placed uppermost, and the medium injected very gently through a rubber catheter introduced into it as far as it will go. Any leaking contrast medium must be removed before the radiographs are taken.

An antero-posterior and a lateral radiograph are not always enough to show the relation of the sinus track to the bone and should be supplemented by oblique or tangential views, aided in some cases by fluoroscopy. A tomogram is often of great help, especially in those cases where the sinus track shows extensive ramifications and it is difficult to see which track is related to the bone or to a sequestrum.

AVOIDANCE OF EXCESSIVE RADIATION

The risk of producing leukaemia following diagnostic radiology for bone disease is probably very slight, but frequent radiographs giving an excessive total dose of radiation should be avoided.

[1] Lipiodol, Neo-Hydriol.   [2] Dionosil.

The risk of an excessive dose to the gonads is probably much greater.* In radiography of the pelvic area, the gonads should when possible be shielded from direct radiation with a circular lead disc or triangular sheet of lead. In patients of both sexes under the age of 40, and in males to a later age, all relatively unnecessary radiography of the lower lumbar spine, pelvis and hips should be avoided. For instance, no uncomplicated case of acute backache or sciatica possibly due to a disc lesion should be radiographed until bed rest or some simple therapeutic procedures have been tried for a reasonable period. The use of a high kilovoltage technique (120–140 kVp) with a reduction in the milliampere seconds is also desirable if the apparatus is available.

* Medical Research Council Report *The Hazards to Man of Nuclear and Allied Radiations*. Cmd. 9780. H.M. Stationery Office, London, 1956; and *Radiological Hazards to Patients*. Second Report of the Committee. H.M. Stationery Office, London, 1960.

12—Bone in Unusual Sites and Calcifications in or Near a Joint

BONE IN MUSCLES AND TENDONS

A bony deposit in a muscle, tendon, joint capsule or joint cavity produces a shadow with an outer white line representing the cortex and an inner criss-cross pattern of fine white lines representing the trabeculae. This bony architecture distinguishes it from a non-specific calcification, which produces a homogeneous or woolly shadow, although occasionally the bony deposit is so dense that the trabecular pattern is invisible.

MYOSITIS OSSIFICANS

A common site for a ossification or a calcification in a muscle is the brachialis just anterior to the lower end of the humerus.

The shadow is separated from the bone by a transradiant zone (Fig. 331), and the lesion commonly follows a known traumatic incident. The shadow is first seen some 2–3 weeks later, and increases in size for another few weeks. Starting as a rather amorphous faint haze, the bone-like architecture is soon apparent. After being stationary for some months, the shadow becomes smaller and may either disappear or persist indefinitely. If removed relatively early there is a strong tendency for the ectopic bone to reform, but if removed later when it has shrunk to some extent, removal may result in a cure of the condition. Post-traumatic myositis is relatively uncommon in other sites, though it may occur in a thigh muscle.

A narrow disc of bone some 1–2 centimetres long is sometimes seen in the ligamentum nuchae, and is usually asymptomatic with no history of trauma.

Fibrodysplasia ossificans progressiva

A rare hereditary disorder occurs in which shadows of ectopic bone are seen in many muscles or tendons. These produce band-like shadows 1–2 centimetres wide with bony architecture extending from the bone into the muscle for some 10 centimetres or more (Fig. 332) and into tendons, particularly in the neck, shoulder girdle, lumbar region, and hip region. They may be so extensive as effectively to stop all movement of the joints. Unlike post-traumatic myositis ossificans, the shadows tend to persist indefinitely. Shortening of the thumb and great toe may be present (*see* Fig. 69).

OSSIFICATION IN A TENDON

Ossification in a tendon near its point of insertion into the bone is common. Since the ossification extends to and joins the bone, it is not always possible to tell whether it started in the tendon and eventually fused to the bone or whether the bone has extended up into the tendon. Common appearances are a $\frac{1}{2}$–1 centimetre narrow pointed projection of bone from the upper posterior angle of the olecranon process of the ulna extending into the triceps tendon, a similar shadow from the upper anterior angle of the patella into the extensor tendon, and another from the upper posterior angle of the calcaneum into the tendo-calcaneus.

These projections are usually asymptomatic and permanent, and are vaguely related to tendon stresses and age. Occasionally a small fragment of ectopic bone is seen either adjacent to the point of insertion of the tendon into the bone, or in the tendon some distance away in a patient with a high level of serum calcium in hyperparathyroidism (Fig. 333).

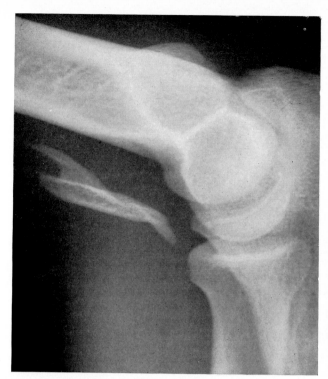

Fig. 331.—Myositis ossificans. Male aged 32 years. Ectopic bone anterior to the humerus. Injury 12 weeks previously.

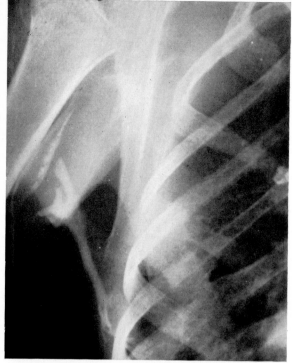

Fig. 332.—Fibrodysplasia ossificans progressiva. Male aged 16 years. Large sheets of ectopic bone in the muscles of the shoulder girdle. Also in neck, lumbar muscles and hip region. Various muscle swellings since age of 2 years. Now stiff neck, jaw, arms. Short proximal phalanx thumb and great toe.

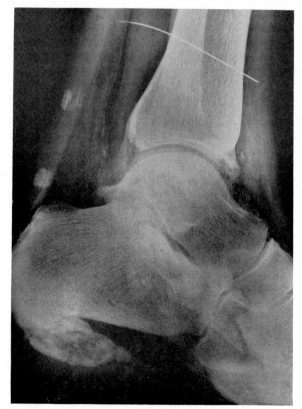

Fig. 333.—Ectopic bone in region of tendo achillis and plantar fascia. Female aged 66 years with hyperparathyroidism. Same case as Fig. 179. Serum Ca. 14·6 mg. per cent; P. 2·2 mg. per cent.

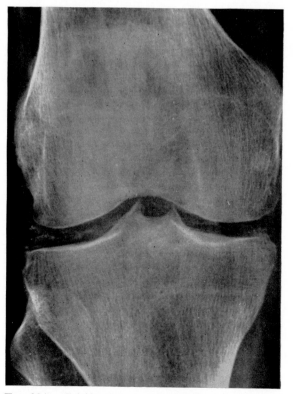

Fig. 334.—Calcifications in the semilunar cartilages of the knee. Female aged 66 years. Hyperparathyroidism. Same case as Fig. 333.

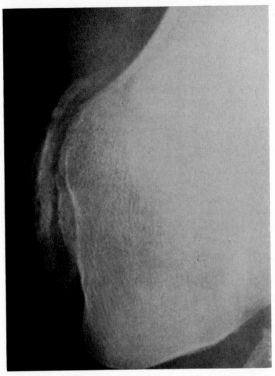

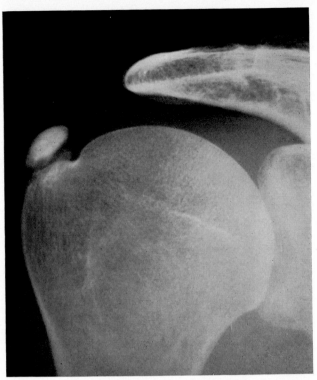

FIG. 335.—Pellegrini Stieda lesion. Male aged 35 years. Ectopic bone starting above medial condyle and extending downwards towards the joint. Pain in knee some weeks. Removal of bone carried out.

FIG. 336.—Calcification in region of the supraspinatus tendon. Male aged 34 years. Pain in the shoulder a few weeks.

CALCIFICATIONS IN STRUCTURES IN OR NEAR A JOINT

CALCIFICATION IN A JOINT CARTILAGE

The joint cartilage most frequently calcified is the semilunar cartilage of a knee joint. A single cartilage may be affected, but more commonly both are calcified and the condition may be bilateral. The size, shape and position of the shadow leave no doubt as to the structure it represents. This change is remarkably uncommon considering the frequency of other metabolic degenerative changes in the knee joint. It may be seen in the elderly, or in a patient with a metabolic disorder with a high level of serum calcium in renal disease with secondary hyperparathyroidism. It may occur in haemachromatosis or in alkaptonuria. It is not in itself productive of symptoms A similar calcification is occasionally seen in a temporo-mandibular joint cartilage.

CALCIFICATION IN A JOINT CAPSULE

A faint opacity adjacent to a joint is sometimes due to deposits of calcium in a diseased joint capsule. It is seen only in the capsule round a shoulder, elbow, hip or knee joint. It is most common in association with a neuropathic arthritis (*see* page 203).

CALCIFICATION IN OR NEAR A JOINT LIGAMENT

A linear calcification is sometimes seen on the medial side of the knee (Pellegrini–Stieda). It begins in the region of the ligament, but also extends considerably above this structure, the upper limit being several millimetres above the lateral or medial condyle (Fig. 335). Unless removal is very complete, the condition tends to recur rapidly.

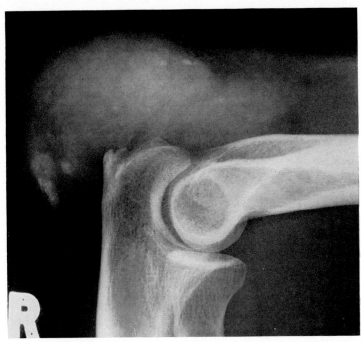

FIG. 337. 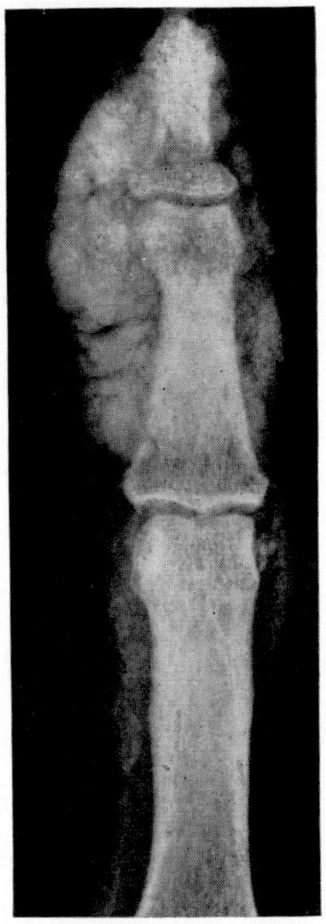   FIG. 338.

FIG. 337.—Gout with calcifications in olecranon bursa. Male aged 49 years. Gout since age of 19 years with attacks every few months, red, hot and painful and relieved by colchicine. Lasts 3 days. Huge swellings, several bursae, and tophi in fingers. Some terminal interphalangeal joints similar to Fig. 325. Serum uric acid 13 mg. per cent.

FIG. 338. Hyperparathyroidism with deposition of calcium in finger tips. Female aged 53 years. Nephritis. Blood urea 500 mg. per cent. Secondary hyperparathyroidism in some bones radiologically and histologically. Calcium carbonate in fingers, pushing tissues aside like an abscess. Calcification in many main arteries and in kidneys. Serum Ca. 9·5; P. 10 mg. per cent. P.M. proof.

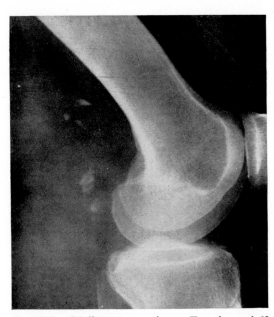

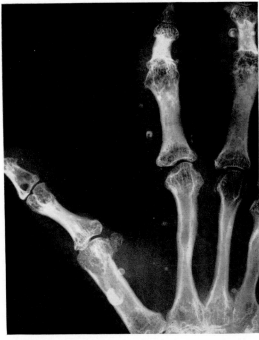

FIG. 339.—Malignant synovioma. Female aged 62 years. Small opacities in region of swelling behind knee, and slight pressure erosion of femur. Swelling noticed 2 years. Histology—synovioma of low malignancy.

FIG. 340.—Maffucci's syndrome. Haemangiomas and chondromas. Female aged 23 years. Swollen hand since the age of 4 years. Skin intact. Small 5 mm. circular shadows in soft parts. Thin metacarpal shaft of second finger, circular transradiant area in terminal phalanx of thumb.

215

CALCIFICATION IN OR NEAR THE SUPRASPINATUS TENDON

A 5–12 millimetre amorphous oval shadow above the lateral third of the head of the humerus is usually due to a calcification in the region of the supraspinatus tendon (Fig. 336). It may easily pass undetected unless a radiograph is taken with the arm in a position of internal rotation, or better still with the patient standing inclined forward 15 degrees for a posterior view. It is most frequently unilateral but is sometimes bilateral, one side often being asymptomatic. The condition may cause considerable pain at one stage, but is usually visible in the radiograph at the time of onset of the pain. The shadow may persist long after the complete relief of the pain. It may disappear spontaneously after some months.

CALCIFICATIONS NEAR THE FINGER JOINTS

Very small, rather indistinct linear or circular calcifications are sometimes seen in the region of the metacarpo-phalangeal or interphalangeal joints. They are easily missed unless carefully looked for. They may be analogous to a supraspinatus tendon calcification, but their exact site is as yet unknown. Known as "peritendinitis calcarea", they may cause some symptoms (Hitchcock and Langton, 1959). Similar shadows may be seen near a hip joint.

Quite different are the more massive calcifications in the pulp of the fingers or in the soft tissues near the distal phalanx commonly seen in diffuse systemic sclerosis and usually associated with absorption of the tip of the phalanx (Fig. 248), but occasionally seen without this bone change.

Gross calcification in the pulp or in the soft tissue around the terminal phalanx may be seen in a metabolic disorder (Fig. 338), particularly in hyperparathyroidism secondary to renal disease, when the calcium may be precipitated in various sites (*see* Figs. 333 and 334).

CALCIFICATION IN TUBERCULOUS SYNOVITIS

A long vertical shadow some 5 millimetres wide may be seen extending up from the region of the ankle joint due to calcification in the synovial disease round a tendon in this region. The underlying tuberculous arthritis may be obvious, or may only be seen after careful inspection of the nearby joints.

CALCIFICATION IN A BURSA OVER A JOINT OR A SYNOVIAL CYST

A semilunar shadow, concave medially and about 1 centimetre long, lying lateral to the head of the humerus will suggest calcification in a subdeltoid bursa. It lies more laterally than a supraspinatus calcification. A smaller, more medial shadow lying under the acromion will suggest a subacromial bursal calcification.

A shadow posterior to the olecranon process is sometimes due to calcification in an olecranon bursa. The site is characteristic and will correspond to a palpable swelling. Calcifications in the olecranon bursa may occur in gout (Fig. 337) with or without the periodic discharge of tophaceous material through the skin.

Calcification is not uncommon in a bursa or bunion lying medial to the great toe joint in association with a hallux valgus. The clinical features are obvious and there may be evidence of infection of the bursa.

Calcification may occur in the neighbourhood of a joint damaged by urate deposits in gout, especially if there is discharge of the tophaceous material from time to time.

A circular linear calcification behind the knee joint, with a diameter of 1–3 centimetres, is seen if there is calcification of a synovial cyst in association with the knee joint.

CALCIFICATIONS IN TUMOURS NEAR BONE

Small calcifications behind the shadow of the patellar ligament are more likely to be in a haemangioma or other innocent tumour than in a bursa or synovial pouch.

Small calcifications behind the knee joint may be loose bodies in a posterior extension of the joint capsule, or may be in a tumour such as a haemangioma or synovioma (Fig. 339). Another name for an innocent synovioma is villo-nodular synovitis.

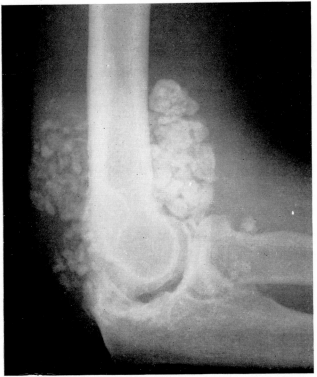

FIG. 341.—Chondromatosis of elbow joint; 5–8 mm. circular calcifications in and around elbow joint. No trabecular structure. Multiple calcified cartilaginous loose bodies in joint.

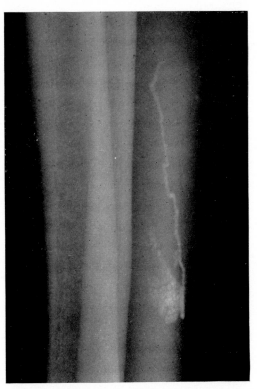

FIG. 342.—Shadow of calcified guinea worm in muscle. Patient resided in part of Africa where the condition was endemic. Asymptomatic.

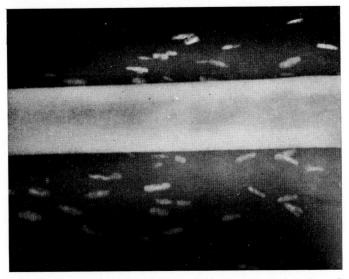

FIG. 343 —Cysticercosis. Male aged 54 years. Posterior view of femur. Small calcifications in muscles of thigh.

A combination of small 3–5 millimetre circular shadows and a well-demarcated transradiant area in a metacarpal or phalanx in the region of the thumb will indicate the combination of a haemangiomatous condition of the soft parts with chondromas in the bone (Maffucci's syndrome—Fig. 340).

CALCIFICATION OR OSSIFICATION IN A JOINT

A bony loose body in a joint may be a sequestrum separated off in a case of osteochondritis dissecans—*see* page 146.

Sometimes multiple opaque loose bodies are seen in a joint. They may arise from hypertrophied synovial fringes, and may consist of calcifying pieces of cartilages or of bone (Fig. 341). The condition is perhaps a benign tumour of synovial membrane and is known as chondromatosis.

CALCIFICATIONS IN MUSCLES

Cysticercosis

Well-demarcated 5–10 mm. oval dense shadows in the muscles may be due to cysticercosis (Fig. 343). There may be only a few or they may be very numerous. There is usually no difficulty in diagnosis, but in the scalp they may be mistaken for an intracerebral calcification, or in the muscles of the chest wall for an intrathoracic lesion. Exact localization of the site of the opacities will generally suffice to avoid such errors.

Guinea worm

A tortuous band-like shadow in a muscle will suggest a calcifying guinea worm (Fig. 342). The patient must have resided in an area where the worm is endemic.

Appendix—Additional Tables

TABLE 2

SUGGESTED CLASSIFICATION OF BONE TUMOURS (*after Lichtenstein*)

Tissue of origin	Benign	Malignant
Cartilage or cartilage connective tissue	Osteochondroma Enchondroma Chondroblastoma Chondromyxoid fibroma	Chondrosarcoma
Osteoblastic	Osteoma Osteoid osteoma Osteogenic fibroma	Osteogenic sarcoma
Non-osteogenic connective tissue	Non-osteogenic fibroma	Fibrosarcoma
	←Giant cell tumours→	
Mesenchymal connective tissue		Ewing's sarcoma
Haematopoietic		Myeloma Leukaemia Lymphoma H.D.
Nerve origin	Neurofibroma and neurilemmoma	
Vascular origin	Haemangioma	H-endothelioma
Notochordal		Chordoma
Basal cell		Adamantinoma

TABLE 3

Blood Chemistry

List of Normal Values (*Department of Pathology, St. Bartholomew's Hospital, London*)

	Plasma or serum mg./100 ml. unless otherwise stated	*m.eq./litre*
Alkali reserve	55–57 vols. CO_2 per cent	24–34 (*acidosis below 24*)
Amylase, diastase	3–10 (Wohlgemuth) units	
Bilirubin	0·1–0·5	
Calcium	9–11	4·0–5·0
Chlorides (as NaCl)	560–620	96–106
Cholesterol (total)	150–250	
Fibrinogen (plasma)	200–400	
Iron (as Fe): Male	80–150 micrograms/100 ml.	
Female	60–120 micrograms/100 ml.	
Phosphatase: Acid	1–3 ⎫ (K-A) units	
Alkaline	3–13 ⎬	
Phosphorus: Adult	2–4	
Child	4–6	
Potassium	17–21	4·0–5·0
Proteins:		
Total g/100 ml.	5·6–8·5	
Albumin g/100 ml.	4·0–6·7	
Globulin g/100 ml.	1·2–2·9	
Pseudocholinesterase	55–120 units	
Sodium	315–350	137–152
Sugar (fasting)	80–120	
Thymol turbidity	1·0–4 units	
Urea	15–40	
Uric acid	1–4·5	
Zinc sulphate turbidity	4–8 units	

TABLE 4

HAEMATOLOGY

List of Normal Values (*Department of Pathology, St. Bartholomew's Hospital, London*)

Red blood cells: men—4·5 to 6·5 millions per cu. mm.; women—3·9 to 5·6 millions per cu. mm.
Haemoglobin: men—14 to 17 grammes per 100 ml. (95–115 per cent Haldane); women—12 to 15·5 grammes per 100 ml. (82–105 per cent Haldane).
White blood cells: 4,000 to 10,000 per cu. mm.
Differential white count (adults):

	per cent	per cu. mm.
Polymorphonuclears	50–70	3,000–6,000
Eosinophils	0·5–3	50–300
Basophils	0–1	0–75
Lymphocytes	20–30	1,000–3,000
Monocytes	3–10	300–600

Counts in infants and children:

	R.B.C.'s millions	W.B.C.'s	Hb (Haldane) per cent	Hb grammes per cent	Polymorphs per cent	Lymphocytes per cent
Birth	6–7	18,000	140	20·7	60	15
2–4 weeks	5·5	12,000	110	16·3	25	50–70
3 months	5·5	8,000	75	11·1	20–30	40–60
1 year	4·5–5	5,000–8,000	75	11·1	20–30	40–60
12 years	5·0–5·5	5,000–8,000	80–100	11·8 14·8	50–60	20–30

Bleeding time: 2 to 5 minutes.
Coagulation time at 37°C.: Dale Laidlaw's method—up to 3 minutes; Lee and White's method—4 to 10 minutes.
Fragility of red cells: haemolysis commences in 0·42–0·46 per cent NaCl and is complete in 0·28–0·32 per cent NaCl.
Packed cell volume (haematocrit value): men—40 to 54 per cent; women—36 to 47 per cent.
Mean corpuscular volume (M.C.V.): 76 to 96 cu. μ.
Mean corpuscular haemoglobin (M.C.H.): 27 to 32 pg.
Mean corpuscular haemoglobin concentration (M.C.H.C.): 32 to 36 per cent.
Mean corpuscular diameter (dry films): 6·6 to 7·7 μ (mean 7·2 μ).
Platelets: 250,000 to 500,000 per cu. mm.
Reticulocytes: 0·5 to 1·5 per cent.
Sedimentation rate (Westergren): men—2 to 5 millimetres in 1 hour; women and children—4 to 7 millimetres in 1 hour.
Volume of blood: 6 to 12 pints, or 3·5 to 7 litres (5 to 10 ml. per 100 grammes of body weight or approx. 1 pint per stone).

TABLE 5

URINE (24-hour Output on a Mixed Diet)

(*Department of Pathology, St. Bartholomew's Hospital, London*)

Calcium (as Ca): up to 300 milligrams per day.
Diastase: 8,000–30,000 (Wohlgemuth) units.
17-ketosteroids: male (20–40) 2–27, mean 14·1; female (18–40) 5–18, mean 10·6.
Some decline with increasing age.
Up to age of 6 years less than 1 mg./day.

TABLE 6

LIST OF MILLI-EQUIVALENTS

To convert milligrams per cent into milli-equivalents per litre, multiply by 10 (to alter the percentage value into litre value) and divide by the weight of one valency of the atom.

Milligrams per cent

Na	divide by 2·3 to obtain milli-equivalent
K	divide by 3·9 to obtain milli-equivalent
Ca	divide by 2·0 to obtain milli-equivalent
Mg	divide by 1·2 to obtain milli-equivalent
Cl	divide by 3·5 to obtain milli-equivalent

For bicarbonate:

Convert volume per cent CO_2 by dividing by 2·2.

TABLE 7

READY RECKONER

Sodium		Chloride		Alkali reserve	
mg. per cent	m.eq./litre	mg. per cent NaCl	m.eq./litre	Vol. per cent	m.eq./litre
290	126	500	85·5	35	16
300	131	520	89	40	18
310	135	540	92	45	20
320	13	550	94	50	22
330	143	560	96	55	25
340	148	570	97·5	60	27
350	152	580	99	65	29
		590	101	70	31
		600	103	75	33·5
		610	104	80	36
		620	105		

10 mg. Na = 4·3 m.eq./1; 10 mg. NaCl = 1·7 m.eq./1; 5 vols. per cent CO_2 = 2·2 m.eq./1.

NORMAL VALUES

Base m.eq./litre		Acid m.eq./litre	
Na	142	HCO_3	27
K	5	Cl	103
Ca	5	HPO_4	2
Mg	3	SO_4	1
		Org. ac.	6
		Protein	16
Total	155	Total	155

References

Adams, P., Davies, G. T., and Sweetnam, P. (1970). "Osteoporosis and the Effects of Ageing on Bone Mass in Elderly Men and Women." *Quart. J. Med.*, N.S. **39**, 601.

Albright, F., and Reifenstein, E. C. (1948). "Ovarian Agenesis" and "Acromegaly". In *The Parathyroid Glands and Metabolic Bone Disease.* London; Baillière, Tindall and Cox.

Allcock, E. A. (1961). "Torulosis." *J. Bone Jt Surg.*, **43B**, 70.

Anderson, C. E., Crane, J. T., Harper, H. A., and Hunter, T. W. (1962). "Morquio's Disease and Dysplasia Epiphysealis Multiplex." *J. Bone Jt Surg.*, **44A**, 295.

Aston, J. N. (1958). "A Case of 'Massive Osteolysis' of the Femur." *J. Bone Jt Surg.*, **40B**, 514.

Baker, S. L., Dent, C. E., Friedman, M., and Watson, L. (1966). "Fibrogenesis Imperfecta Ossium." *J. Bone Jt Surg.*, **48B**, 804.

Barnes, R. (1956). "Aneurysmal Bone Cyst." *J. Bone Jt Surg.*, **38B**, 301.

Barnett, E., and Nordin, B. E. C. (1960). "The Radiological Diagnosis of Osteoporosis—A New Approach." *Clin. Radiol.*, **11**, 166.

Beadle, O. A. (1931). *Spec. rep. ser. med. Res. Coun.* No. 161. London; H.M. Stationery Office.

Beisel, W. R., Zerzan, C. J., Rubini, M. E., and Blythe, W. B. (1958). "Phosphaturesis: A Direct Renal Effect of Tri-iodothyronine." *Amer. J. Physiol.*, **195**, 357.

Bourne, G. H. (1956). *The Biochemistry and Physiology of Bone.* New York; Academic Press.

Brailsford, J. F. (1948). "The Serious Limitations and Erroneous Indications of Biopsy in the Diagnosis of Tumours of Bone." *Proc. R. Soc. Med.*, **41**, 225.

Branco, F., and Horta, J. da S. (1958). "Notes on a Rare Case of Essential Osteolysis." *J. Bone Jt Surg.*, **40B**, 519.

Bywaters, E. G. L. (1950). "Jaccoud Type Arthritis." *Brit. Heart J.*, **12**, 101.

—— and Ansell, B. W. (1958). "Arthritis Associated with Ulcerative Colitis." *Ann. rheum. Dis.*, **17**, 169.

Caffey, J. (1957). "Some Traumatic Lesions in Growing Bones other than Fractures." *Brit. J. Radiol.*, **30**, 225.

—— (1958). "Achondroplasia of Pelvis and Lumbosacral Spine." *Amer. J. Roentgenol.*, **80**, 449.

Calvé, J. (1925). "A Localized Affection of the Spine Suggesting Osteochondritis of the Vertebral Body, with the Clinical Aspect of Pott's Disease." *J. Bone Jt Surg.*, **7**, 41.

Charters, A. D. (1957). "Local Gigantism." *J. Bone Jt Surg.*, **39B**, 542.

Cockshott, P., and MacGregor, M. (1959). "The Natural History of Osteomyelitis Variolosa." *J. Fac. Radiol.*, **10**, 57.

Collins, D. H. (1949). *The Pathology of Articular and Spinal Disease.* London; Edward Arnold.

Cooke, A. M. (1955). "Osteoporosis." *Lancet*, **18**, 877, and **19**, 929.

Cozens, L. (1961). "The Developmental Origin of Spondylolisthesis." *J. Bone Jt Surg.*, **43A**, 180.

Davis, A. G. (1961). "Yaws." In *Tropical Radiology.* Ed. by H. Middlemiss. London; Heinemann.

Dent, C. E. (1957). "Steatorrhoea and Hypoparathyroidism." *Lancet*, **1**, 1196.

—— and Friedman, M. (1964). "Hypophosphataemic Osteomalacia with Complete Recovery." *Brit. med. J.*, **1**, 1676.

—— and Harris, H. (1956). "Hereditary Forms of Rickets and Osteomalacia." *J. Bone Jt Surg.*, **38B**, 204.

—— and Hodson, C. J. (1954). "The Radiological Appearances Associated with Certain Metabolic Bone Diseases." *Brit. J. Radiol.*, **27**, 605.

Devas, M. B. (1958). "Stress Fractures of the Tibia in Athletes." *J. Bone Jt Surg.*, **40B**, 227.

—— (1963). "Stress Fractures in Children." *J. Bone Jt Surg.*, **45B**, 528.

Doyle, F. (1966). "Some Quantitative Radiological Observations in Primary and Secondary Hyperparathyroidism." *Brit. J. Radiol.*, **39**, 161.

—— (1972). "Involutional Osteoporosis." In *Clinics in Endocrinology and Metabolism.* Philadelphia and London: Saunders.

Durie, E. B., and MacDonald, L. (1961). "Cryptococcosis (Torulosis) of Bone." *J. Bone Jt Surg.*, **43B**, 68.

Dwinnell, L. A., Dahlin, D. C., and Ghormley, R. K. (1954). "Parosteal (Juxtacortical) Osteogenic Sarcoma." *J. Bone Jt Surg.*, **36A**, 732.

Engelmann, G. (1929). "Ein Fall von Osteopathia hyperostotica (sclerotisans) multiplex infantalis." *Fortschr. Röntgenstr.*, **39**, 1101.

Evans, D. L. (1958). "Legg–Calvé–Perthes' Disease—A Study of Late Results." *J. Bone Jt Surg.*, **40B**, 168.

—— and Lloyd-Roberts, G. C. (1958). "Treatment in Legg–Calvé–Perthes' Disease—A Comparison of In-patient and Out-patient Methods." *J. Bone Jt Surg.*, **40B**, 182.

Evans, J. A. (1954). "Roentgen Observations of Aging Chest." *J. Amer. Geriat. Soc.*, **2**, 772.

Fényes, I., and Zoltán, L. (1959). "Calvé's Disease; Does it Exist? The Question of its Aetiology." *Brit. J. Radiol.*, **32**, 394.

Fett, H. C., and Russo, V. P. (1959). "Osteoid Osteoma of a Cervical Vertebra." *J. Bone Jt Surg.*, **41A**, 948.

Forbus, W. D., and Bestebreurtje, A. M. (1946). "Coccidioidomycosis: A Study of 95 Cases of the Disseminated Type, with Special Reference to the Pathogenesis of the Disease." *Milit. Surg.*, **99**, 653.

Fripp, A. T. (1958). "Vertebra Plana." *J. Bone Jt Surg.*, **40B**, 378.

Golding, F. C. (1959). "Appearances after Certain Orthopaedic Procedures." In *A Textbook of X-ray Diagnosis.* Ed. by S. C. Shanks and P. J. Kerley. London; Lewis.

Gorham, L. W., and Stout, A. P. (1955). "Massive Osteolysis. Its Relation to Haemangiomatosis." *J. Bone Jt Surg.*, **37A**, 985.

REFERENCES

Griffiths, D. L., and Moynihan, F. J. (1963). "Multiple Epiphyseal Injuries ('Battered Baby' Syndrome)." *Brit. med. J.*, **2**, 1558.

Gulledge, W. H., and White, W. (1951). "Engelmann's disease." *J. Bone Jt Surg.*, **33A**, 793.

Hancox, H. (1956). "The Osteoclast." In *The Biochemistry and Physiology of Bone*. Ed. by G. H. Bourne. New York; Academic Press.

Harris, W. H., Dudley, H. R., and Barry, R. J. (1962). "The Natural History of Fibrous Dysplasia." *J. Bone Jt Surg.*, **44A**, 207.

Havard, C. W. H., and Bodley Scott, R. (1959). "Urticaria Pigmentosa." *Quart. J. Med.*, **28**, 459.

Hawkins, T. D. (1959). "Changes in Tuberose Sclerosis." *Brit. J. Radiol.*, **32**, 157.

Hill, L. C. (1957). "Systemic Lupus Erythematosus." *Brit. med. J.*, **2**, 655.

Hitchcock, E. R., and Langton, L. (1959). "Peritendinitis Calcarea." *J. Fac. Radiol.*, **10**, 86.

Hitchcock, H. A. (1940). "Progression of Displacement in Spondylolisthesis." *J. Bone Jt Surg.*, **22**, 1.

Hubble, D., (1956). "Cretinism with Vertebral Changes." *Brit. med. J.*, **1**, 875.

Jaffe, H. L., and Lichtenstein, L. (1942a). "Non-osteogenic Fibroma of Bones." *Amer. J. Path.*, **18**, 205.

— — (1942b). "Chondroblastoma." *Amer. J. Path.*, **18**, 969.

— — (1949). "Chondromyxoid Fibroma." *Arch. Path.*, **45**, 541.

— — and Portis, R. B. (1940). "Giant Cell Tumour of Bone." *Arch. Path.*, **30**, 993.

Kellgren, J. H., Ball, J., and Bier, F. (1959). "Clinical Significance of Rheumatoid Serum Factor." *Brit. med. J.*, **1**, 523.

Kho, K. M., Wright, A. D., and Doyle, F. H. (1970). "Heel Pad Thickness in Acromegaly." *Brit. J. Radiol.*, **43**, 119.

Kodicek, E. (1972). "Recent Advances in Vitamin D Metabolism." In *Clinics in Endocrinology and Metabolism*, p. 305. London; Saunders.

Leffmann, R. (1959). "Congenital Dysplasia of the Hip." *J. Bone Jt Surg.*, **41B**, 689.

Leri, A., and Joanny, J. (1922). "Une affection non décrite des os: hyperostose en coulée sur toute la longeur d'un membre ou 'melorheostose'." *Bull. Soc. méd. Hôp. Paris*, **46**, 1141.

Lichtenstein, L. (1952). *Bone Tumours*. (See Fig. 22, chondroblastoma.) London; Kimpton.

Looser, E. (1920). "Über pathologische Formen von Infraktionen und Callusbildungen bei Rachitis und Osteomalakie und anderen Knochenerkrankungen." *Zbl. Chir.*, **47**, 1470.

McGavran, M. H., and Spady, H. A. (1960). "Eosinophilic Granuloma of Bone." *J. Bone Jt Surg.*, **42A**, 979.

McKusick, V. A. (1966). *Heritable Disorders of Connective Tissue*. 3rd edn. St. Louis; C. V. Mosby.

McLean, F. C. (1956). "The Parathyroid Glands and Bone." In *The Biochemistry and Physiology of Bone*. Ed. by G. H. Bourne. New York; Academic Press.

Martin, D. S., Jones, R. R., and Durham, N. C. (1941). "Systemic Blastomycosis." *Surgery*, **6**, 939.

Maudsley, R. H., and Stansfeld, A. G. (1956). "Non-osteogenic Fibroma." *J. Bone Jt Surg.*, **38B**, 714.

Mikity, V. G., and Jacobson, G. (1958). "Progressive Diaphyseal Dysplasia (Engelmann's Disease)." *J. Bone Jt Surg.*, **40A**, 206.

Milkman, L. A. (1934). "Multiple Spontaneous Idiopathic Symmetrical Fractures." *Amer. J. Roentgenol.*, **32**, 622.

Milner, S. M., and Baker, S. L. (1958). "Disappearing Bone." *J. Bone Jt Surg.*, **40B**, 502.

Morgan, D. B., Spiers, F. W., Pulvertaft, C. N., and Fourman, P. (1967). "The Amount of Bone in the Metacarpal According to Age and Sex." *Clin. Radiol.*, **18**, 101.

Mustard, W. T., and Duval, F. W. (1959). "Osteoid Osteoma of Vertebrae." *J. Bone Jt Surg.*, **41B**, 132.

Paterson, D. E. (1961). "Bone Changes in Leprosy." In *Tropical Radiology*. Ed. by H. Middlemiss. London; Heinemann.

Platt, R. (1959). "Some Consequences of Renal Inadequacy." *Lancet*, **1**, 159.

Pritchard, J. J. (1956). "The Parathyroid Glands and Bone." In *The Biochemistry and Physiology of Bone*. Ed. by G. H. Bourne. New York; Academic Press.

Pugh, G. D. (1954). *Roentgenologic Diagnosis of Diseases of Bone*. Baltimore; Williams and Wilkins.

Rosen, S. von (1962). "Diagnosis and Treatment of Congenital Dislocation of the Hip in the Newborn." *J. Bone Jt Surg.*, **44B**, 284

Schintz, H. R., Baensch, W. A., Friedl, E., and Uehinger, E. (1951). *Roentgen Diagnostics*. Vol. 1. English translation by James T. Case. London; Heinemann.

Scott, R. Bodley (1956). "Lipoid Storage Diseases and Non-lipoid Histiocytosis." *Practitioner*, **177**, 148.

Shanks, S. C., and Kerley, P. J. (1959). *A Text-book of X-ray Diagnosis*, Vol. 4. 3rd ed. London; Lewis.

Shephard, E. (1956). "Multiple Epiphyseal Dysplasia." *J. Bone Jt Surg.*, **38B**, 458.

Sherman, M. S. (1952). "Psoriatic Arthritis," *J. Bone Jt Surg.*, **34A**, 831.

Simon, G. (1956). *Principles of Chest X-ray Diagnosis*. London; Butterworths.

Sissons, H. A. (1956). "Osteoporosis of Cushing's Syndrome." *J. Bone Jt Surg.*, **38B**, 418.

Stanbury, S. W. (1957). "Azotaemic Renal Osteodystrophy." *Brit. med. Bull.*, **13**, 57.

— (1972). "Osteomalacia." In *Clinics in Endocrinology and Metabolism*, p. 239. London; Saunders.

Steinbach, H. L., and Russell, W. (1964). "Measurement of Heel Pad Thickness as an Aid to Diagnosis in Acromegaly." *Radiology*, **82**, 418.

Südeck, P. (1900). Quoted by Sweetapple (1949).

Sweetapple, H. (1949). "Südeck's Atrophy." *Med. J. Aust.*, **2**, 581.

Thiemann, H. (1909). Quoted by Schinz and his colleagues (1951). P. 737. *Röntgenstr. Fortschr.*, **14**, 79.

Watson, W. (1951). "Simultaneous Multisection Tomography." *Radiography*, **17**, 221.

— (1953). "Simultaneous Multisection Tomography." In *Modern Trends in Diagnostic Radiology (Second Series)*. Ed. by J. W. McLaren. London; Butterworths.

Whitaker, P. H. (1959). "Tuberose Sclerosis." *Brit. J. Radiol.*, **32**, 152.

Williams, R. E. (1959). "Osteochondrosis." In *A Text-book of X-ray Diagnosis*, Vol. 4, p. 367. 3rd ed. Ed. by S. C. Shanks and P. J. Kerley. London; Lewis.

Woodhouse, N. J. C., Doyle, F. H., and Joplin, G. F. (1971). "Vitamin D Deficiency and Primary Hyperparathyroidism." *Lancet*, **2**, 283.

Ziedes des Plantes, B. G. (1933). "Planigraphie." *Fortschr. Röntgenstr.*, **47**, 407.

Index